Handbook of Breast MRI

Handbook of Breast MRI

Jeremy Price
The Canberra Hospital and ACT Breast Screen, Canberra, Australia

CAMBRIDGE
UNIVERSITY PRESS

CAMBRIDGE UNIVERSITY PRESS
Cambridge, New York, Melbourne, Madrid, Cape Town,
Singapore, São Paulo, Delhi, Tokyo, Mexico City

Cambridge University Press
The Edinburgh Building, Cambridge CB2 8RU, UK

Published in the United States of America by Cambridge University Press, New York

www.cambridge.org
Information on this title:
www.cambridge.org/9780521139663

First published 2012

Printed in the United Kingdom at the University Press, Cambridge

A catalog record for this publication is available from the British Library

Library of Congress Cataloging-in-Publication Data
Price, Jeremy, 1956–
Handbook of breast MRI / Jeremy Price.
p. ; cm.
Includes bibliographical references and index.
ISBN 978-0-521-13966-3 (pbk.)
I. Title.
[DNLM: 1. Breast Diseases--diagnosis--Handbooks. 2. Magnetic Resonance Imaging--methods--Handbooks. WP 39]

618.190754--dc23

2011040526

ISBN 978-0-521-13966-3 Paperback

For SWC, who never for a moment doubted it would happen – the fact is it never would have happened without you.

Contents

Preface

In the last decade, breast MRI has firmly established its place as a mainstream imaging technique, with providers experiencing rapid growth, particularly in high-risk screening and in the preoperative assessment of patients with known breast cancer.

It really is a great time to get involved. The great pioneers of breast MRI have worked tirelessly in the 25 years since contrast-enhanced breast MRI began, so that the key elements of technique and interpretation are now well understood. With high-gradient-strength MRI machines and technical advances in breast coil design, image quality has improved immeasurably, while computer-aided detection systems make the task of reporting breast MRI studies much quicker and easier.

With the advent of commercially available MRI-guided vacuum-assisted biopsy systems, the problem of how to biopsy lesions shown only by MRI has at last been effectively overcome. There is now a clear need for more radiologists to gain expertise in breast MRI diagnosis and in intervention to meet the steadily increasing demand.

In recent years, some important questions in breast MRI have been answered, most notably with many prospective trials demonstrating the superior sensitivity of MRI over x-ray mammography in women at increased risk of breast cancer. It has further been established that MRI outperforms mammography not only in revealing invasive cancer, but also in detecting ductal carcinoma in situ (DCIS). Consequently, the role of breast MRI in high-risk screening is now unchallenged. Conversely, the answers to other questions have become less clear, with the role of breast MRI in preoperative planning now particularly controversial.

Innovations in many other clinical arenas are also poised to make their impact on existing paradigms in breast cancer management. Gene expression profiling has provided important new insights into the pathogenesis of the heterogeneous group of diseases which make up breast cancer. The prospect of an improved understanding of the pathologic spectrum of breast cancer also offers enticing possibilities for a more tailored approach to surveillance and therapeutic options according to individual risk. There is good reason to believe that MRI will be at the forefront of the imaging techniques used to further exploit these advances.

This book aims to assist radiologists seeking to add breast MRI to their skill set. Some may be familiar with MRI but not breast imaging, while others may be experienced breast imagers but not well-versed in MRI. Either way, there may be reluctance to embark on a technique renowned for its steep learning curve. If reading this book makes that learning curve a little easier to negotiate, it will have fulfilled its goal. For those who decide that breast MRI is not for them, at least they should have gained an insight into a technique that is now a routine diagnostic tool in breast imaging.

Acknowledgements

Thanks to my clinical colleagues and to all those women who have trusted me during the breast MRI learning experience. Special thanks go to Independent Property Group whose generous donation made our 16-channel coil possible and to ACT Chief Minister Katy Gallagher for her support. Thanks to Professor Paul Gatenby for authorizing use of images from The Canberra Hospital; to Dianne Lane and all the MRI Technologists, Clerical Staff and Nurses; to my radiology colleagues Dr. Ann Harvey and Professor Graham Buirski; to Dr. Huw Llewellyn, Anita Davenport, Rally Vella, Matthew Shilling, Linda Warwick and our radiology trainees whose many excellent questions forced me to organize my thoughts! Finally, thanks to the several luminaries of breast MRI who were so generous with their time in answering my own questions, and in offering encouragement and advice.

Glossary

Absolute and relative risk: Absolute risk is the chance of breast cancer developing over a stated time period, e.g., 20% in 10 years. Lifetime risk is an absolute risk provided life expectancy is defined, e.g., 70 years or 85 years. Relative risk is the increase in breast cancer risk above average, e.g., 2-fold relative risk for a woman with a first degree relative affected by breast cancer.

Adjuvant therapy: Use of chemotherapy or endocrine therapy after primary surgical treatment and radiation therapy (RT), with the aim of eradicating any distant micrometastatic cancer (not clinically evident but with a reasonable likelihood that it may be present). "Adjuvant! Online!" is a web-based algorithm which assesses multiple risk factors to assist in selecting endocrine therapy and/or chemotherapy, offering estimates of the % benefits of different treatment options.

Brachytherapy: Use of a radiation source at short range (as opposed to teletherapy), by inserting isotopes into the tissues.

Clustered microcysts: Tiny 2–3 mm cystic lesions which on ultrasound (US) are anechoic with thin septations and no solid component. Histologically, clustered microcysts correlate with dilated acini in fibrocystic change.

Comedonecrosis: Originally a gross macroscopic description of the oozing of creamy pus-like necrotic material from the cut ends of ducts at the surface of ductal carcinoma in situ (DCIS) specimens. The term implies high- or intermediate-grade DCIS with central duct necrosis and is often associated with casting calcifications on x-ray mammography (XRM).

Desmoplastic reaction: Reactive fibrosis around an invasive cancer resulting in spiculations, which contain relatively few tumor cells. The host reaction may reflect an attempt to wall-off the pathologic process, and often indicates a relatively slow tumor growth pattern, so that spiculated cancers tend to be low-grade lesions. Desmoplasia also occurs with DCIS (usually high-grade, possibly because low-grade DCIS is so indolent that no host reaction is induced). The differential for mammographic density associated with malignant calcifications is between desmoplastic reaction and focal invasion.

Disease-free survival: Patient alive and with no recurrence found at given number of years (in trials, usually assessed at multiples of 5 years).

Ductal intraepithelial neoplasia (DIN): Recently proposed term encompassing both atypical ductal hyperplasia (ADH) and DCIS which recognizes the difficulty in making this distinction histologically. The term also avoids the word "carcinoma" in the definition of a pathologic process which (in pure form) has no metastatic potential and is not life-threatening.

Ductoscopy: Surgical technique in which major ducts at the nipple are examined internally with a micro-endoscope. Actively discharging ducts are usually relatively large and easy to cannulate, but even small ducts involved by DCIS produce tiny amounts of fluid which can reveal their location on the nipple surface. These ducts can then be carefully dilated sufficient to accommodate the micro-endoscope. Intraluminal disease can then be directly demonstrated allowing an accurate segmental approach to surgical excision.

Early-stage breast cancer (EBC): Cases with the potential for surgery to be curative, corresponding to TNM (tumor-node-metastasis) Stage I to II disease (tumor < 5 cm diameter with either palpable but not fixed nodes, or < 10 pathologically involved axillary nodes, and no skin or chest wall involvement). Even a tumor > 5 cm in diameter may fall within this definition provided there is no axillary lymphadenopathy (TNM Stage IIB). There is no universally agreed definition of EBC and some would include tumors > 5 cm diameter with positive nodes (Stage IIIA) in this category.

Endocrine therapy: Treatment designed to inhibit the progression of hormone receptor-positive tumors. The term is preferred to "hormone therapy" which could then be confused with "hormone replacement therapy".

Epidermal growth factor receptor (EGFR): Also known as human epidermal growth factor receptor type 1 (HER1), an immunohistochemistry (IHC) marker often positive in basal-like cancers and considered a potential target for research into treatment of BRCA1-linked breast cancers.

Extensive intraductal component (EIC): Histologic term used for an invasive ductal carcinoma (IDC) exhibiting DCIS as a prominent feature within the main tumor mass, and extensively in surrounding tissue. The term also included an extensive area of predominantly DCIS with foci of microinvasion. The term has largely been superseded by more emphasis on measuring overall lesion size and the importance of obtaining clear surgical margins in excision specimens.

Gene expression profiling: Cancers show marked alteration in cell function, reflecting an ability to "switch on or off" genes which generate enzymes driving the innumerable metabolic pathways. In cancer cells, these genetic changes are usually geared towards self-replication, but nevertheless the profile of genes expressed gives a "gene signature" which can define the tumor type. This is also termed molecular pathology because tumor evaluation is made at the level of molecule production.

Hormone replacement therapy (HRT): Substitution of normal endogenous female hormones with exogenous hormones after menopause.

Immunophenotype: Immunohistochemical staining characteristics determined using antibodies to label specific protein antigens expressed by tumor cells, e.g., cytokeratins, estrogen receptor (ER), progesterone receptor (PR), Ki-67.

Isolated tumor cells: Single tumor cells, clusters of fewer than 200 tumor cells or clusters of not more than 0.2 mm diameter in a single histologic cross-section (either routine histology or IHC).

Ki-67 index: Ki-67 is an immunohistochemical marker which has emerged as a reliable indicator of tumor cell proliferation, and is a strong predictor of the biologic aggressiveness of cancers. The Ki-67 index is the percentage of tumor nuclei which stain positive. Recently a Ki-67 threshold value of 15% has been used to differentiate between luminal A and B molecular subtypes as defined by the gold standard of gene expression profiling. The Ki-67 index also shows promise in predicting which DCIS cases may behave unfavorably.

Laser capture microdissection (LCM): Technique by which specific cell clusters can be retrieved from a formalin-fixed paraffin-embedded slide. For example, LCM can be used to extract an area of DCIS from associated invasive breast cancer and surrounding normal tissue. A gel layer placed over the slide surface is sensitized by a laser pulse to make it sticky, so that the target cells become adherent. This technique allows evaluation of gene expression profiles of breast cancer samples without the need for fresh-frozen tissue.

Lobular intraepithelial neoplasia (LIN): Recently proposed, and not yet widely accepted term including both atypical lobular hyperplasia (ALH) and lobular carcinoma in situ (LCIS) which recognizes the difficulty in making this distinction histologically and avoiding the word "carcinoma" in the definition.

Locally advanced breast cancer (LABC): Cases not amenable to cure by local surgery alone but not demonstrably metastatic, corresponding to TNM Stage III disease (tumor < 5 cm diameter but with fixed axillary or pathologically 10 or more axillary lymph nodes, or involving skin with ulceration or nodules, or involving chest wall).

Lymphovascular invasion (LVI): Histologic infiltration of venules or lymphatics by invasive cancer indicating an aggressive tumor with high risk of metastatic disease. Although considered to be an independent poor prognostic indicator, there is wide observed variation in the reported incidence of LVI from 5% to 50%. Perineural invasion is sometimes associated and has a similar implication.

Microarray-comparative genomic hybidization CGH: Microarray-based comparative genomic hybridization, a gene expression profiling technology using DNA microarrays ("gene chips"). The technique allows the analysis of thousands of DNA–mRNA reactions in a grid system, yielding data which are interpreted using software algorithms to define tumor genotype (see also tissue microarray).

Microdochectomy: Surgical technique for solitary pathologic duct discharge, used particularly when an intraduct papilloma has been demonstrated close to the nipple–areolar complex (NAC), as a means to minimize the extent of resection. After cannulation of the discharging duct, methylene blue is then injected with excision of the outlined duct system.

Microinvasion: Term used in relation to DCIS where microscopic invasive foci are present which measure less than 1 mm in diameter. As the extent of DCIS increases, so the likelihood that areas of microinvasion are present also rises. Microinvasion is also more likely with high-grade DCIS.

Micrometastases: Term used in pathologic TNM (pTNM) staging for histologically identified nodal metastases > 0.2 mm but < 2 mm in diameter. A micrometastasis of < 0.2 mm is not considered to be an involved node (Appendix 3).

Minimal breast cancer: Invasive cancer smaller than 10 mm diameter on pathology corresponding to T1ab in the TNM classification.

Multifocal and multicentric cancer: Multifocality is commonly used to describe an invasive cancer with one or more additional satellite tumors present within 2–3 cm of the index lesion. Multicentricity is used where additional invasive cancer or DCIS is found at least 2–3 cm remote from the index lesion or in another quadrant. However, definitions vary with regard to the required distance between tumors, with some considering lesions to be multicentric only when there is as much as 5 cm of separation. The key management implication is that multifocal disease may still be amenable to breast-conserving therapy (BCT) while multicentric involvement is likely to require mastectomy.

Neoadjuvant systemic therapy (NST): The use of chemotherapy or endocrine therapy prior to surgery, aiming to shrink large tumors to make the resection easier. In some cases, down-staging of the tumor may make breast conservation possible.

Overall survival: Patient alive at given number of years after initial diagnosis of breast cancer. For clinical trial evaluation, mortality is usually assessed at multiples of 5 years and must be defined as either breast cancer-related or attributable to other causes.

p53: This protein, produced by the TP53 (tumor protein 53) gene has an important role in preventing cell proliferation after DNA damage and in initiating cell death if DNA repair is impossible. Mutations in the TP53 gene occur in a variety of tumors, including up to 40% of breast cancers, and high levels correlate with high-grade disease and poorer prognosis. The overexpression of p53 protein can be identified by IHC staining and is frequently a feature of basal-like, human epithelial growth factor receptor type 2 (HER2)-positive cancers and luminal type B cancers. A heritable mutation in TP53 is also responsible for Li-Fraumeni syndrome.

pTNM: Pathologic TNM staging, additional to clinical TNM classification. The content is similar for tumor and metastases, but differs significantly for nodal status due to the incorporation of results of sentinel lymph node biopsy (SLNB), IHC and molecular studies (Appendix 3).

Recurrence: Return of clinical disease after primary treatment for breast cancer can be classified as (i) local: confined to the ipsilateral breast, mastectomy scar or chest wall, (ii) regional: ipsilateral axillary, supraclavicular, internal mammary nodes or (iii) distant metastases: contralateral or other remote nodes, bone, brain, lung, liver, pleura, peritoneum, viscera.

Resection margins: Specimens from local excision are orientated by marking with surgical sutures or clips by an agreed convention (often Short suture Superior, Medium suture Medial, Long suture Lateral). On receipt in pathology, the exposed margins are painted with different colored inks allowing clearance measurements to be made in millimeters from histologic sections. Where ink is seen contacting cancer cells (either invasive or DCIS), positive margins are reported and further excision is usually performed (shaving of the involved cavity wall). Obtaining clear margins is very important prognostically and influences choice of adjuvant therapy. For a pure invasive cancer only, a margin of even 1 mm may be accepted, but because the limits of DCIS are more difficult to define histologically, acceptable margins are variable defined from 3 to 10 mm, provided RT is to be given.

Signal-to-noise ratio (SNR): Apart from high spatial resolution, good image contrast is the other fundamental factor in producing good breast magnetic resonance imaging (MRI) images. Image contrast is all about getting the maximum signal into the pixels, and to be visible at all, the signal level has to be distinguishable from *background noise*. The greater the SNR, the more options there are for magnetic resonance imaging (MRI) "trade-offs," using the inherent signal advantage to increase spatial resolution or shorten sequence times. In breast MRI, intravenous contrast is used to further enhance T1 signal of the malignant lesions we want to identify. Other ways to increase SNR for breast MRI studies include increasing field strength, using dedicated multichannel phased array coil design and parallel imaging.

Tissue microarray (TMA): Technique originally developed for IHC assays whereby hundreds of tiny (~1 mm) tissue sections are arrayed on a glass slide for evaluation of antibody–antigen-based staining reactions. The technology has evolved for gene expression profiling of tumors using "gene chips" (microarray-CGH) in which thousands of DNA–mRNA reactions can be evaluated to define tumor genotype. Nevertheless, IHC markers are required to establish immunophenotype as a surrogate for genetic alterations.

TNM staging: The Tumor-Node-Metastasis international clinical staging system for breast cancer was originally produced in 1958 by the UICC (Union Internationale Contre le Cancer, also known as the International Union Against Cancer or Union for International Cancer Control). A similar system was then published in 1977 by the AJCC (American Joint Committee on Cancer). Differences in the two systems were eliminated in 1987 so that both are now equivalent (Appendix 3).

Van Nuys prognostic index: An index proposed in 1996 for predicting the risk of local recurrence of DCIS, based on a score for the three most important indicators being size of DCIS, margin status and the histopathologic nuclear grade.

Abbreviations

ACR	American College of Radiology
ACRIN	American College of Radiology Imaging Network
ACS	American Cancer Society
ADC	apparent diffusion coefficient
ADH	atypical ductal hyperplasia
AI	aromatase inhibitor
AJCC	American Joint Committee on Cancer
ALCL	anaplastic large-cell lymphoma
ALH	atypical lobular hyperplasia
ALND	axillary lymph node dissection
APBI	accelerated partial breast irradiation
ATEC	Automated Tissue Excision and Collection
BCT	breast-conserving therapy
BI-RADS	Breast Imaging Reporting Data System (ACR, USA)
BMI	body mass index
BOADICEA	Breast and Ovarian Analysis of Disease Incidence and Carrier Estimation Algorithan
BPM	bilateral prophylactic mastectomy
BSE	breast self-examination
CAD	computer-aided detection
CAPSS	columnar alteration with prominent apical snouts and secretions
CBE	clinical breast examination
CC	craniocaudal (standard mammographic view)
CGH	comparative genomic hybridization
CISH	chromogenic in situ hybridization
CMF	cyclophosphamide, methotrexate, 5-fluorouracil
CNB	core needle biopsy
COMICE	COmparative effectiveness of MR Imaging in breast CancEr (UK Trial)
CT	computed tomography
DCIS	ductal carcinoma in situ
DD	differential diagnosis
DIEP Flap	deep inferior epigastric perforator flap
DIN	ductal intraepithelial neoplasia (term including ADH and DCIS)
DMIST	Digital Mammography In Screening Trial (ACRIN trial)
DWI	diffusion-weighted imaging
EBC	early-stage breast cancer (Stages 0–II)
EBCTCG	Early Breast Cancer Trialists' Collaborative Group
EGFR	epidermal growth factor receptor (HER1)
EIC	extensive intraductal component
EORTC	European Organisation for Research and Treatment of Cancer
ER	estrogen receptor
FAC	5-fluorouracil, anthracycline (doxyrubicin), cyclophosphamide
FDA	Food and Drug Administration (USA)
FDG	18F Fluorodeoxyglucose
FEC	5-fluorouracil, epirubicin (specified anthracycline), cyclophosphamide
FISH	fluorescence in situ hybridization
FNA/FNAB/ FNAC	fine-needle aspiration/biopsy/ cytology
FOV	field of view (MRI parameter)
FSE	fast spin echo, aka TSE = turbo spin echo (MRI sequence)
GFR	glomerular filtration rate
GI	gastrointestinal
HER1	human epidermal growth factor receptor type 1 (EGFR)
HER2	human epidermal growth factor receptor type 2 (HER2/neu, c-erbB2)
HIBCRIT	HIgh Breast Cancer Risk ITalian Study (Italian trial)
HRT	hormone replacement therapy
IBIS	International Breast Intervention Study
IBMC	International Breast MRI Consortium
IDC	invasive ductal carcinoma
IHC	immunohistochemistry
ILC	invasive lobular carcinoma
IMC	internal mammary chain (internal thoracic nodes)
IR	inversion-recovery (MRI sequence)
ISH	in situ hybridization
ITCs	isolated tumor cells
IVF	in vitro fertilization
LABC	locally advanced breast cancer (Stage 3)
LCIS	lobular carcinoma in situ
LIN	lobular intraepithelial neoplasia (term including ALH and LCIS)
LIQ	lower inner quadrant
LMP	last menstrual period
LOQ	lower outer quadrant
LVI	lymphovascular invasion
MARIBS	Magnetic Resonance Imaging Breast Screening (UK trial)
MIP	maximum intensity projection
MLO	mediolateral oblique (standard mammographic view)

MONET	MR mammography Of Nonpalpable brEast Tumors (Dutch trial)
MRI	magnetic resonance imaging
MRISC	Magnetic Resonance Imaging Screening (Dutch trial)
MRS	magnetic resonance spectroscopy
MSK	musculoskeletal
NAC	nipple–areolar complex
NBOCC	National Breast and Ovarian Cancer Center (Australia)
NOS	not otherwise specified (IDC of no special type)
NPV	negative predictive value
NSABP	National Surgical Adjuvant Breast and Bowel Project
NSF	nephrogenic systemic fibrosis
NST	neoadjuvant systemic therapy
PARP	poly (ADP-ribose) polymerase
PASH	pseudoangiomatous stromal hyperplasia
PCR	pathologic complete response
PET	positron emission tomography
PPV	positive predictive value
PR	progesterone receptor (also PgR)
RCT	randomized controlled trial
RECIST	Response Evaluation Criteria in Solid Tumors
RODEO	ROtating Delivery of Excitation Off-resonance (MRI sequence)
ROI	region of interest
RR	relative risk
RRSO	risk-reducing salpingo-oophorectomy
RT	radiation therapy
RT-PCR	reverse transcriptase polymerase chain reaction
SER	signal enhancement ratio
SERM	selective estrogen receptor modulator
SLNB	sentinel lymph node biopsy
SNAC	Sentinel Node versus Axillary Clearance (Australian trials)
SNR	signal-to-noise ratio (MRI parameter)
SPAIR	SPectral Adiabatic Inversion Recovery (MRI sequence)
STIR	Short Tau Inversion Recovery (MRI sequence)
TAC	taxane, anthracycline, cyclophosphamide
TARGIT	TARGeted Intra-operative RT
TDLU	terminal duct-lobular unit
TNM	tumor, node, metastasis (tumor staging system)
TRAM flap	transverse rectus abdominis musculocutaneous flap
TUS	targeted ultrasound (also directed or second-look ultrasound)
UIQ	upper inner quadrant
UK	United Kingdom
UOQ	upper outer quadrant
US	ultrasound
USA	United States of America
USPIO	ultrasmall superparamagnetic iron oxide
VAB	vacuum-assisted biopsy
VIBE	Volumetric Interpolated Breath-hold Examination (MRI sequence)
VOI	volume of interest
WHO	World Health Organization
WLE	wide local excision, aka lumpectomy, partial mastectomy
XRM	x-ray mammography

Chapter 1

Basics of breast MRI

Chapter outline

- What's so great about breast MRI anyway?
- The evolution of contrast-enhanced breast MRI
- What you need to get started
- Patient preparation prior to scanning
- Technical considerations in protocol design

What's so great about breast MRI anyway?

Magnetic resonance imaging is unique in combining excellent soft tissue contrast and exquisite anatomic detail together with an ability to differentiate chemical composition through T1 and T2 relaxation effects. Fluid in a cyst, fatty tissue and fibroglandular breast parenchyma are readily distinguished on spin-echo T1- and T2-weighted sequences by virtue of their different signal characteristics. Other MRI techniques, such as IR can be used to suppress signal from specific tissues, commonly the bright signal from fat, to make pathologic findings more conspicuous (Table 1.1).

In the breast though, it is the additional information obtained from using intravenous gadolinium as a contrast-enhancing agent that is the key to the success of MRI in cancer detection. Tumoral angiogenesis is associated with both increased vascularity and abnormal leaky capillaries, and it is by this mechanism that invasive cancers show enhancement on MRI, with much higher sensitivity than conventional XRM.

Table 1.1 Basic signal characteristics in breast MRI

	T1 signal	T2 signal
Cyst fluid	LOW (dark)	HIGH (bright)
Fatty tissue	HIGH (but dark with IR)	HIGH (but dark with IR)
Fibroglandular tissue	INTERMEDIATE (gray)	INTERMEDIATE (gray)
Invasive cancer/DCIS	HIGH (after gadolinium)	INTERMEDIATE (gray)

Initial evidence for the superiority of MRI in cancer detection derived from a number of prospective trials, published in the mid 2000s, where MRI was used in addition to XRM for screening women at high risk on the basis of known or suspected genetic susceptibility [1–4]. Across these studies, breast MRI had more than double the sensitivity of XRM, leading to the 2007 ACS recommendation that annual MRI be added to routine surveillance for women with an estimated lifetime breast cancer risk of 20–25% or more [5]. Equally impressive in the screening setting was the NPV of up to 97–99% [1, 3, 6]. A normal screening breast MRI study, then offers an unprecedented ability to exclude the presence of invasive breast cancer.

In recent years it has also become clear that state-of-the-art MRI achieves overall higher sensitivity for DCIS than does XRM [7]. In one review reflecting current breast MRI techniques, only 7/222 (~3%) of all malignant lesions failed to enhance, with MRI achieving 98% sensitivity for invasive cancer and 90% for DCIS [8].

Why does MRI perform better than XRM?

On XRM in a fatty breast, stellate cancers are seen as white stars on a dark background, and lesion detection is a relatively simple task. On XRM in a dense breast, the task is to detect the same white stars but now against a white background. This is so difficult that we train ourselves to detect a subtle architectural disturbance around a stellate mass, rather than the mass itself.

Lesion detection in dense breast tissue becomes even more difficult for non-spiculated masses and for diffusely infiltrating cancer types such as ILC, which may show minimal or absent architectural change. Not surprisingly, the sensitivity of XRM falls dramatically in dense breasts, with even extensive invasive cancers sometimes escaping detection.

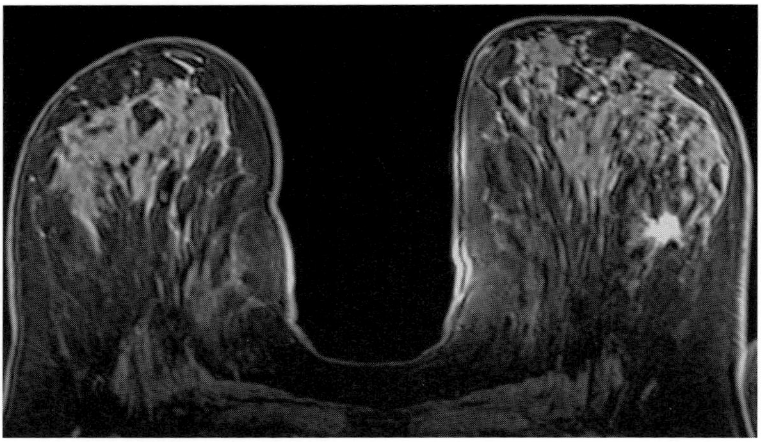

Fig. 1.1 Enhancing invasive cancer: On this early post-contrast fat-suppressed T1-weighted image, the stellate left breast IDC is highly conspicuous due to intense enhancement. Breast fat has been rendered dark by using IR fat suppression, while the dense fibroglandular breast tissue shows intermediate (gray) signal.

On contrast-enhanced breast MRI, nearly all invasive cancers are rendered conspicuously bright white, regardless of the density of the surrounding tissue (Fig. 1.1). This excellent lesion visibility, unaffected by even extreme breast density, is perhaps the most instantly impressive feature of breast MRI.

Another major advantage of MRI over XRM lies in the image acquisition. With XRM, mechanical compression of the breast is used to convert a 3D object into a single composite 2D image in each of two planes. An MRI scan renders the whole breast volume as stacks of tomographic slices down to a millimeter thick, and images can be obtained in any desired plane. For the patient, this eliminates the need for mechanical compression which is at least unpleasant for many women, and intolerable for some. Meanwhile, for the radiologist, the benefit is that MRI images are not subject to the composite effects of XRM, where density throughout the breast is summated on a single image. Summation effects are a major factor both in obscuring cancers, and in creating spurious findings which simulate cancer.

The combination of excellent soft tissue contrast and tomographic imaging offered by MRI, unaffected by breast density, translates into much more accurate delineation of tumor size and extent. Demonstrating multifocal, multicentric and contralateral disease was among the first established applications of breast MRI. Of all available imaging techniques, MRI provides the best correlation with surgical histopathology. This ability to accurately define disease extent makes MRI the gold standard for preoperative imaging assessment for breast cancer.

Since MRI uses only magnetism and radiofrequency impulses to produce the image, there is no ionizing radiation required. This is a particular advantage in the context of breast cancer screening, where examinations are regularly repeated over many years. Since the risks of radiation-induced cancer are much more of a concern in younger women, who generally also have denser breasts, MRI is potentially well-suited for screening in this group.

Will breast MRI replace mammography?

Despite its many advantages, MRI is not a panacea for breast imaging, and nor is it a replacement for XRM. Rather it is another diagnostic tool which, like any other, needs to be applied judiciously for optimum cost–benefit. To begin with, breast MRI is much more expensive than XRM and is not yet as widely available. Radiologists skilled in breast MRI are in short supply, and even for those with experience, interpreting an MRI study with in excess of 1000 individual images is a far more time-consuming exercise than reading a standard two-view mammogram. These logistic and financial considerations alone will ensure that MRI is not about to replace XRM any time soon. That said, as breast MRI becomes more commonplace it is possible that MRI could eventually supersede XRM as a primary screening technique [9].

An important clinical reason why XRM and MRI are still generally regarded as complementary rather than competing techniques relates to the detection of DCIS. Microcalcification, the key XRM sign of DCIS, is not visible on MRI. However, experience has shown that DCIS is very frequently present without microcalcification on XRM and can often be identified by MRI.

Nevertheless, some DCIS (particularly low-grade disease), may be occult on MRI, and yet readily detected on XRM by the presence of microcalcification. Probably about 15–25% of all DCIS cases will be occult on MRI, but up to half may be shown only by MRI. Consequently, it is recommended that MRI and XRM continue to be used in combination for most purposes.

Despite this, in the setting of high-risk screening at least, it may be that the days of XRM are numbered. The recent multicenter EVA trial from Germany found that the addition of XRM, as compared to MRI alone, only marginally raised the cancer yield from 15 to 16 per 1000 screens [10]. The use of XRM in these usually young women with familial breast cancer may be difficult to justify if similar findings are confirmed in other studies.

The strengths and weaknesses of MRI compared to XRM are summarized in Table 1.2. MRI is, of course, not possible where there is a contraindication such as the presence of a cardiac pacemaker, neurostimulator device or non-MRI-compatible cerebral aneurysm clip or heart valve (Table 1.3). Other magnetic or metallic devices, including coronary or other vascular stents, inferior vera cava filters and some breast-expander type implants may also be unsafe for MRI due to the risk of movement. Patients are screened for all metallic devices as any of these can result in significant heating due to eddy currents created by the magnetic field. Up to 5% of women may be unsuited to breast MRI for various other reasons, including severe claustrophobia [2, 4].

Table 1.2 Breast MRI compared with XRM

Strengths
No ionizing radiation required
High sensitivity for breast cancer, including DCIS
No uncomfortable compression required
Multiplanar acquisition, with whole breast volumetric data
Performance unaffected by breast density
Superior imaging–histopathologic correlation of disease extent
Weaknesses
More costly and less widely available
Takes longer to perform and interpret
Does not directly show microcalcification
Requires intravenous contrast injection of gadolinium
Not possible where MRI is contraindicated, e.g., pacemaker
Not tolerated by up to 5% of patients, e.g., severe claustrophobia

Table 1.3 Some common contraindications to MRI

Cardiac pacemaker
Implantable cardioverter defibrillator
Cochlear implant
Other implanted electromagnetic device, e.g., neurostimulator, insulin pump
Ferromagnetic or unknown cerebral aneurysm clip
Metallic ocular foreign body

The requirement for an intravenous injection of contrast for breast MRI is a further drawback, although the risk of a serious adverse reaction or death due to gadolinium is much lower than with iodinated contrast media. Based on worldwide experience from over 200 million doses of gadolinium chelates, the incidence of anaphylactoid reaction is estimated to be less than 1 in 100 000 injections.

Recently, a rare but severe and sometimes fatal adverse effect of gadolinium chelates has emerged as a new disease, known as nephrogenic systemic fibrosis (NSF). This condition is confined to patients with either severe acute or end-stage chronic renal failure, with exposure to gadolinium as a trigger event (Appendix 1). Fortunately, NSF has little impact on the performance of breast MRI studies, provided that severe kidney disease is excluded.

What about the low specificity of MRI?

A major criticism which is regularly levelled at breast MRI is that it has low specificity with "too many false positives" but this is really a misconception, with its roots buried in history. In the early days of breast MRI, the initial hope was that enhancement might equate with malignancy. When this soon proved not to be the case, the presence of any enhancement which was not due to cancer was considered to be a false-positive result.

Today though, with the accumulated knowledge and technologic advances over the past two decades, the position is quite different. The presence of enhancement on breast MRI is now just the starting point for a systematic analysis from which most non-malignant causes can be correctly excluded. Despite this reality, there is a continuing perception that MRI still generates an unacceptably high proportion of false-positive results.

False-positive rates must also be gauged in the context of overall accuracy. In evaluating diagnostic tests, it is important to appreciate the inherent relationship between sensitivity and specificity. The expected trade-off for achieving very high sensitivity, a characteristic of breast MRI, is a reduction in specificity. In effect, as the threshold is lowered to include more abnormal results (true positives), so questionable findings tend to be included, leading to more false-positive results. Recent evidence suggests that the overall specificity of MRI at least equals that of XRM, with much higher sensitivity.

For clinical purposes, the PPV (percentage of cases in which the prediction of a positive result proves to be correct) is often a more useful indicator of false-positive rates than specificity (Appendix 2). Ultimately, the best indicator of specificity in breast imaging is to evaluate the benign to malignant ratio in cases where biopsy is performed (this ratio closely relates to PPV, e.g., benign to malignant biopsy ratio of 3:1 equates to a PPV for biopsy of 25%). In the setting of prospective high-risk screening, MRI has achieved results as good as or better than XRM, with biopsy ratios of about 1:1 (PPV of 50%) typically reported [1, 3, 10].

When the role of MRI in lesion characterization is considered, data from the multicenter IBMC trial 6883 suggest that MRI actually performs rather better than XRM. In this prospective study across 18 tertiary level institutions in the USA, Canada and Germany, women with suspicious lesions on conventional imaging were evaluated by MRI prior to biopsy. The study showed superior specificity for MRI with a PPV of 72% compared with 53% for XRM [11].

At this point, having established the key strengths and weaknesses of breast MRI, and hopefully having at least begun to dispel the myth of low specificity, we can move on to review the historical development of breast MRI. This is not mere idle nostalgia, as understanding the key steps in the evolution of breast MRI allows for a much better appreciation of the techniques currently used when performing and interpreting these studies.

The evolution of contrast-enhanced breast MRI

Spin-echo images of the breast were among the very first clinical MRI studies ever performed, and were obtained even before the brain and spine were studied. However, early experience suggested that the presence of breast cancer was not reliably demonstrated, and interest faded. The breakthrough came when invasive cancers were shown to enhance

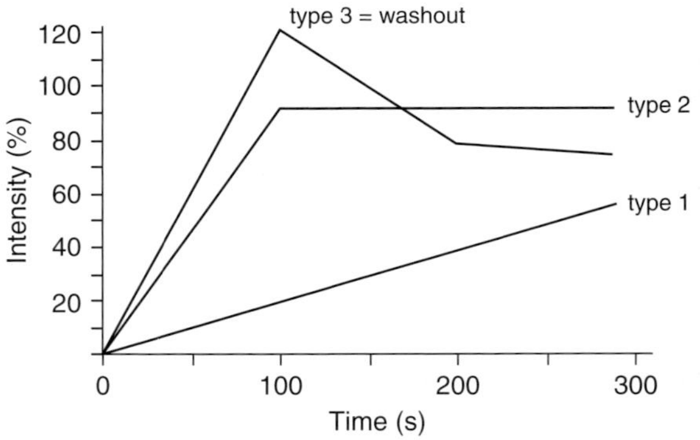

Fig. 1.2 Time–intensity curves: The slow-rising type 1 curve shown here is typical for normal background enhancement of fibroglandular tissue. The majority of invasive cancers show intense enhancement in the early phase (within 2 minutes from injection), and display either a plateau (type 2) or washout (type 3) curve. A washout kinetic curve has a high PPV for malignancy.

after intravenous injection of gadolinium, as first reported in a small preliminary study of 20 patients by Heywang *et al.* in 1986 [12]. All 14 invasive cancers and a single fibroadenoma showed significant enhancement, while benign proliferative changes enhanced only slightly or not at all. Image subtraction was used to improve visibility of a 1.5 cm cancer in a dense breast.

It soon became clear that some benign lesions, particularly fibroadenomas, often showed significant enhancement, and investigators then began to focus on how to better differentiate malignant from benign pathology [13]. With the development of fast gradient-echo T1-weighted sequences, scanning the breast using a dynamic technique looked promising. In 1989, Kaiser and coworkers showed that invasive cancers typically showed signal increase in the order of 100% (i.e., a doubling of *signal intensity*) within the first 2 minutes after contrast injection [14]. It was then hoped that *enhancement rate* might be used to differentiate malignant from benign lesions. The concept of repeating a series of dynamic post-contrast scans was also developed. Using a defined ROI, it was possible to plot the enhancement course of a lesion over several minutes as a *time–intensity* or *kinetic curve* (Fig. 1.2).

Compromising on spatial versus temporal resolution

Normal fatty breast tissue posed a significant problem because abnormal enhancement was difficult to distinguish from background bright fat signal on T1-weighted images. This had to be overcome either by adding an IR pulse for *fat suppression* or by using *subtraction* technique. Each of these options had drawbacks – subtraction was vulnerable to motion artifact while applying fat suppression carried a significant time penalty. Dynamic scans needed to be completed in 1–2 minutes to capture characteristics of the time–intensity curve. A choice then had to be made between rapidly repeated scans with multiple time points (only easily achievable with subtraction), and the more time-consuming fat-suppressed sequences which offered better resolution but limited scope for repetition.

Meanwhile, it was clear that a potential strength of MRI was the ability to show small invasive cancers by virtue of their enhancement, but to detect small lesions required thin slices and a large matrix size. These conflicting requirements severely tested the limits of the available MRI technology and further compromises had to be made. While European equipment vendors opted for bilateral breast coils, manufacturers in the USA favored the use of single breast coils to reduce the FOV and improve resolution.

These technical limitations resulted in the development of two broad schools of thought, alternatively emphasizing either spatial or temporal resolution. In Europe, bilateral, dynamic, subtracted breast MRI became popular, while on the other side of the North Atlantic, unilateral, high spatial resolution techniques with active fat suppression were favored [15]. For some years, there was debate as to whether the morphology of a mass or its signature on the time–intensity curve was ultimately the better predictor of malignancy.

Unfortunately, the time–intensity curves seen with invasive cancers showed considerable overlap with benign lesions. More importantly, not all invasive cancers showed rapid contrast uptake, with a small proportion displaying only weak or delayed enhancement. At the same time, of course, not all cancers showed stellate morphology, with well-circumscribed and very small lesions being particularly difficult to characterize. No matter which approach to diagnosis was favored, a significant number of cases were indeterminate.

Another approach to characterizing a mass was to perform a dynamic scan limited to the lesion itself. By examining a small volume of tissue, it was possible to achieve both high temporal resolution with multiple time points and high spatial resolution. However, because this technique required two contrast studies (one to identify the lesion and another to characterize it), practical value was limited, and it was never widely adopted for routine use.

Gradually key morphologic features which could reliably distinguish benign from malignant lesions emerged. In 1997, using a specially designed coil and imaging a single breast to optimize resolution, Nunes and colleagues described a morphology-based interpretation model featuring signs with high NPV in excluding malignancy, which formed the framework for currently used diagnostic algorithms [16].

Combining morphologic and kinetic elements

In a landmark study in 1999, Kuhl *et al.* examined the kinetic curves of 266 enhancing lesions, considered to be suspicious for malignancy on the basis of rapid early-phase contrast enhancement alone or suggestive morphology [17]. Patients with only typically benign slow initial enhancement were excluded. The lesions were then evaluated on enhancement rate, taking a threshold of above 80% as malignant, while the effect of applying the three kinetic curve types in the post-initial or delayed phase was also examined (Fig. 1.3). Among those lesions showing a type 1 curve, 94% were benign and only 6% malignant. Of those with a type 2 curve, 64% were malignant and 36% benign and with a type 3 curve, 87% were malignant and 13% were benign. This confirmed a clear relationship between curve type and overall likelihood of malignancy although with marked overlap for type 2 curves (Fig. 1.4).

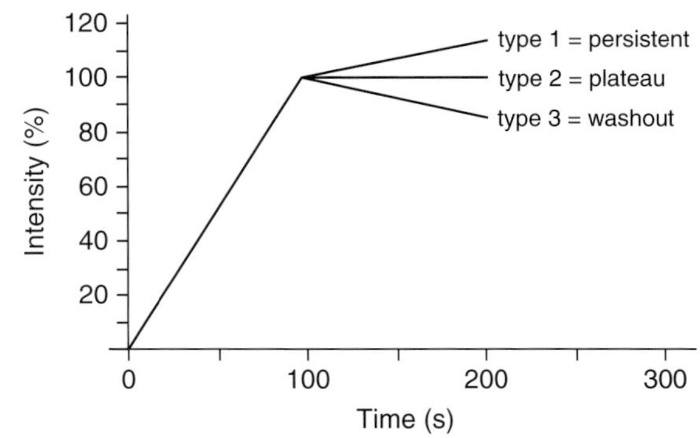

Fig. 1.3 Time–intensity curves: For lesions with moderate to rapid initial-phase enhancement, three basic curve types can be defined based on kinetic behavior in the delayed, post-initial or late phase. The type 3 curve is strongly associated with malignancy.

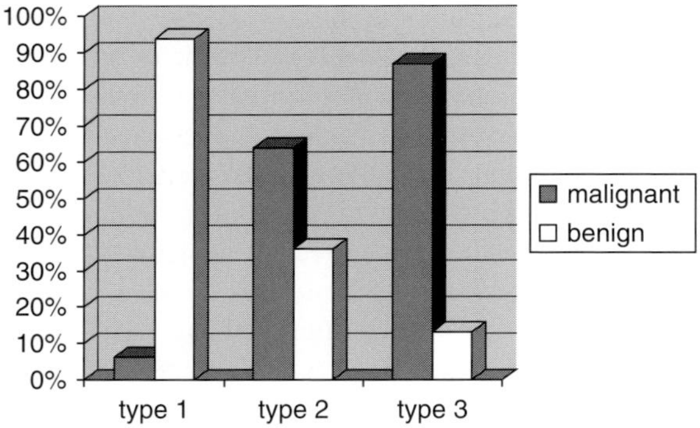

Fig. 1.4 Using late-phase enhancement to improve specificity: Histogram showing proportion of benign and malignant lesions by kinetic curve type in the study by Kuhl *et al.* [17].

Furthermore, if rapid initial enhancement of 80% above baseline alone was used to predict malignancy, sensitivity was 91% but with specificity of only 37% and PPV of 47%. By adding a simple qualitative assessment of curve type (type 2 or type 3 curve taken to predict malignancy), sensitivity stayed at 91%, while specificity increased to 83% with a PPV of 77%.

Kuhl *et al.* emphasized that where morphology indicated malignancy, kinetic curves were non-contributory. However, with probably benign morphology, performing a kinetic curve was of value as a type 1 curve might be used to allow follow-up rather than biopsy. A type 3 curve was considered to be an absolute indication for biopsy with an 87% PPV for malignancy. However, lack of washout did not imply that a lesion was not malignant, and it was emphasized that even a slow-rising type 1 curve could occur with invasive lobular or low-grade scirrhous invasive ductal cancers.

After Kuhl and coworkers had demonstrated the potential for kinetic curves to improve specificity, the value of the three types of time–intensity curve became widely accepted. The type 1 or *persistent* curve (enhancement steadily increasing after the initial phase) was usually benign. The type 2 or *plateau* curve (flattening out in the late phase) was sometimes malignant. The type 3 curve (rapid initial phase followed by late-phase *washout*, in which the intensity of enhancement reduced) was strongly associated with malignancy. Morphologic and dynamic features could then be combined in the diagnostic algorithm. Lesion morphology is evaluated first and takes precedence over kinetics, so for example a stellate mass is considered to be malignant until proven otherwise, regardless of the enhancement curve type.

Subsequently, the multicenter IBMC trial provided further insight into the relative contributions of morphologic and dynamic criteria in a much more selected patient population. In that trial, all patients had known suspicious lesions on conventional imaging requiring biopsy prior to performing MRI [18]. A cohort of women underwent both a high spatial resolution 3D breast MRI study and a further separate high temporal resolution 2D dynamic study of the lesion with scans every 15 seconds for 5 minutes.

In the IBMC study, 26% of cancers had a type 1 curve, making it clear that a type 1 curve could not be used to exclude malignancy [18, 19]. Meanwhile 76% of lesions with a type 3 curve proved to be malignant, with washout kinetics conferring ~5-fold increased likelihood of malignancy compared to persistent kinetics. A type 3 curve also had high specificity (~90%), confirming this as a key malignant sign and indicating that combined morphologic and kinetic interpretation models should yield the best results [18].

Kinetic curves are particularly valuable as a discriminator for mass lesions which are indeterminate on morphologic criteria alone (circumscribed or slightly irregular). In such cases, dynamic assessment can assist in deciding which lesions can be managed by interval follow-up and which may require biopsy (Fig. 1.5).

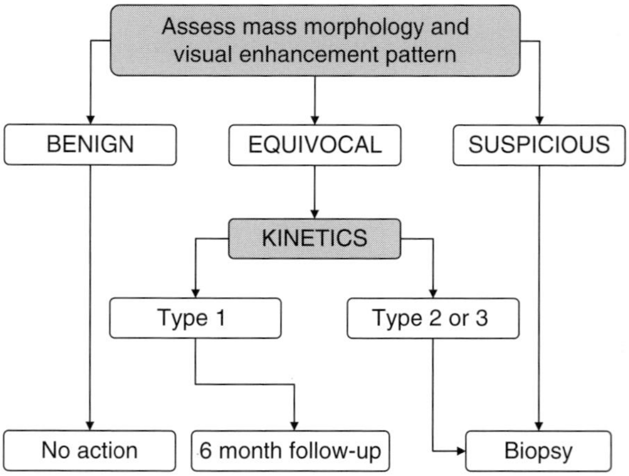

Fig. 1.5 Diagnostic algorithm for a mass: For a mass with unequivocally benign morphology, a kinetic assessment is often not necessary. Where mass morphology is equivocal, kinetics can be used as a "tie-breaker" to decide between early follow-up and biopsy, because a type 1 curve adds support for a benign diagnosis. For a mass with suspicious morphology, biopsy is required regardless of kinetics.

MRI-only lesions, targeted ultrasound and MRI-guided intervention

Another major initial problem was how to manage an abnormality shown only by MRI, the so-called *MRI-only lesion*, when MRI-compatible biopsy systems had not yet been developed. Fortunately, in instances where an invasive cancer was present, the lesion could often be identified on a *second-look* or *targeted ultrasound* (TUS), by focusing attention to the location of the MRI abnormality. Biopsy could then be performed under US guidance. For lesions not shown by TUS, a "watchful waiting" policy had to be adopted, with interval follow-up MRI usually first at 6 and then at 12 months.

The introduction of MRI-compatible hookwires with an acceptably low level of metal artifact and good mechanical strength was the first major advance in the management of MRI-only lesions. Surgical excision could then be offered when suspicious MRI findings warranted a histologic diagnosis. However, the watchful waiting approach was still widely used for small "unidentified breast objects" or "enhancing incidental lesions," which appeared to have a generally low likelihood of malignancy.

For many years, there was no satisfactory and widely available direct MRI-guided biopsy technique. Early experience with MRI-guided core biopsy was promising but the technique was unreliable for retrieving small MRI targets. Then, during the late 1990s, the technique of MRI-guided VAB emerged, pioneered in Europe by Heywang-Köbrunner and coworkers. This proved to be a viable alternative to MRI-guided hookwire localization and gained rapid acceptance. Establishing a method to biopsy most lesions without the need for surgical intervention effectively overcame the last major barrier to the development of breast MRI as a routine imaging technique.

Detection of DCIS by MRI

As experience increased and resolution steadily improved, it became clear that DCIS could be identified on MRI, although sensitivity was variable, with a reported range of 40–100%. One factor contributing to variability was the difficulty in distinguishing DCIS from other non-mass enhancement patterns seen with normal hormonal stimulation and proliferative fibrocystic change.

Furthermore, TUS often showed no abnormality with DCIS, which likely contributed to DCIS underdiagnosis in the absence of MRI-guided intervention techniques. This combination of factors explains why reported rates of MRI diagnosis of DCIS were initially often low.

Gradually, key features of distribution and morphology of enhancement were established which were helpful in differentiating DCIS from benign processes, while kinetics proved to be of limited value. Encouraging results for DCIS detection emerged from the prospective high-risk screening trials, notably the single-center Canadian and German studies, although the number of DCIS cases was small [1, 3].

In 2005, Menell and coworkers reported a retrospective review of pure DCIS in 33 breasts in which the sensitivity of MRI was 88% compared with only 27% for XRM [20]. High-resolution scanning was considered to be a major factor in this dramatically improved sensitivity compared to previous studies on DCIS detection by MRI. Soon after, Kuhl *et al.* reported a prospective study of 167 women with pure DCIS in which MRI sensitivity was 92% and XRM sensitivity 56% [21]. Notably, MRI performed best with biologically aggressive disease – among 89 women with high-grade DCIS, MRI sensitivity was 98%, with only about half of these cases detected by XRM.

Developing a common language: the ACR Lexicon

Another factor which undoubtedly hindered the development of breast MRI was the absence of standardized terminology to describe abnormal findings. This made it difficult to compare published work from different institutions and to disseminate information. In 2003, the introduction of an MRI Lexicon into the ACR BI-RADS system addressed this issue, providing a framework of key descriptors for breast MRI findings [22].

That the Lexicon was so rapidly and widely adopted around the world is a testament to its success in promoting mutual understanding throughout the breast MRI community. Nevertheless, the Lexicon was designed as a "work in progress" intended to evolve as its concepts are tested in clinical practice and accordingly the recent 2011 revision featured some significant changes.

Indications for breast MRI

So having understood the principles of breast MRI, the next question is when exactly should we apply this technique in the context of existing paradigms

Table 1.4 Clinical indications for referral for breast MRI

Screening of high-risk women
Preoperative staging for extent of known cancer
Equivocal lesion on XRM, US or clinical examination
Complex or dense breast with repeated equivocal mammograms
Positive axillary node with no breast primary evident
Scar versus tumor recurrence
Positive margins after resection to delineate residual disease
Monitoring response to neoadjuvant chemotherapy
Prior to accelerated partial breast irradiation
Breast implants for leakage and/or cancer detection

for managing breast disease? The list of recognized clinical indications for contrast-enhanced breast MRI given in Table 1.4 covers a wide range, but for the purposes of more detailed discussion in later chapters these can be conveniently divided into four groups.

High-risk screening

Used for routine surveillance in women at increased risk of breast cancer, usually on the basis of a strong family history, MRI detects many mammographically occult cancers. Accordingly, cancers are identified at an early stage, with a better prospect of surgical cure. The high sensitivity and high NPV of MRI are key strengths in this role.

Preoperative tumor staging

In a patient with known cancer, MRI aims to map local tumor extent as accurately as possible by showing multifocal, multicentric or contralateral disease. Of all available imaging techniques, MRI shows the best correlation with histopathologic disease extent, making it a potentially valuable tool in surgical planning. Findings impacting surgical management are found in up to 30% of women with newly diagnosed breast cancer, and the reported yield of contralateral breast cancer is around 3–5%. It is then, not surprising that preoperative MRI assessment of breast cancer is routine in some centers.

Problem-solving applications

This group covers a diverse range of situations which are not strictly related to either screening or tumor staging. Instead, MRI is used to clarify a specific clinical or radiologic question. The use of MRI to monitor neoadjuvant chemotherapy is also included in this heading.

Breast implants

Non-contrast MRI has long been used in the diagnosis of implant failure, although this role can be expected to wane with the advent of newer and more durable silicone implants. Contrast-enhanced MRI has a potential role in cancer detection in women with augmented breasts, where mammography is compromised.

What you need to get started

Over the 25 years since contrast-enhanced breast MRI began, technologic advances have made it possible for modern MRI systems to successfully combine rapid dynamic imaging with excellent spatial resolution, and demand for breast MRI has burgeoned. There is now a choice of several commercially available options for MRI-guided biopsy, and a steadily increasing number of radiologists are becoming engaged in breast MRI. So, what do you need to be able to join them?

MRI machine: field strength and gradient strength

In most instances, breast MRI is an addition to an existing installed system. A 1.5T system is widely considered as the minimum standard, because high SNR is a fundamental requirement and proportionately reduced at lower field strengths. In theory, doubling field strength doubles the SNR, with the option to obtain either better spatial resolution or shorter scan times.

While 3.0T magnets have been increasingly used for breast MRI, there are trade-offs for higher SNR, notably problems with obtaining homogeneous fat suppression. The consensus is that breast MRI at 3.0T does not offer major benefits over 1.5T for routine purposes, but may be an advantage for some adjunctive techniques, particularly MRS and DWI.

Spatial information in MRI is encoded by manipulating magnetic gradients in the transverse x- and y-axes, and along the bore of the magnet (the z-axis), using three sets of gradient coils. The time to achieve maximum gradient strength is the *rise-time* or *slew rate*. This is important, because how rapidly the gradients can be switched on and off dictates how fast a sequence can be performed. Recent MRI machines permit maximum gradient strengths of up to 50 mT/m (milliTesla per meter) to be reached in times as short as 200 microseconds [23]. Strong gradients with fast rise-times are particularly important for breast MRI because of the need for both high spatial and high temporal resolution in post-contrast dynamic 3D gradient-echo sequences.

For new installations purely for breast MRI, Aurora Imaging Technology (North Andover, MA, USA) have pioneered the production of fully dedicated breast MRI systems with design optimized for maximum patient comfort and ease of access for interventional procedures. The 1.5T Aurora system uses Spiral RODEO, a sequence which employs spiral k-space sampling and combines excellent image quality with extremely rapid examination times.

Other vendors offer new MRI systems which are configured as "dedicated" breast machines, but these are really modifications of standard designs as opposed to Aurora's single-purpose concept. One potential advantage of a machine like the Siemens Espree Pink is that it can be converted back to a general purpose MRI scanner should demand for breast MRI turn out to be less than anticipated.

Breast coils

A dedicated breast coil is essential and must include the capability to perform MRI-guided interventions, unless a prior arrangement is made for biopsies to be performed at an alternative site. Unlike standard surface coils, dedicated breast coils employ phased-array technology, in which arrays of elements (individual small coils) are used in combination. Array coil design, with each element examining only a small volume of tissue, means less noise is contributed to the composite final image than if a single large surface coil had been used. As a result, a larger region can be examined with improved SNR. Each element has its own receiver channel, with 4-, 8- and recently 16-channel coils now available. These multichannel coils, with increasingly superior SNR, allow for either higher resolution or shorter scan times and have the additional advantage of supporting parallel imaging (see later).

When selecting a breast coil, in addition to the vendors own products, be sure to consider the options offered by companies such as Invivo (Orlando, FL, USA) and Sentinelle Medical (Toronto, ON, Canada), now owned by Philips and Hologic respectively. For MRI machines made by GE, Sentinelle market the Vanguard Breast MR Auxiliary Table, which is in essence a fully detachable integrated imaging and intervention trolley. With two of these units, patients can be cannulated and positioned before being taken into the magnet room, greatly improving workflow efficiency in centers with high throughput. The Sentinelle Vanguard, table-top systems (for GE, Siemens and Toshiba MRI machines) incorporate patented Variable Coil Geometry, which allows adjustment of the lateral elements for different breast sizes.

Access to conventional breast imaging

As will be seen in Chapter 3, access to conventional imaging, particularly high-resolution US (broadband probes ranging up to at least 10–12 MHz), is essential for optimal management of lesions revealed by breast MRI. Targeted ultrasound is the first consideration for workup of suspected mass lesions, which can often be identified and biopsied without resorting to more invasive and costly MRI-guided interventional methods. Similarly, additional mammographic views are sometimes needed, particularly in the context of identifying microcalcification which may then be easier to biopsy using x-ray stereotactic technique.

MRI-guided biopsy capability

As MRI is so much more sensitive compared to XRM, MRI-only lesions will be encountered which cannot be localized by any other technique. Therefore, it is essential to be able to obtain histologic tissue samples using MRI-guided intervention. At the minimum this means having the capability to position an MRI-compatible hookwire in a suspicious lesion to allow surgical excision. However, the standard of care is to use VAB as a minimally invasive means of obtaining a histologic diagnosis in the majority of cases.

There is now a range of VAB systems on offer which are compatible with MRI machines from all major vendors. Most of these have floor-based vacuum-generating units which remain outside the magnet room, with lengthy plastic tubing supplying the biopsy handpiece. The Bard Vacora system is a fully self-contained handheld device with the advantages of being both less expensive and readily portable, allowing easy transfer between locations. Although it lacks the vacuum power and sophistication of the floor-based systems, the Bard Vacora is an attractive option for low-volume breast MRI sites, and still provides much larger tissue samples than traditional 14-gauge CNB. Features of VAB systems are discussed in detail in Chapter 4.

Where there are several MRI sites performing relatively small numbers of diagnostic breast MRI studies, it may be possible for one or more selected centers to purchase the necessary equipment and develop expertise in MRI-guided VAB. The other sites can then send cases for MRI biopsy to the larger center, allowing concentrated experience and more cost-effective utilization of equipment.

The option of a CAD system

With the large amount of volumetric data requiring analysis, workstation review is now mandatory, and commercially available CAD systems such as DynaCAD or Cadstream offer several advantages. Full synchronization of multiple data sets allows instant and accurate correlation of possible lesions on different sequences. The ability to generate time–intensity curves "on-the-fly" is an invaluable timesaver as is user-friendly color-mapping which can be toggled on and off the images as required. Using such features, a suspicious finding can be pinpointed with the cursor, immediately viewed on multiple sequences for evaluation of signal characteristics and morphology, then kinetically assessed in just a few moments.

Even with minimal movement, subtracted images benefit significantly from the application of pixel-shift software to improve misregistration artifacts. While such software packages can be costly add-ons when purchased from some MRI vendors, sophisticated autoregistration software is fully integrated into commercially available CAD systems. When it is considered that a CAD system provides a purpose-built reporting station and registration software, the combined savings go a long way towards paying for the investment. Many CAD systems also offer reporting templates using BI-RADS terminology which assist in providing rapid dictation in an appropriate synoptic format. This provides both consistency in reporting style and further time-savings. Accordingly, if a significant workload is anticipated, a CAD system is well worthwhile just because it makes reading and reporting so much faster. Finally, increasingly sophisticated biopsy modules can facilitate MRI-guided interventions, reducing the risk of targeting errors. Before dismissing CAD as an expensive luxury, be sure to carefully compare functionality and overall cost offered by MRI vendors versus commercial CAD systems (Table 1.5).

Perhaps the main pitfall of using a CAD system is the risk of becoming overly reliant on color maps for lesion identification. The arbitrary nature of the threshold settings must be understood – there is no absolute cutoff below which cancer does not occur. Keep in mind that color-mapping is only ever an adjunct, not a primary diagnostic technique, and that

Table 1.5 Advantages of dedicated MRI CAD system

Synchronized display of multiple sequences with 3D reformats in any plane
Color-mapping parametric overlay for overview of kinetics
On-the-fly kinetic curve display using ROI defined by cursor
Automatic correction of misregistration in subtracted images
Faster reporting – automated reports using BI-RADS
Automated biopsy guidance software
3D volume-rendering useful for neoadjuvant treatment monitoring

morphology always "trumps" kinetics. Furthermore, while CAD may aid in distinction between invasive cancers and benign masses, it is not helpful in differentiating DCIS from other benign changes [24, 25].

Patient preparation prior to scanning

Once the basic requirements to start an MRI service are in place, the next step is to plan how best to schedule patients and manage workflow on a daily basis. Magnet time is a valuable commodity to be used as efficiently as possible. Even with a small number of cases, workflow is greatly improved by having a session set aside for breast MRI cases rather than fitting them in to general MRI lists. This avoids time wasted in changing coils and allows a system for optimum throughput to be developed. After completing clerical work, recording essential clinical information (Table 1.6) and performing MRI safety checks, cannulation can be performed in an anteroom so the next patient is ready for scanning immediately the previous patient is completed.

Table 1.6 Essential clinical information for breast MRI studies

First day of LMP or date of cessation of periods
Possible or known current pregnancy or lactation
Drug history – HRT, SERMs (tamoxifen), any anticoagulant agents
Any current symptoms – lump, nipple discharge
Personal history (previous biopsy, previous cancer history, available pathology details)
Dates and availability of previous imaging (MRI, mammogram, US, biopsy)
If previous breast cancer, details of location, date and whether RT given
Family history of breast and ovarian cancer with ages at diagnosis

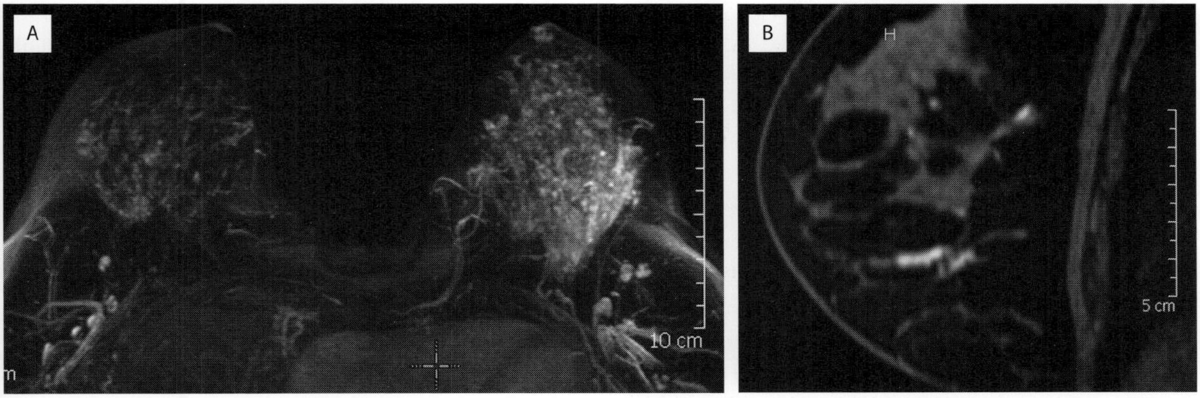

Fig. 1.6 Hormonal effects: (A) MIP image (composite 3D rendering of subtracted data), from MRI study performed in young woman on day 22 of her cycle, shows marked diffuse enhancement in left breast and only mild changes on the right. A repeat study on day 10 of the next menstrual cycle was completely normal with virtually "empty" breasts bilaterally. (B) Asymmetric focal linear-ductal enhancement seen in postmenopausal woman on HRT, which resolved completely on a repeat study 8 weeks after stopping HRT.

Biologic factors in cancer detection

In planning workflows, the fundamental objective of demonstrating breast cancer with maximum sensitivity and specificity should always be kept in mind. Even with state-of-the-art equipment the best results can only be achieved by careful attention to technique at every stage of the process. To identify the smallest possible invasive cancers (5 mm or less) and to detect and characterize DCIS, high-resolution imaging is a key requirement. Still more fundamental though is to ensure that an adequate contrast injection enters the patient's circulation and that she is able to keep still while the images are acquired! After all, cancer detection by MRI relies on ensuring that an adequate contrast volume and rate of injection are used, so that rapid enhancement (more likely to be pathologic) can be distinguished from usually slow-enhancing parenchyma.

Even for the detection of invasive cancer, MRI is not perfect, with reported failure rates in the range of 2–8% [8, 18, 26, 27]. Low-grade IDC, tubular cancers and pure or mixed ILC are the most common pathologic types,[28, 29] and are usually missed because they tend to enhance more slowly than high-grade cancers. Accordingly, even if a satisfactory bolus of contrast is delivered, it may be impossible to differentiate these slowly enhancing cancers from the normal surrounding breast tissue. This problem is amplified if the normal parenchyma itself shows unusually marked contrast uptake, commonly due to hormonal stimulation (cyclical in premenopausal women or to HRT after menopause). Such hormonal changes can cause false-positive MRI findings of asymmetric focal or diffuse enhancement (Fig. 1.6).

Furthermore in a small subset of ~10% of usually premenopausal women, a symmetrical diffuse distribution of strong early enhancement may be seen, even when MRI is performed in the second week of the cycle. Obscuration by strong *background enhancement* is the leading cause of cancers missed by MRI (Table 1.7).

Background enhancement is to MRI what breast density is to XRM, i.e., the major cause of reduced sensitivity. Just as breast density is graded in XRM reports using the BI-RADS system (Table 1.8), so

Table 1.7 Causes of invasive cancers missed by MRI

Technical factors (~20%)
Faulty injection technique
Motion artifact
FOV too small (cancer at periphery of breast)
Surgical clip artifact
Biologic factors (~80%)
Strong background enhancement
Small tumor size, including DCIS with small invasive foci
Diffuse infiltrative tumor growth pattern (more frequently with ILC)
Slow or non-enhancing low-grade IDC, ILC or mixed types, tubular cancer

Shimauchi *et al.* [8], Schnall *et al.* [18], Schnall and Orel [19], Heywang-Köbrunner *et al.* [26], Teifke *et al.* [27], Linda *et al.* [28], Ghai *et al.* [29].

Table 1.8 BI-RADS classification of breast density

BI-RADS	Descriptive definition
Class 1	Almost entirely fat
Class 2	Scattered fibroglandular densities
Class 3	Heterogeneously dense
Class 4	Extremely dense

Table 1.9 BI-RADS classification of background enhancement

BI-RADS	Descriptive definition
Class 1	Absent or minimal
Class 2	Mild
Class 3	Moderate
Class 4	Marked

background enhancement on MRI is graded in a similar manner (Table 1.9). However, it is important to appreciate that MRI background enhancement and XRM density are not the same. An XRM dense breast may show absent or minimal enhancement, while a fatty breast can sometimes show marked background enhancement on MRI. The pathologic nature of background enhancement is not yet clear, but it may relate to increased vascularity from exaggerated hormonal effects on glandular breast tissue. Whatever the exact mechanism, in common with mammographic density, there is emerging evidence that MRI background enhancement is itself a significant risk factor for breast cancer development.

Another factor well known to obscure cancers on breast MRI is the use of excessive compression to immobilize the breast. Due to the abnormal nature of tumor angiogenesis, vascular flow to a cancer can be selectively reduced even though normal breast tissue remains well perfused. This is because the abnormal small vessels in the tumor circulation have thin walls which lack the usual fibro-elastic tissue, and are therefore much more easily occluded.

Scheduling issues

Premenopausal women

For routine screening MRI and most problem-solving applications, premenopausal women should ideally be booked between days 5 and 15 from the first day of the menstrual cycle. For clinically urgent cases such as newly diagnosed breast cancer for staging, booking according to the menstrual cycle may not always be acceptable. Clinical colleagues need to be aware of the risks of increased false-positive rates and potentially lower sensitivity if scans in premenopausal women are performed with suboptimal timing. In any event, it is strongly advisable to avoid the fourth (premenstrual) week of the cycle.

Postmenopausal women

While it is not essential to stop HRT prior to the MRI scan, in occasional instances where confusing enhancement is encountered it will be necessary to perform a follow-up scan after 6–12 weeks off HRT.

Irregular cycles or previous hysterectomy

A problem is posed where the time of the ovarian cycle cannot be reliably assessed. The usual pragmatic approach is to perform the MRI study, and if unacceptable background enhancement is an issue, to repeat it 2 weeks later hoping to coincide with a more favorable part of the cycle. However, this still results in significant cost and inconvenience for those women. A more elegant solution has been described by Ellis who showed that in women with irregular cycles or who have had a hysterectomy but retained their ovaries, background enhancement can be minimized by performing the MRI scan when serum progesterone is <4.7 nmol/L, corresponding to the normal follicular phase [30]. A baseline blood sample is drawn when the woman is ready to book in, and if the serum progesterone level is too high, it is then repeated 3–5 days later. Most women require only one or two blood samples to be drawn and the principle can be applied in other similar clinical situations (Table 1.10).

Pregnancy

Breast MRI should be avoided during pregnancy unless clinically urgent. Although there are no known harmful effects of MRI itself, the fetus should not be exposed to gadolinium, particularly during organogenesis in the first trimester. The referring clinician and patient should also be made aware that hormonal effects in pregnancy make interpretation of the breast MRI study more difficult.

Table 1.10 Use of serum progesterone <4.7 nmol/L for timing breast MRI

Naturally irregular cycles, e.g., perimenopausal status
Irregular cycles due to contraceptive measures
Hysterectomy with retained ovaries
Chemotherapy-induced perimenopausal status

Lactation

Increased diffuse contrast uptake is typically seen, compromising MRI interpretation, so routine studies are ideally deferred for 6 weeks after ceasing lactation. This may be relaxed in the case of high-risk women due for annual screening, as an MRI study even with slightly reduced sensitivity is preferable to no MRI at all. When a clinically urgent study is required, some mothers may prefer to express and discard breast milk for 24 hours after the gadolinium injection.

Claustrophobia

Where the MRI system permits, positioning the patient feet-first in the magnet can significantly reduce claustrophobia. Otherwise, time should be allowed for premedication with the oral anxiolytic lorazepam (Ativan, Wyeth) at a dose of 0.5–2.0 mg 30–60 minutes prior, while an additional sublingual dose is an option during lengthier biopsy procedures.

Cannulation and gadolinium injection

A cannula of no less than 20 g caliber is recommended, routinely placed at the elbow in the median cubital vein to give the most direct route to the axillary vein. If a peripheral vein has to be used, this should be noted as it may affect the kinetic curve. In patients who have had previous breast cancer treatment (particularly ALND or RT) the contralateral arm should be used for cannulation whenever possible to avoid the risks of lymphedema and cellulitis.

Injection rates of 2–3 ml/s are required for optimal bolus effect and using a power injector gives the most consistent results. For hand injection the contrast bolus is given over 5–10 seconds. Either way, it is essential to follow with a 20 ml saline flush at the same rate. Even with the most standardized injection technique, keep in mind that considerable variability has to be expected due to physiologic factors like heart rate and stroke volume. There is usually no need for a delay to allow for circulation time before commencing the first post-contrast sequence, as acquisition time is at least 1 minute. For some 3D gradient-echo sequences, the MRI vendors may recommend a delay of 20–25 seconds so that the contrast peak coincides with the center of k-space sampling, which optimizes image contrast.

The standard clinical dose of gadolinium is 0.1 mmol/kg. The concentration of gadolinium used in commercially available preparations is 0.5 mmol/ml so 1 ml of gadolinium is required for every 5 kg of body weight. As the usual ampoule size is 10 ml this is the correct dose for a 50 kg person, while the dose for a 100 kg person is 2 ampoules or 20 ml. As the approximate weight range for most women having breast MRI is 50–100 kg, the usual dose range is 10–20 ml.

While some have advocated doubling the standard dose of gadolinium for MRI studies in the hope of improving lesion detection, more is not necessarily better. One report found that gadobenate dimeglumine (MultiHance, Bracco, Milan, Italy) gave best results at a dose of 0.1 mmol/kg, compared with halved and doubled doses of 0.05 mmol/kg and 0.2 mmol/kg respectively [31]. Larger doses may even cause increased background enhancement of normal tissue, reducing sensitivity and potentially causing false-positive findings.

Recent evidence for gadobenate as the contrast medium of choice for breast MRI comes from the multicenter DETECT trial [32]. In this blinded crossover study, 151 women alternately received both gadobenate and gadopentetate dimeglumine (Magnevist, Schering, Berlin, Germany), in otherwise identical MRI studies. Across three readers, the study showed significantly higher malignant lesion detection rates of 92–94% for gadobenate versus 80–83% for gadopentetate. Futhermore, specificity was also significantly improved using gadobenate, which gave PPVs in the range of 77–91% versus 61–81% for gadopentetate [32].

Positioning the patient prior to scanning

While the first post-contrast T1 series is completed within about 90 seconds, the multiple repeated acquisitions required for a dynamic study result in a total scan time of several minutes. Accordingly, minimizing movement is vital, particularly if subtraction technique is used. Not only can movement obscure small lesions on subtracted scans, but misregistration artifact can cause spurious enhancement which mimics pathology. Making the patient as comfortable as possible prior to starting the dynamic scan, and explaining exactly when to stay still are key factors to achieve movement-free studies (Table 1.11).

Folds in patient gowns may tighten and act as a tourniquet, which is not only uncomfortable but can interfere with the injection. Therefore gowns must be removed as the patient is positioned on the table. Each breast is placed into the coil-well with the nipple directed straight down to preserve topography.

Table 1.11 Tips for patient positioning

Remove gown – eliminates possibility of tourniquet effect
Position breasts – nipple should be pointing straight down
Check midline position and craniocaudal extent of tissue within the coil
Use light side-to-side compression with additional coil padding if desired
Position head in cradle support
Position arms – avoid "loop" if arms above head to prevent radiofrequency burns
Check patient is comfortable – offer padding under the legs
Explain the noises from the sequences and when they MUST keep still

Recent 16-channel coils with enclosed designs (necessary to accommodate the extra elements) restrict external access to the breast, so the required position needs to be explained to the woman. The technologist should check that tissue is not folding or spilling outside the coil, and can assist in gently easing the breasts into the coil from above. It is important to ensure the patient is in the midline and that craniocaudal centering is satisfactory, and does not include excessive abdominal fat below the inframammary fold.

It is still a case of "one size fits all" for most breast coils, and various means have been tried to prevent movement in patients of often widely differing body habitus. For smaller breasts, padding can be used to fill the dead space around each breast if desired. For pendulous breasts, some suggest using a sheet as a sling support, while others recommend women wear a T-shirt but both these measures tend to distort breast shape. Immobilizing compression plates (built in to many current coil designs) are effective but should be only gently applied to avoid occluding the vascular supply of a cancer.

Current coil designs all have head-supports, but additional padding may be helpful for the arms, which need to be stably positioned, usually above the head rather than by the sides. The main disadvantage of the latter is that because the arms are lateral to breast tissue, aliasing (wrap-around) artifact can be an issue. However, placing the arms by the sides may be preferred to improve coverage in smaller breasts, counteracting the tendency for breasts tissue to be pulled out from the coil with the arms above. Note also that when the arms are placed above the head, they should not be in contact with each other, as forming a "loop" has the potential for a radiofrequency burn to occur.

Pressure on the sternum is a problem with some coils, but can be alleviated by adding a customized midline thin strip of dense foam padding. Placing a pillow under the legs is also recommended to improve overall patient comfort and compliance during scanning.

Technical considerations in protocol design

Essential technical requirements for breast MRI are listed in Table 1.12. To help in understanding how these factors relate to scanning protocols, some theoretical background to MRI is now briefly presented.

Signal-to-noise ratio and parallel imaging

A key factor in obtaining high-quality MRI is getting high SNR into the image matrix. The more *signal* there is for each *voxel*, the more options you have available for "trade-offs" to increase spatial resolution or shorten scan times. For breast MRI, SNR can be maximized using the combination of high-field-strength magnets and multichannel phased array coils. Another technical trick which can be used to increase signal acquired per unit time is *parallel imaging*.

This technique first appeared commercially as Philips SENSE technology but other vendors have adopted the concept (Table 1.13). The key is to speed up the process of image acquisition by making more efficient use of multichannel array coils. Instead of all channels gathering the same information, two different data sets can be acquired at the same time, i.e., in parallel, and then subsequently combined into one image. This then effectively doubles the acquisition speed (*acceleration factor* of 2), apart from time

Table 1.12 Essential technical requirements for breast MRI

Field strength 1.5T or greater with fast rise-times
Dedicated bilateral breast coil with biopsy capability
Include non-contrast T2-weighted pulse sequence
Include 3D contrast-enhanced T1-weighted gradient-echo sequence
Contrast injection of 0.1 mmol/kg at 2–3 ml/s
Minimum dynamic three time points with temporal resolution of 60–90 seconds
Subtraction, homogeneous fat suppression, or combination of both
Thin sections of 3 mm or less, with 1 mm ideal for isotropic reformatting
Pixel size (in-plane resolution) of less than 1 mm

Table 1.13 Acronyms used for parallel imaging techniques

SENSE = SENSitivity Encoding (Philips)
iPAT = integrated Parallel Acquisition Technique (Siemens)
GRAPPA = GeneRalized Autocalibrating Partially Parallel Acquisition (Siemens)
ASSET = Array Spatial Sensitivity Encoding Technique (General Electric)
SPEEDER = No acronym! (Toshiba)
SMASH = SiMultaneous Acquisition of Spatial Harmonics (generic)
Auto-SMASH = Automatic SMASH (generic)
PPA = Partially Parallel Array (generic)

allowed for a very short pre-scan calibration sequence. For acceleration factors greater than 2–3, significant aliasing (wrap artifact) arises and the SNR advantage reduces.

For breast MRI, parallel imaging opened up the possibility of synchronous sagittal acquisition of dynamic scans. Previously, using sagittal acquisition for dynamic scans meant scanning each breast separately so that the vital first minute after contrast was missed on one side. With parallel imaging, both breasts could be scanned synchronously, rapidly and with good spatial resolution. Consequently some centers adopted bilateral sagittal acquisition as routine. However, the speed advantage of using parallel imaging without significant loss of image quality is equally applicable to axial scan protocols.

Coverage, field of view and spatial resolution

Optimizing images is all about trade-offs using the available signal, with high resolution and large FOV presenting conflicting requirements. The FOV must be just large enough to include all breast tissue and the axillary regions but no larger, as including surrounding space simply "wastes" pixels and reduces spatial resolution.

Using the smallest possible FOV means a smaller matrix size can be applied to achieve the required submillimeter in-plane resolution. For axial imaging of both breasts an FOV of 32–36 cm gives adequate anatomic coverage and using a 448 × 448 matrix gives pixel sizes of 0.5–0.7 mm, affording excellent image in-plane resolution.

Slice thickness is the other key determinant of resolution, because to reliably detect a 3 mm lesion requires at least an equal and preferably a smaller slice thickness, although this inevitably reduces SNR in each voxel. Nevertheless, with current MRI systems and 3D gradient-echo T1 sequences, it is possible to routinely achieve bilateral dynamic breast MRI studies with submillimeter in-plane resolution, 1 mm slice thickness, 1 minute temporal resolution and yet still preserve adequate SNR.

Demonstration of the axillary regions was poor with early coil designs due to various issues including cardiac pulsation artifact, wrap-around (aliasing) effects and poor signal. Both cardiorespiratory movement and wrap artifacts arise in the phase-encoding direction, which should be set left–right for axial imaging and head–feet for sagittal acquisition (but never anterior–posterior as this would propagate artifact over the breasts). Recent 16-channel breast coil designs incorporate additional elements which cover the axillary regions, boosting SNR and allow high-resolution virtually artifact-free imaging of the lymph nodes.

Imaging of only one breast in the axial plane with a small FOV leads to wrap-around artifacts from the contralateral breast, and is not recommended. However, for unilateral sagittal imaging of the dependent breast an FOV as small as 20 cm may be adequate and there should be no outside tissue to interfere. For sagittal acquisition with some breasts it is possible to further reduce scan time, without loss of resolution, using a rectangular FOV (with fewer steps in the time-dependent phase-encoding direction).

Suppressing fat signal in T1-weighted images

On a non-fat-suppressed T1-weighted image, fat has by far the brightest tissue signal and tops the range of signal intensity display. With the addition of IR fat suppression, fat signal is reduced to zero, which greatly expands the contrast range which can be displayed (*scaling effect*). When gadolinium is added, areas of enhancement top the scale and become conspicuous against the dark background of suppressed fat signal.

The alternative method of removing bright fat signal from T1-weighted images is using subtraction technique which "compares" pre- and post-contrast images and displays the difference, giving an accurate map of enhancement, provided there is no movement in between. While subtraction was originally applied to pre- and post-contrast non-fat-suppressed T1-weighted images, it can also be used

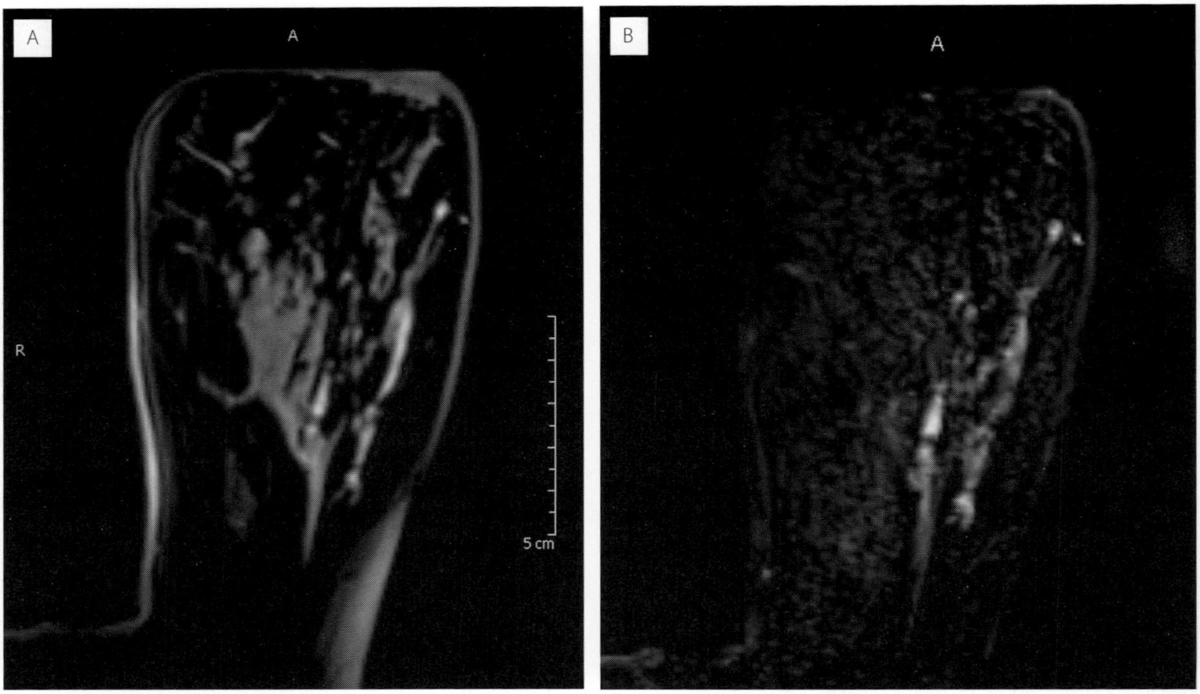

Fig. 1.7 Subtraction technique: On post-contrast fat-suppressed image (A) linear contrast is difficult to appreciate against intermediate signal fibroglandular parenchyma, but on subtracted image (B) the linear-ductal pattern of this extensive high-grade DCIS (which was non-calcified and occult to XRM) is clearly demonstrated.

with fat-suppressed T1-weighted images. One advantage of adding subtraction is in instances where fat suppression is inhomogeneous – because the exact same artifact arises on both pre- and post-contrast images, it is removed by image subtraction.

Furthermore, even with fat suppression applied, it can be challenging to detect subtle enhancement on a background of fibroglandular breast tissue which itself displays intermediate (gray) signal (Fig. 1.7). Given that adding subtraction technique to fat-suppressed T1-weighted images carries no acquisition time penalty, can overcome issues relating to inhomogeneous fat suppression and improves conspicuity of some subtle lesions, it seems worthy of routine use.

More about kinetic curves

Whereas CT scanners can be exactly calibrated with phantoms, and *absolute* measurements of tissue density made using Hounsfield units (water 0 HU, fat −100 HU, blood pool ~40 HU and so on), this is not the case for MRI systems. Instead, signal intensities of different tissues can only be compared *relative* to each other. To evaluate the effect of gadolinium in breast MRI, increase in T1 signal intensity *relative* to baseline pre-contrast signal intensity is used to calculate *relative signal intensity* or *relative enhancement*, expressed as a percentage using the formula below.

Kinetic curves, then, are a plot of relative signal intensity against time from injection. Fundamentally, relative enhancement is greatly dependent on the amount and rate of delivery of the contrast injection, and on the exact design of the T1-weighted sequence used. Therefore, where units of signal intensity are displayed on the y-axis of a kinetic curve, these are arbitrary, specific to that MRI system and to the particular pulse sequence.

$$\text{Relative enhancement} = \frac{SI_{\text{contrast}} - SI_{\text{baseline}}}{SI_{\text{baseline}}} \times 100$$

As a result, all possible factors should be standardized in scanning protocols, so that at least breast MRI studies performed on the same MRI system are closely comparable. Nonetheless, for practical purposes, the y-axis is more meaningful when converted from arbitrary units into % signal intensity.

Initial or early phase of contrast uptake (wash-in)

The early or *initial phase* refers to contrast uptake or *wash-in* during the first 2 minutes after injection. Rate of enhancement can be classified as slow, moderate or rapid. Terms such as "mild" and "intense" tend to be used interchangeably with "slow" and "rapid," referring to the peak intensity reached during the initial phase. In other words, if contrast uptake is rapid, the curve rises steeply in the initial phase and a high peak relative signal intensity or peak relative enhancement will be reached.

So if the initial pre-contrast signal was 600 arbitrary units and this increased to a peak of 1500 after contrast, this would be a peak relative enhancement of (1500–600)/600 = 150%. This can be used to measure *wash-in rate* or *peak enhancement velocity* as signal increase per unit time. In practice, it is more convenient to simply evaluate the level of enhancement at a constant time, often the first post-contrast time point at 60–90 seconds after injection.

As a guide, enhancement of up to 50% above baseline signal intensity in a given ROI can be considered slow or mild, from 50% to 100% is intermediate or moderate, and anything above 100% would qualify as rapid or intense.

Post-initial or delayed phase of contrast uptake (washout)

The post-initial, late or delayed phase refers to the period beyond 2 minutes from injection. Normal parenchyma typically shows low levels of enhancement (below 50%) with a gradual continuous rise in signal intensity throughout the duration of the study. Assuming a lesion shows at least moderate enhancement (wash-in of 50–100%) during the initial phase, one of three things can happen. If the curve continues to rise, albeit at a slower rate, it is a type 1 or *persistent* curve. If it levels off it is a type 2 or *plateau* curve and if it goes down, it is a type 3 or *washout* curve (Fig. 1.3).

The type of kinetic curve can also be expressed as the signal enhancement ratio (SER), which compares early-to late-phase enhancement (see formula). It is this ratio which is used to derive the standard color maps used by CAD systems, with SER > 1 indicating washout kinetics (coded red), SER = 1 defining a plateau curve (coded green), and SER < 1 indicating persistent kinetics (coded blue). Typically malignant kinetic criteria comprise a peak enhancement velocity (or peak early-phase enhancement) of > 80–90% and SER of 1 or greater (combination of rapid wash-in and either plateau or washout)

$$\text{Signal enhancement ratio} = \frac{SI_{early} - SI_{baseline}}{SI_{delayed} - SI_{baseline}}$$

Dynamic sequence options

While the first post-contrast T1-weighted sequence must be performed within 2 minutes from injection in order to capture the peak for a rapidly enhancing lesion, reducing the time below 1 minute is unnecessary. So, once temporal resolution of 1–2 minutes is achieved (60–90 seconds is ideal), all MRI factors should be arranged so as to optimize spatial resolution [33].

Furthermore, while traditional protocols repeated the same T1 sequence at equal intervals across the dynamic series, e.g., a 70 second scan performed 6 times in 7 minutes, some newer protocol designs aim to make better use of available time by accepting fewer time points. In fact, to distinguish the three kinetic curve types requires only two post-contrast time points (baseline pre-contrast scan, first time point before 2 minutes to capture the enhancement peak, second time point in delayed phase to distinguish plateau from washout curves).

One possible approach then is to perform a high-resolution 3D T1-weighted morphology-based scan with about double the acquisition time, during the third and fourth post-contrast minutes followed by a final delayed-phase kinetic scan. Although fewer time points are available, the basic kinetic curve shape can still be defined and is all that is required for practical purposes. Meanwhile, a "free" high-resolution morphologic scan has been obtained.

Another option for post-contrast scans is to use rapid breath-hold dynamic 3D fat-suppressed acquisitions such as Siemens VIBE.

Deciding on a protocol

So to summarize, key requirements in technique are (i) adequate volume and rate of contrast injection, (ii) minimal movement artifact, (iii) high-resolution images and (iv) a minimum three-time-point dynamic sequence. It is also important to keep overall examination time as short as possible for better patient compliance in keeping still and to maximize patient throughput.

As Table 1.14 shows, the minimum protocol would be a fat-suppressed T2-weighted sequence followed by one pre- and two post-contrast T1-weighted dynamic scans. Using an isotropic 3D gradient-echo acquisition ensures high-quality multiplanar reformatted images, obviating the need for further planes of acquisition after contrast. As has been mentioned, using parallel imaging, direct sagittal acquisition is an option. However, a compelling argument for using standard axial acquisitions is that symmetry of enhancement between the breasts across the dynamic series is much easier to appreciate.

Direct sagittal acquisition of post-contrast images may be considered when there is only one breast, or for assessment of extent of unilateral known DCIS. In these circumstances, a non-dynamic high-resolution direct sagittal acquisition using a smaller FOV of 20–24 cm has the advantage of clearly demonstrating the typical segmental or ductal distribution of DCIS enhancement extending towards the nipple.

The axial fat-suppressed T2-weighted sequence is also a useful "screening" sequence for unexpected pathology, particularly metastatic disease in the context of breast cancer staging, and some advocate adding a coronal STIR sequence to include the whole chest and upper abdomen for these cases.

For those who prefer to include a non-fat-suppressed FSE T2-weighted series (for assessing signal in masses) a sagittal acquisition allows for comparison with the mammographic MLO view, which can help when correlating areas of asymmetric density or architectural distortion. Some advocate using non-fat-suppressed T1-weighted images for similar reasons, and this sequence may also show minimal artifact from titanium marker clips to better advantage.

Table 1.14 Suggested sequences for routine breast MRI studies

Axial non-contrast fat-suppressed IR T2-weighted sequence (for cysts and masses)
Axial non-contrast fat-suppressed IR T1-weighted sequence (mask for subtractions)
Minimum of 2 × axial IR T1-weighted post-contrast dynamic sequences (for kinetic curve type)
Intercalated high-resolution axial IR T1-weighted 3D gradient-echo sequence (for morphology)
Optional sagittal non-contrast FSE T2-weighted sequence (for cysts and masses)
Optional whole-body STIR (for staging indications)
Optional DWI sequences (b-values of 0 and 600–800) and MR spectroscopy
Optional T2-weighted water-suppressed "silicone-only" sequence for silicone implant screen

Magnetic resonance spectroscopy

Research into proton (1H) MRS has shown that a choline peak is present in most breast cancers but absent in normal breast tissue. Studies using single-voxel analysis at 1.5T report sensitivity in the range of 70–100%, although small lesion size (< 10–15 mm) is still a limiting factor for masses [34, 35]. Furthermore, MRS is less reliable for non-mass enhancement as DCIS may not always exhibit a choline peak. Nevertheless, MRS has potential to improve specificity and could help reduce the number of mass lesions requiring biopsy. Reduction in the choline peak also appears to be a sensitive and early indicator of response to neoadjuvant chemotherapy. However, thus far MRS has not been widely incorporated into routine clinical practice.

Diffusion-weighted imaging

Diffusion-weighted imaging is familiar to MRI users as an extremely sensitive technique for the detection of early cerebral infarction, where it can give a clear positive result within hours of the clinical onset of acute stroke. More recently the technique has also proven valuable in tumor imaging at many sites in the body.

Image contrast in DWI depends on the degree to which molecules are free to move randomly in the tissues, i.e., by diffusion. Watery tissues with very mobile molecules give lower signal intensity, while solid, hypercellular, rigid tissues with restricted molecular diffusion (more characteristic of malignancy) give stronger signal. Cancers, then, typically show *restricted diffusion* which gives bright signal on DWI. Tissues with inherent high T2 signal also display bright signal on DWI, a confounding effect called *T2 shine-through*.

The degree of diffusion-weighting is defined by b-values, expressed in units of mm^2/s, with T2 shine-through effects being lessened for higher b-values. Data from two image sets with different b-values are needed to calculate the ADC, which can then be displayed as an ADC map for comparison with other imaging sequences. Restricted diffusion gives a low ADC value (bright on the DWI sequence but dark on the ADC map) and allows distinction from T2 shine-through (bright on both DWI and ADC map). For easy interpretation and direct comparison with other sequences, the ADC values displayed in the parametric map can be color-coded [36]. In defining a ROI on an ADC map, care must be taken to exclude cystic or necrotic parts of a mass which may not accurately represent its histologic nature.

For practical application then, prior to the contrast-enhanced study two DWI data sets are needed to produce an ADC map, with echo-planar imaging used to allow rapid acquisition. For one data set, a b-value of 0 is used, while for the other b-values in the range of 600–800 mm^2/s appear to be optimal for the breast [36, 37], although b-values of up to 1500 mm^2/s have been used to improve visual assessment of lesion extent.

There is overlap between ADC values for benign and malignant lesions and sensitivity and specificity for malignancy depend on where the ADC threshold is set. Most studies have used an ADC cutoff of $1.1–1.3 \times 10^{-3}$ mm^2/s, with lower values indicating malignancy. However, ADC values are slightly higher for DCIS (mean $1.3–1.4 \times 10^{-3}$ mm^2/s), with thresholds for malignancy below $1.6–1.8 \times 10^{-3}$ mm^2/s required to give an overall sensitivity of 95–100% [36, 38]. Fibroadenomas typically show an ADC value of ~1.4 while mucinous cancers are the usual malignant outliers with ADC values of 1.7–1.8 mm^2/s [39, 40].

The addition of DWI significantly increases specificity, even for small lesions (< 1 cm), with one study finding that its use could have avoided biopsy in one-third of benign cases [36]. Other recent studies have also confirmed high accuracy for DWI in differentiating benign from malignant lesions, even for non-mass enhancement [41, 42].

The potential to improve lesion characterization makes DWI a useful addition to routine scanning, while it also has value in determining tumor extent, including monitoring response to neoadjuvant chemotherapy [39]. Finally, the combination of high sensitivity and acceptable specificity offered by DWI raises the exciting prospect that it could even be developed for use as a non-contrast screening sequence.

MULTIPLE CHOICE QUESTIONS

1.1 Answer true or false to the following statements
- A. The negative predictive value of a normal breast MRI for invasive cancer exceeds 90%.
- B. A type 2 kinetic curve (plateau) in a mass can be confidently classified as benign.
- C. A type 3 kinetic curve (washout) in a mass is strongly associated with malignancy.
- D. For invasive cancers missed by MRI, strong background enhancement is a major factor.
- E. In breast MRI, spectroscopy at 3.0T is widely used as a routine screening technique.

1.2 Answer true or false to the following statements
- A. A strength of MRI is its ability to directly demonstrate microcalcification in DCIS cases.
- B. Bilateral breast MRI studies using a slice thickness of 6 mm give adequate spatial resolution.
- C. Abnormal vessels associated with tumor angiogenesis usually have thick muscular walls.
- D. Neither breast density nor background enhancement are risk factors for breast cancer.
- E. Breast MRI can be useful in distinguishing between a surgical scar and local recurrence.

See page 189 for answers.

References

1. Warner E, Plewes DB, Hill KA, *et al*. Surveillance of BRCA1 and BRCA2 mutation carriers with magnetic resonance imaging, ultraound, mammography and clinical breast examination. *JAMA* 2004; **292**: 1317–25.
2. Kriege M, Brekelmans CTM, Boetes C, *et al*. Efficacy of MRI and mammography for breast-cancer screening in women with a familial or genetic predisposition. *N Engl J Med* 2004; **351**: 427–37.
3. Kuhl CK, Schrading S, Leutner CC, *et al*. Mammography, breast ultrasound, and magnetic resonance imaging for surveillance of women at high familial risk for breast cancer. *J Clin Oncol* 2005; **23**: 8469–76.
4. Leach MO, Boggis AK, Dixon AK, *et al*. Screening with magnetic resonance imaging and mammography of a UK population at high familial risk of breast cancer: a prospective multicenter cohort study (MARIBS). *Lancet* 2005; **365**: 1769–78.
5. Saslow D, Boetes C, Burke W, *et al*. American Cancer Society

guidelines for breast screening with MRI as an adjunct to mammography. *CA Cancer J Clin* 2007; **57**: 75–89.

6. Lehman C, Gatsonis C, Kuhl CK, *et al.* MRI evaluation of the contralateral breast in women with recently diagnosed breast cancer. *N Engl J Med* 2007; **356**: 1295–303.
7. Kuhl CK, Schrading S, Wardelmann E, *et al.* Magnetic resonance imaging versus mammography for diagnosing ductal carcinoma in situ. *J Clin Oncol, 2007 ASCO Annual Meeting Proceedings (Post-Meeting Edition)* 2007; **25**(189): 1504.
8. Shimauchi A, Jansen SA, Abe H, *et al.* Breast cancers not detected at MRI: review of false-negative lesions. *AJR Am J Roentgenol* 2010; **194**: 1674–9.
9. Hall FM. The rise and impending decline of screening mammography. *Radiology* 2008; **247**: 597–601.
10. Kuhl C, Weigel S, Schrading S, *et al.* Prospective multicenter cohort study to refine management recommendations for women at elevated familial risk of breast cancer: the EVA trial. *J Clin Oncol* 2010; **28**: 1450–7.
11. Bluemke DA, Gatsonis CA, Chen MH, *et al.* Magnetic resonance imaging of the breast prior to biopsy. *JAMA* 2004; **292**: 2735–42.
12. Heywang SH, Hahn D, Schmidt H, *et al.* MR imaging of the breast using gadolinium-DTPA. *J Comp Assist Tomogr* 1986; **10**: 199–204.
13. Heywang SH, Wolf A, Pruss E, *et al.* MR imaging of the breast with Gd-DTPA: use and limitations. *Radiology* 1989; **171**: 95–103.
14. Kaiser WA, Zeitler E. MR imaging of the breast: fast imaging sequences with and without Gd-DTPA. Preliminary observations. *Radiology* 1989; **170**: 681–6.
15. Kuhl CK. Concepts for differential diagnosis in breast MR imaging. *Magn Reson Imaging Clin N Am* 2006; **14**: 305–28.
16. Nunes LW, Schnall MD, Orel SG, *et al.* Breast MR imaging: interpretation model. *Radiology* 1997; **202**: 833–41.
17. Kuhl CK, Mielcareck P, Klaschik S, *et al.* Dynamic breast MR imaging: are signal intensity time course data useful for differential diagnosis of enhancing lesions? *Radiology* 1999; **211**: 101–10.
18. Schnall MD, Blume J, Bluemke DA, *et al.* Diagnostic architectural and dynamic features at breast MR imaging: multicenter study. *Radiology* 2006; **238**: 42–53.
19. Schnall M, Orel S. Breast MR imaging in the diagnostic setting. *Magn Reson Imaging Clin N Am* 2006; **14**: 329–37.
20. Menell JH, Morris EA, Dershaw DD, *et al.* Determination of the presence and extent of pure ductal carcinoma in situ by mammography and magnetic resonance imaging. *Breast J* 2005; **11**: 382–90.
21. Kuhl CK, Schrading S, Bieling HB, *et al.* MRI for diagnosis of pure ductal carcinoma in situ: a prospective observational study. *Lancet* 2007; **370**: 485–92.
22. D'Orsi CJ, Bassett LW, Berg WA, et al. *BI-RADS Breast Imaging Reporting and Data System, Breast Imaging Atlas*, 4th edn. Reston, VA, American College of Radiology, 2003.
23. Hendrick RE. *Breast MRI Fundamentals and Technical Aspects*. New York, Springer, 2008.
24. Wang LC, Demartini WB, Partridge SC, *et al.* MRI-detected suspicious breast lesions: predictive values of kinetic features measured by computer-aided evaluation. *AJR Am J Roentgenol* 2009; **193**: 826–31.
25. Arazi-Kleinman T, Causer PA, Jong RA, *et al.* Can breast MRI computer-aided detection (CAD) improve radiologist accuracy for lesions detected at MRI screening and recommended for biopsy in a high-risk population? *Clin Radiol* 2009; **64**: 1166–74.
26. Heywang-Köbrunner SH, Bick U, Bradley WG, *et al.* International investigation of breast MRI: results of a multicenter study (11 sites) concerning diagnostic parameters for contrast-enhanced MRI based on 519 histopathologically correlated lesions. *Eur Radiol* 2001; **11**: 531–46.
27. Teifke A, Hlawatsch A, Beier T, *et al.* Undetected malignancies of the breast: dynamic contrast-enhanced MR imaging at 1.0 T. *Radiology* 2002; **224**: 881–8.
28. Linda A, Zuiani C, Girometti R, *et al.* Unusual malignant tumors of the breast: MRI features and pathologic correlation. *Eur J Radiol* 2010; **75**: 178–84.
29. Ghai S, Muradali D, Bukhanov K, *et al.* Nonenhancing breast malignancies on MRI: sonographic and pathologic correlation. *AJR Am J Roentgenol* 2005; **185**: 481–7.
30. Ellis RL. Optimal timing of breast MRI examinations for premenopausal women who do not have a normal menstrual cycle. *AJR Am J Roentgenol* 2009; **193**: 1738–40.
31. Knopp MV, Bourne MW, Sardanelli F, *et al.* Gadobenate dimeglumine-enhanced MRI of the breast: analysis of dose response and comparison with gadopentetate dimeglumine. *AJR Am J Roentgenol* 2003; **181**: 663–76.
32. Martincich L, Faivre-Pierret M, Zechmann CM, *et al.* Multicenter, double-blind, randomized, intraindividual crossover comparison of gadobenate dimeglumine and gadopentetate dimeglumine for breast MR

imaging (DETECT Trial). *Radiology* 2011; **258**: 396–408.

33. Kuhl CK, Schild HH, Morakkabati N. Dynamic bilateral contrast-enhanced MR imaging of the breast: trade-off between spatial and temporal resolution. *Radiology* 2005; **236**: 789–800.
34. Bartella L, Morris EA, Dershaw DD, *et al.* Proton MR spectroscopy with choline peak as malignancy marker improves positive predictive value for breast cancer diagnosis: preliminary study. *Radiology* 2006; **239**: 686–92.
35. Tozaki M, Fukuma E. ^{1}H MR spectroscopy and diffusion-weighted imaging of the breast: are they useful tools for characterizing breast lesions before biopsy? *AJR Am J Roentgenol* 2009; **193**: 840–9.
36. Partridge SC, Demartini WB, Kurland BF, *et al.* Quantitative diffusion-weighted imaging as an adjunct to conventional breast MRI for improved positive predictive value. *AJR Am J Roentgenol* 2009; **193**: 1716–22.
37. Pereira FPA, Martins G, Figueiredo E, *et al.* Assessment of breast lesions with diffusion-weighted MRI: comparing the use of different b values. *AJR Am J Roentgenol* 2009; **193**: 1030–5.
38. Woodhams R, Matsunaga K, Iwabuchi K, *et al.* Diffusion-weighted imaging of malignant breast tumors. The usefulness of apparent diffusion coefficient (ADC) value and ADC map for the detection of malignant breast tumors and evaluation of cancer extension. *J Comput Assist Tomogr* 2005; **29**: 644–9.
39. Woodhams R, Kakita S, Hata H, *et al.* Identification of residual breast carcinoma following neoadjuvant chemotherapy: diffusion-weighted imaging – comparison with contrast-enhanced MR imaging and pathologic findings. *Radiology* 2010; **254**: 357–66.
40. Woodhams R, Kakita S, Hata H, *et al.* Diffusion-weighted imaging of mucinous carcinoma of the breast: evaluation of apparent diffusion coefficient and signal intensity in correlation with histologic findings. *AJR Am J Roentgenol* 2009; **193**: 260–6.
41. Partridge SC, Mullins CD, Kurland BF, *et al.* Apparent diffusion coefficient values for discriminating benign and malignant breast MRI lesions: effects of lesion type and size. *AJR Am J Roentgenol* 2010; **194**: 1664–73.
42. Yabuuchi H, Matsuo Y, Kamitani T, *et al.* Non-mass-like enhancement on contrast-enhanced breast MR imaging: lesion characterization using combination of dynamic contrast-enhanced and diffusion-weighted MR images. *Eur J Radiol* 2010; **75**: e126–32.

Chapter 2

Imaging-related anatomy and pathology

Chapter outline

- Introduction
- Breast anatomy
- Basic mammography and breast ultrasound
- Review of breast histopathology
- Molecular classification of breast cancer
- Mammographic correlates of pathologic subtypes
- Mammographic correlates of molecular subtypes

Introduction

While a basic level of knowledge is assumed, this chapter offers a brief review of breast anatomy, conventional breast imaging and breast pathology as useful background information to subsequent chapters. Over the last decade, the new molecular classification of breast cancer has assumed increasing clinical importance and has improved our understanding of pathogenesis. There is a developing appreciation of the concept that tumor biology may be more important in determining clinical outcomes than tumor burden. The concept of a broad division into low-grade and high-grade pathways of breast cancer development has important implications for management at a time when it is increasingly recognized that over diagnosis and overtreatment are significant issues in breast cancer screening programs. Some correlations between mammographic appearances and tumor pathology are highlighted, which are particularly pertinent in relation to BRCA gene mutation carriers, a high-risk subgroup where the use of screening MRI is becoming routine.

Breast anatomy

For clinical purposes, the breast is divided into four quadrants: upper inner (UIQ), upper outer (UOQ), lower inner (LIQ) and lower outer (LOQ). The *nipple–areolar complex* (NAC) and *subareolar region* are distinct (Fig. 2.1). In the UOQ, glandular tissue

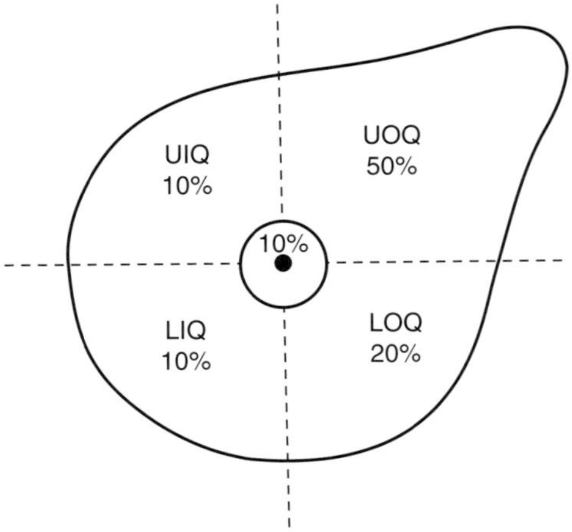

Fig. 2.1 Schematic of breast quadrants: Approximate percentages for the incidence of invasive cancers by quadrant are shown.

extends superolaterally as the *axillary tail (of Spence)*. To describe the depth of a lesion seen on imaging, the breast can be divided into three zones – subareolar (anterior), glandular (middle) and retroglandular (deep).

The regional lymph node drainage, with division of the axillary nodes into levels I, II and III is shown in Fig. 2.2. Only level I (low) axillary lymph nodes, lying lateral to pectoralis minor, are visible on XRM. The mid-axillary or level II nodes lie posterior to pectoralis minor, with interpectoral (Rotter's) nodes also included in this group. The level III (high) axillary nodes, lying medial to pectoralis minor and below the clavicle, are also termed the *apical* or *infraclavicular* nodes.

Embryologically, the breast buds form by infolding of epidermal tissue. As breast development begins at puberty, further growth and division occurs to form each duct system (segment or lobe). In fact, each lobe or segment is lined by cells which have divided and proliferated from the same cluster of cells at the nipple surface. Segments show wide variation in size

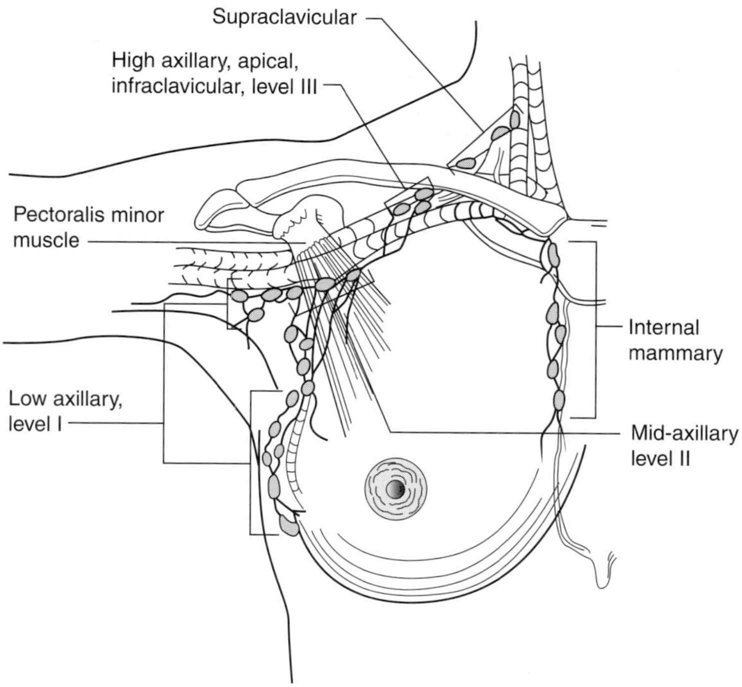

Fig. 2.2 Schematic of lymph node anatomy: Used with the permission of the American Joint Committee on Cancer (AJCC), Chicago, Illinois. The original source for this material is the *AJCC Cancer Staging Manual*, Seventh Edition (2010) published by Springer Science and Business Media LLC, www.springerlink.com.

and may extensively ramify and interdigitate. Usually only 2–3 very extensive duct systems drain over two-thirds of the breast and these tend to be distributed peripherally, with smaller more compact lobes centrally [1]. While 12–20 milk ducts may open at the nipple, many are blind-ending and non-functional or drain very small lobes and as few as 7–12 duct systems may be clinically relevant in the context of breast cancer risk.

The major ducts subdivide down into terminal ducts and the many blind-ending ductules or acini that make up each lobule. The terminal duct and lobule together comprise the TDLU, and it is here that a great majority of pathologic processes first arise. In fact, the only common lesion thought to originate from a large true duct rather than from the TDLU itself, is the solitary intraduct papilloma [2].

Histologically, the ducts and lobules are lined by a double layer of cuboidal or columnar epithelium, with major extralobular ducts also showing prominent surrounding elastic tissue. The two layers, an inner secretory luminal cell layer and a distinct outer myopeithelial cell layer are surrounded by the basement membrane (Plate 1). The myoepithelial cells are sometimes referred to as basal cells, because they contact the basement membrane. It is breaching of the basement membrane by malignant cells which distinguishes in situ disease from invasion microscopically.

As mentioned earlier, the lobes of the breast develop from clusters of epidermal cells at the nipple. It follows from this that if the original population of epithelial cells (derived from a single stem cell) were defective and predisposed to malignant transformation, the entire lobe could develop with an unstable epithelium ("sick lobe theory") [3]. Such a developmental hypothesis would account for the segmental distribution of DCIS and for the occurrence of multifocal or multicentric invasive cancers, which may be arising in the same segment even if widely separated, when the ramification of lobes is considered [4].

Basic mammography and breast ultrasound

X-ray mammography

The standard mammographic views are the MLO and the CC (Fig. 2.3). The MLO view is designed to parallel the obliquely oriented pectoralis major

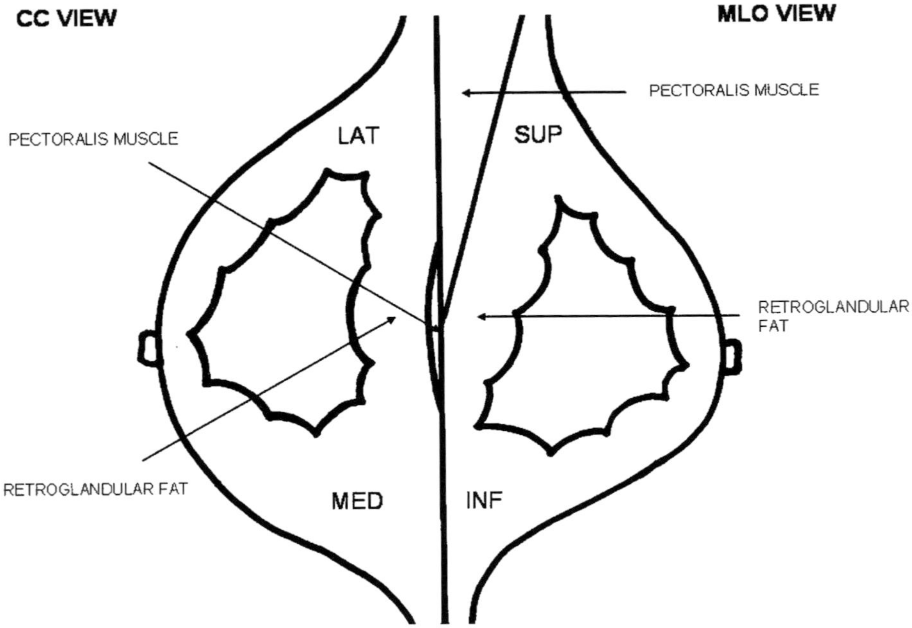

Fig. 2.3 Schematic of basic mammographic anatomy: The retroglandular fat, subareolar zone and medial breast on the CC view are important review areas for subtle cancers.

muscle to maximize inclusion of the overlying breast tissue, including the axillary tail. Supplementary true lateral views are sometimes taken, particularly for localizing a possible lesion. Due to geometric distortion, a laterally placed lesion will appear lower in position on the true lateral view than on the MLO, while a medially placed lesion will appear higher (mnemonic: Lateral = Lead falls, Medial = Muffins rise).

On XRM, certain locations are known to commonly harbor cancers. About 50% of all invasive cancers arise in the UOQ, and may project onto the retroglandular fat on the MLO view (Fig. 2.3). This obliquely oriented band of fat density parallel to the pectoralis muscle has been dubbed the "Milky Way," because it is here that stellate lesions are found in abundance. It is well known that subtle cancers, easily overlooked on XRM, are frequently located in the medial quadrants of the breast, in the subareolar zone and in the retroglandular fat, making these important review areas (Table 2.1). The MLO view does not display the medial half of the breast well, so careful viewing of the CC view is particularly important to detect a subtle medially placed lesion.

Most significant mammographic abnormalities, where cancer is a consideration in the differential diagnosis, can be classified as either (i) stellate lesions (masses which display spiculated margins), (ii) circumscribed or irregular masses or (iii) microcalcifications. Most masses on XRM are also identified sonographically and can then be biopsied using US guidance if required. On the other hand, microcalcifications are usually not readily identified by US and require biopsy using x-ray stereotactic techniques. Asymmetric density and/or architectural distortion on XRM are relatively non-specific findings which may also represent malignancy.

Table 2.1 Mammographic review areas for possible subtle cancers

"Milky Way" (retroglandular fat seen anterior to pectoralis muscle on MLO)
Retroglandular zone (retroglandular fat) also known as "no-man's land"
Medial half of the breast – involutes early so usually predominantly fatty
Retroareolar zone – complex and dense area, requires careful evaluation
Axillary region – occasionally a suspicious node may be identified
Inframammary fold – easily overlooked and worthy of routine review

Mammographic masses

Masses in breast imaging can be thought of most simply as circumscribed, irregular or stellate. It is the nature of the margins and not the shape of a mass which carries the most important diagnostic implications. In mammographic workup, *coned compression* views are used to displace overlying tissues which cause confusing *summation shadowing* in order to clarify the nature of mass margins or to interrogate an area of asymmetric density and/or architectural distortion.

A mass which has spiculated margins is usually an invasive cancer. Indeed, the gamut of possible benign spiculated lesions in the absence of any previous surgical intervention is limited (Table 2.2). Masses with irregular margins are suspicious, while circumscribed masses are usually benign with cysts and fibroadenomas by far the most common (Table 2.3). The *halo sign* in mammography describes the appearance of a hyperlucent rim around a circumscribed mass due to *mach effect* (visual physiology). While even a partial halo sign has a high PPV for benignity, this largely reflects the fact that cysts and fibroadenomas greatly outnumber circumscribed cancers. It is important to be aware that some invasive cancers are circumscribed and may even exhibit the mammographic halo sign. Furthermore, seemingly rather paradoxically, these may be high-grade cancers with a rapid growth pattern which often arise in the same young population of women who also frequently harbor cysts and fibroadenomas (Fig. 2.4).

Table 2.2 Differential diagnosis of stellate lesion

IDC NOS (often low grade, if spiculation is prominent)
ILC, pure or mixed types (e.g., tubulo-lobular)
Tubular cancer
Radial scar or complex sclerosing lesion (size > 1 cm)
Post-surgical or post-biopsy scar
Sclerosing adenosis
Atypical fat necrosis

Table 2.3 Differential diagnosis of circumscribed mass

Cyst
Fibroadenoma (rarely develop after age 40 years)
Intramammary lymph node
Benign papilloma
Grade 3 IDC NOS
Intracystic (encapsulated) papillary carcinoma
Mucinous carcinoma (usually present > 60 years)
Medullary carcinoma (often present < 50 years)
Phyllodes tumor (rare, large/rapid growth)
Juvenile ("giant") fibroadenoma (rare, large/rapid growth)

Mammographic microcalcifications

Microcalcifications (as opposed to obviously benign macrocalcifications) may be either benign or malignant and exhibit distinct patterns which can be broadly correlated with histopathology. To elucidate the nature of microcalcifications, *magnification* views are performed in orthogonal planes (CC and lateral). Calcifications which can be localized to the skin on a tangential view are invariably benign. Other microcalcification patterns which can confidently be classified as benign include the following:

(i) Classic "teacup" forms on a lateral mammogram view are due to dependent layering of "milk of calcium" (suspension of calcium oxalate within dilated lobular acini or microcysts), corresponding to fibrocystic change (blunt duct adenosis, columnar cell change) (Fig. 2.5).
(ii) Scattered, rounded, well-defined "pearl-like" calcifications are solid casts of dilated lobular acini or microcysts, characteristic of "burnt-out" fibrocystic or "involutional-type" (postmenopausal) changes.
(iii) Intraductal or periductal well-defined linear or lucent-centered sausage-shaped calcifications are distinctive for *mammary duct ectasia (periductal or plasma cell mastitis)*, particularly when bilateral and widespread. However, focal and unilateral ductal calcification suggestive of periductal mastitis should be regarded with suspicion.

Malignant microcalcification patterns:

(i) Most casting forms (linear or branching calcification of necrotic material forming casts within the ducts) are malignant (~95%) and usually due to high-grade DCIS with comedonecrosis (Fig. 2.5).
(ii) Granular forms ("crushed stones" or "broken glass") frequently represent DCIS (~60%). Marked pleomorphism (variation in form,

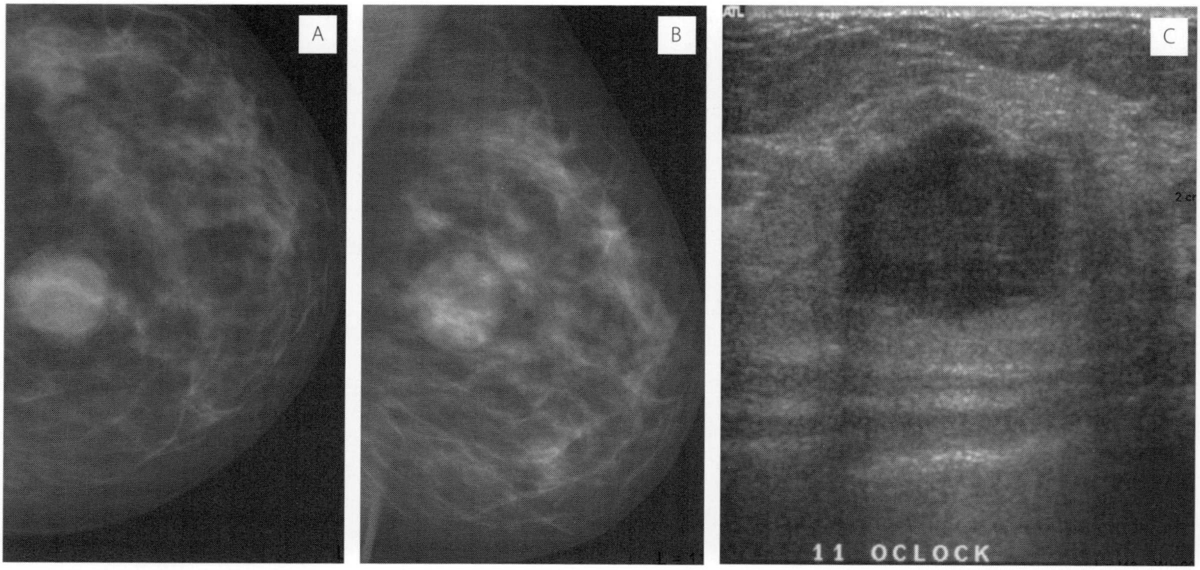

Fig. 2.4 Circumscribed cancer: (A) Left MLO and (B) CC mammogram views in a 39-year-old woman show well-circumscribed mass with partial halo sign, located in the retroglandular zone. Ultrasound image (C) shows a homogeneous hypoechoic rounded mass with posterior acoustic enhancement, but the margins are angular. Biopsy showed grade 3 IDC with medullary features which was ER, PR and HER2 negative. The patient was referred for genetic testing, but no BRCA mutation was identified.

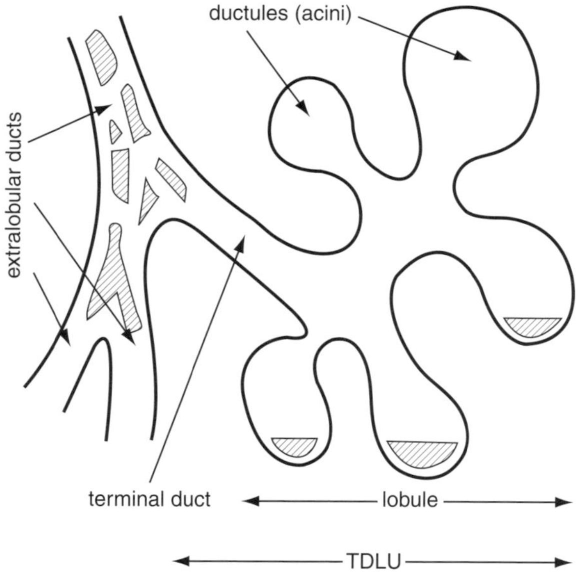

Fig. 2.5 Schematic of TDLU: The lobule shows adenosis with dilated acini and associated benign layering "teacup"-type calcifications due to milk of calcium. In contrast, casting calcifications typical of DCIS with comedonecrosis are shown in the extralobular ducts.

size and density of individual calcific particles) increases suspicion of malignancy, but distinction from benign fibrocystic change is frequently impossible without biopsy. In addition to morphology, distribution is important, with bilateral changes or scattered calcifications favoring benignity, while clustered calcifications have to be regarded with greater suspicion. The decision to biopsy should always be based on the "worst-looking" individual microcalcifications, not the most predominant type.

(iii) Powdery, amorphous or "cotton wool" calcifications are frequently benign (typically sclerosing adenosis), but can also be seen with ADH and low-grade DCIS. A *segmental distribution* of the calcifications (corresponding to an anatomic segment), increases the suspicion of malignancy.

Most DCIS present as mammographic microcalcification and only a minority (< 10%) have clinical features of nipple discharge or a palpable mass. Ultimately, any new cluster of microcalcification (other than layering "teacup" forms) will usually require x-ray stereotactic biopsy. The incidence of DCIS has risen dramatically in recent decades due to increased diagnosis through XRM screening programs, and now represents at least 20% of new breast cancer diagnoses.

As DCIS becomes more extensive, the risk that areas of microinvasion may be present increases. For a cluster of DCIS microcalcification measuring

< 10 mm in diameter, invasion is demonstrated histologically in about 20–25%, rising to over 40% for larger clusters [5, 6]. Invasion is also more likely to be present with high-grade DCIS (~35%) than low-grade DCIS (< 15%) [5].

Breast sonography

Ultrasound is widely used as an adjunctive technique to XRM to clarify the nature of a mass and as a means to allow biopsy. Ultrasound can reliably define most simple cysts as benign (Table 2.4), although small deeply situated cysts, those with low-level internal echoes or thickened walls (*complicated cysts*) and clustered microcysts can be difficult to characterize and may require aspiration. Where there is a definite solid component (*complex cyst*), a histologic diagnosis is required, although dependent debris can mimic an intracystic mass.

For solid masses, Stavros has established key sonographic features which indicate malignancy (Table 2.5) [7, 8]. The signs with the highest sensitivity for cancer relate to surface characteristics, i.e., are seen at the interface between the lesion and surrounding tissue (*angular margins, spiculation*, the *thick echogenic halo* and *microlobulation*). The thick echogenic halo is usually a variant of spiculation, where the spicules are too fine to be fully resolved by US, although in a minority of cases the halo is due to an inflammatory reaction with peritumoral edema [8]. Five sonographic signs stand out as combining acceptable sensitivity and high PPV for invasive cancer, with *angular margins* as the single most accurate sign (Table 2.6).

Microlobulations (1–2 mm diameter rounded surface projections) often signify DCIS with expanded ducts and cancerization of lobules, particularly when seen in combination with other DCIS signs of *duct extension, branch pattern* and calcification. Microlobulations can also occur in benign lesions, particularly fibrocystic change with clustered microcysts [8]. As an isolated finding, microlobulation is a relatively "soft" malignant sign with a low PPV for malignancy. Duct extension is usually a single large projection from a tumor mass into a central duct oriented towards the nipple, while branch pattern refers to multiple smaller projections into peripheral ducts directed away from the nipple [8].

Table 2.4 Sonographic features of simple cyst

Circumscribed round or ovoid shape
Uniformly thin smooth wall
Anechoic contents
Posterior acoustic enhancement
Edge-shadowing artifact

Table 2.5 Malignant US features of solid nodules (Stavros criteria)

Surface characteristics
Angular margins
Spiculation
Thick echogenic halo
Microlobulation
Shape characteristics
Taller than wide
Duct extension
Branch pattern
Internal characteristics
Shadowing
Marked hypoechogenicity
Calcifications

Table 2.6 Best sonographic signs of invasive cancer (Stavros criteria)

Angular margins: ~90% sensitivity, 60% PPV
Spiculations/echogenic halo: ~70% sensitivity, 80% PPV
Taller-than-wide shape: ~50% sensitivity, 75% PPV
Marked hypoechogenicity: ~50% sensitivity, 65% PPV
Acoustic shadowing: ~50% sensitivity, 60% PPV

In the Stavros algorithm, for a lesion to be classified as BI-RADS 3 (risk of malignancy less than 2%) there must be no malignant signs, plus one of the following three benign discriminators must be met:

(i) mass or palpable ridge which is purely and intensely hyperechoic
(ii) complete thin echogenic capsule plus ovoid wider-than-tall shape
(iii) complete thin echogenic capsule plus < 4 gentle lobulations.

It should be clear from this that most sonographically solid masses require biopsy, the commonest exceptions being a ridge of normal fibroglandular parenchyma and a classical fibroadenoma, while a typically benign-appearing intramammary lymph node can also be safely classified as BI-RADS 2.

Review of breast histopathology

Fibrocystic change

This term encompasses a spectrum of benign conditions representing histopathologic responses to hormonal imbalance (ER/PR ratio). As such, fibrocystic change is really just an exaggeration of normal cyclical changes, seen in the glandular tissue and stroma of perhaps half of premenopausal women. Arguably the term is too imprecise to be of any real clinical value, [2] but it is nevertheless entrenched in common usage. Fibrocystic changes are uncommon after menopause except in women who are on HRT. Subdivision is made into proliferative fibrocystic change (*adenosis* and *ductal hyperplasia*) or non-proliferative (*fibrosis* and *tension cysts* formed by obstruction of TDLUs).

Adenosis

This includes hyperplastic processes with proliferation of the glandular components of breast tissue (acinar or tubular structures of the TDLU). One common and important subtype is *sclerosing adenosis*, where adenosis is accompanied by marked stromal fibrosis, which can result in architectural distortion. Another subtype, associated with dilated acini and microcyst formation, has been called *blunt duct adenosis* but is now classified in the category of *columnar cell lesions*.

Ductal hyperplasia

This encompasses the traditional spectrum of ductal proliferative changes from normal to benign *usual ductal hyperplasia* progressing through ADH to frank DCIS (Fig. 2.6). However, evidence from molecular studies suggests that usual duct hyperplasia is, in fact, probably not a direct precursor of ADH and DCIS. Although usual ductal hyperplasia is a benign proliferative lesion, it is associated with a small generalized increase in breast cancer risk of 1.5- to 2-fold [2].

Columnar cell lesions

Synonyms include CAPSS (columnar alteration with prominent apical snouts and secretions), blunt duct adenosis and columnar metaplasia. Often found in biopsies of mammographic microcalcification, CAPSS lesions without atypia (*columnar cell change, columnar cell hyperplasia*) are benign. If cytologic atypia (*CAPSS with atypia, flat epithelial atypia*) is present, histologic features of coexisting lobular neoplasia, ADH or low-grade DCIS should be sought. It is now thought that CAPSS lesions are an important non-obligate precursor stage in the development of low-grade DCIS and low-grade invasive carcinoma. As such, some experts recommend excision in the presence of CAPSS with atypia after biopsy of microcalcifications, to avoid sampling errors.

Benign breast masses

Adenoma

The *tubular adenoma* is related to fibroadenoma but lacks the fibrotic stroma (the key differentiating feature). These are uncommon and present in younger women as a circumscribed mass, while *lactating adenoma* arises only in pregnancy or post-partum.

Fibroadenolipoma

These uncommon benign hamartomas are readily diagnosed on imaging by the distinctive but variable fatty component in a sharply circumscribed mass. Predominantly fatty lesions resemble lipomas. However, those with more fibrous stroma are difficult to characterize.

Fibroadenoma

Extremely common, often multiple masses, presenting in younger women and only very rarely arising as

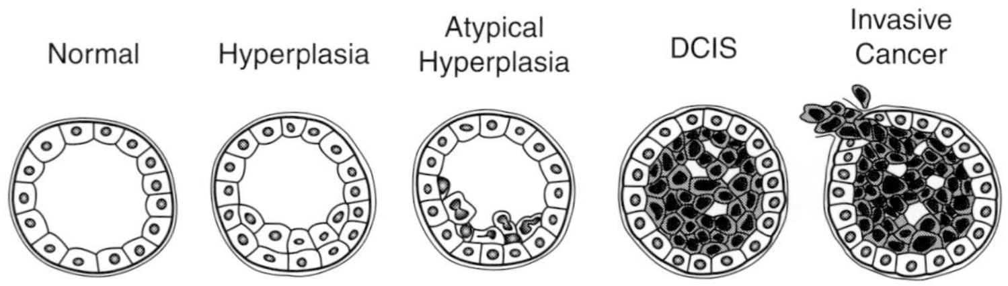

Fig. 2.6 Traditional "stepwise" model of IDC pathogenesis: Evidence from molecular studies now suggests that this traditional model of breast cancer development may be flawed, and that ADH is in fact a precursor lesion only for low-grade DCIS. Used with the permission of Dr. Susan Love Research Foundation [103].

new lesions after menopause. Depending on maturity, they range from myxoid to grossly sclerosed (fibrotic) masses and may develop the classical "popcorn calcification." Women who have fibroadenomas have a slightly increased 1.5- to 2-fold increased risk of breast cancer.

Complex fibroadenoma

Fibroadenomas which contain within them proliferative changes such as ductal hyperplasia or sclerosing adenosis are termed *complex fibroadenomas*. While such complex fibroadenomas are benign and not premalignant, they reportedly confer a 3- to 4-fold relative risk of breast cancer.

Fibroadenomatoid hyperplasia

Fibroadenomatoid change describes focal changes in the breast similar to those seen in a fibroadenoma but with no discrete mass. Coarse calcification is often a presenting mammographic feature leading to stereotactic biopsy.

Juvenile fibroadenoma

These rare lesions are also known by the purely descriptive term of *giant fibroadenoma*, and present as rapidly growing circumscribed benign masses usually before age 30 years and often in teenagers. Lesions show marked hypercellularity, and can be thought of as the counterpart of phyllodes tumor in postmenopausal women.

Phyllodes tumor

These account for ~1% of primary breast tumors, and present as rapidly growing circumscribed masses usually after menopause. Clefts and leaf-like projections in cystic spaces are seen characteristic in larger lesions. Most are benign, about 20% borderline and 20% malignant. Malignant lesions are locally invasive with distant metastases occurring uncommonly, usually to lung or bone, while axillary nodal metastases are rare [2].

Fat necrosis

Usually results from surgery or blunt trauma such as a seat-belt injury, although in ~50% of cases there is no clear history of injury. Fat necrosis can closely mimic malignancy both clinically and on conventional imaging, appearing as an irregular or stellate mass.

Pseudoangiomatous stromal hyperplasia

Usually seen either in premenopausal women or in older women on HRT, PASH may present as a clinically palpable or a mammographic mass. Although benign, lesions are hormonally stimulated, often multifocal and may recur after excision. On XRM and US the mass is usually at least moderately well defined and non-calcified. Lesions vary from a few millimeters (increasingly found incidentally on pathology) up to several centimeters when clinically apparent. Although the condition is not premalignant or a risk factor for cancer, the lesions are usually excised, in part because of the potential for histologic confusion with angiosarcoma.

Chronic mastitis

Term used for common occurrence of chronic inflammation associated either with cyst rupture and release of secretions into surrounding breast stroma, or a similar but usually more widespread periductal process with inflammation, fibrosis and sometimes characteristic linear calcifications (*secretory, periductal* or *plasma cell mastitis*). Granuloma formation may be a feature.

Subareolar abscess

Also known as SMOLD (squamous metaplasia of lactiferous ducts or Zuska's disease), this uncommon condition results from leakage of keratinaceous debris into stroma causing a foreign body reaction, although secondary infection and abscess formation often occur [2]. Recurrence and chronicity with development of fistulae are typical and effective treatment requires complete surgical excision. The condition is strongly associated with a smoking history. The presentation of a subareolar mass with nipple retraction can closely mimic malignancy.

Diabetic mastopathy

Usually seen in premenopausal type 1 (insulin-dependent) diabetics and less commonly with type 2 diabetes, patients present with one or more painless hard masses which are usually indistinguishable from invasive cancer clinically. The terms *lymphocytic mastopathy* or *sclerosing lymphocytic lobulitis* may be preferred to reflect occurrence of the condition even in non-diabetics, probably on an autoimmune basis, sometimes in association with conditions such as Hashimoto's thyroiditis. Histopathology shows dense keloidal fibrosis and a lymphocytic infiltrate. Lesions may be bilateral, recurrent or both in over 60% of cases [9]. On XRM only non-specific density may be seen, while US often shows strong acoustic shadowing due to fibrosis [9, 10].

Granulomatous mastitis

Uncommon idiopathic condition of young women, usually presenting as a mass clinically, sometimes after a recent pregnancy. An asymmetric density is typical on XRM with an irregular hypoechoic mass with tubular extensions on US, while axillary lymphadenopathy and skin thickening are further features which mimic malignancy [11]. On histology, the granulomas are characteristically lobulocentric. Differential diagnosis includes other granulomatous conditions (foreign body reaction, chronic mastitis, infections and even sarcoid).

Conditions associated with increased cancer risk

Several breast lesions merit special consideration because their presence in biopsy specimens may imply an increased risk of future development of breast cancer. In the case of precursor lesions the risk may be predominantly in the affected breast, often in the region of the original percutaneous or excision biopsy, as is the case with ADH/DCIS and with lobular neoplasia, to be discussed shortly.

However, a number of more innocuous lesions, including fibroadenomas, are also associated with an increased risk which is generalized to both breasts. In fact, a history of previous breast biopsy can in itself be considered a risk factor, because it is usually proliferative lesions which arouse suspicion on imaging and lead to a biopsy being performed. Table 2.7 summarizes relative and absolute risks associated with the various pathologic entities to be considered.

Table 2.7 Estimated risks of subsequent cancer after a "high-risk" biopsy result

	Relative risk	Absolute risk
Fibrocystic change (non-proliferative)	×0	~2% at 15 years
Fibroadenoma	×1.5–2	
Usual ductal hyperplasia	×1.5–2	
Solitary papilloma	×2	~4% at 15 years
Radial scar	×2	
Sclerosing adenosis	×2–3	
Multiple papillomas without atypia	×3	~6% at 15 years
Complex fibroadenoma	×3–4	
Atypical ductal hyperplasia	×4–5	~8–10% at 15–20 years
Multiple papillomas with atypia	×7	
Lobular neoplasia	×6–10	~15–20% at 15–20 years
DCIS (risk of progression to invasion)	×8–10	~30–60% at 10 years

Papillary lesions

At least half of solitary benign intraduct papillomas arise centrally (within 2 cm of the NAC) and may present with nipple discharge, often in women under age 50 years. Origin from the duct wall, a frond-like growth pattern into the duct lumen, and a fibrovascular core are characteristic pathologic features, but there is a wide spectrum of papillary lesions showing such appearances. These range from benign intraduct papillomas, through papillomas with ADH or DCIS (more frequent with multiple peripheral papillomas), to *encapsulated* or *intracystic papillary carcinoma* and *intraductal papillary carcinoma* (considered equivalent to DCIS if fully contained within the cyst or duct) and finally to frankly invasive papillary carcinoma. Familiarity with the range of imaging appearances of papillary lesions is important for accurate pathologic correlation [12, 13]. Masses are commonly circumscribed and may show a halo sign, while calcification, either benign or malignant, is present in ~25% of papillary lesions [13].

Where multiple core biopsies show a solitary benign papilloma with corresponding benign radiologic appearances, findings are often considered to be concordant. However, when atypia (ADH) arises in a papilloma, it may only involve small focal areas of the lesion, so that biopsy can be unreliable. Furthermore DCIS or even invasion may be present in the adjacent breast tissue at the periphery of a histologically benign-appearing lesion where only the center is sampled by CNB [12]. Accordingly, a number of studies have concluded that histologically "benign" papillomas should be excised in the light of significant upgrade rates to atypia or malignancy of 14–38% [14–16]. Of note, upgrade to DCIS or IDC at excision may occur even where complete lesion removal has been documented by 11-gauge VAB technique with a benign concordant result [15]. Nevertheless, vacuum-assisted removal of benign papillomas has been suggested as a possible alternative to surgical excision [17].

After finding atypia in a papilloma, there is a reported 7.5-fold increased risk of developing cancer, usually in the same breast, suggesting that this is probably a precursor lesion [18]. Other reports suggest a generalized 4- to 5-fold increased risk after a diagnosis of solitary papilloma with atypia, approximately equal for both breasts and similar to ADH found in isolation [2, 19]. A solitary papilloma without atypia confers a 1.5- to 2-fold generalized increased risk of subsequent breast cancer [18, 19]. The risk is about 3-fold for multiple peripheral papillomas, rising to 7-fold when atypia is present [19].

Radial scar

Synonyms: sclerosing duct hyperplasia, sclerosing adenosis with pseudoinfiltration. Radial scars over 1 cm are referred to as complex sclerosing lesions. Histologically, these lesions show a central fibroelastotic zone with radiating entrapped tubular structures accompanied by adenosis and cysts peripherally. The tubular structures show preservation of both cell layers (luminal and myoepithelial) in contrast to tubular carcinoma where the myopeithelial layer is lost, making this an important distinguishing feature.

On XRM, radial scars present as stellate lesions with sheaves of long spicules but no apparent central mass giving the classic "black star" appearance [20]. Radial scars are typically planar, and often better seen on only one mammographic projection, but such variation in conspicuity is also common with small invasive cancers [21]. While XRM appearances may suggest the diagnosis, histology is always required. In one series of 22 mammographically suspected radial scars 40% showed malignancy at surgical excision (4 invasive ductal NOS, 2 tubular cancers, 1 ILC and 2 DCIS) [22]. Although initially thought to be uncommon, it appears that microcalcification is frequently associated with radial scars and may even be the only XRM finding [23–25].

When a radial scar is suspected on XRM, either CNB or VAB are now preferred to surgical excision as the initial diagnostic procedure, because if cancer is diagnosed on imaging-guided biopsy, the patient can receive definitive surgery. When radial scar is confirmed histologically, there is a significant incidence of associated carcinoma on excision biopsy, which is more frequent with larger lesions. In one pathologic study, associated cancer was found in 30% of radial scars > 6 mm in diameter compared with less than 3% for smaller lesions [18]. In that series, the cancers were most often located at the periphery of radial scars, which has implications for core biopsy technique to ensure that sampling is not directed only at the center of the lesion. Hence, surgical removal is widely recommended, although incidental pathologically detected small radial scars which appear completely removed by CNB or VAB may be the exception to this rule.

It is possible that referral bias may have falsely elevated the incidence of cancer associated with radial scar [24]. In a series of 75 screen-detected radial scars, Cawson *et al.* found a 7% incidence of DCIS and no invasive cancer, although ADH was present in 57% of all surgically excised lesions [26]. It has been proposed that excision may not be necessary for all radiologically diagnosed lesions if they have been adequately sampled by multiple core biopsies [23]. Cawson *et al.* suggested only mammographic follow-up for concordant biopsy results with no atypia, but emphasized the need for wide sampling with at least 5–8 passes using 14-gauge CNB. Reporting on experience with 157 radial scars diagnosed by CNB (65) or VAB (92), Brenner *et al.* found an incidence of cancer of 28% at excision when biopsy showed atypical hyperplasia compared with only 4% if there was no atypia [27]. Brenner *et al.* concluded that surgical excision might be avoided if at least 12 cores were obtained showing no atypical hyperplasia and there was mammographic–histologic concordance [27]. In a further study of imaging-diagnosed radial scars without atypia, Linda *et al.* found a 5% upgrade rate to malignancy after stereotactic VAB, and a 9% upgrade rate after US-guided 14-gauge CNB [28].

In summary, it may be possible to avoid surgical excision of radial scars in selected patients where multiple VAB samples have shown no atypia, as the risk of an upgrade appears to be only ~5%.

The finding of a radial scar on biopsy is also a generalized marker of increased breast cancer risk, independent of other background pathologic features such as usual ductal hyperplasia [29]. From their series of predominantly incidental small pathologic radial scars (median size < 5 mm) Jacobs *et al.* found an associated 2-fold increase in relative risk for subsequent breast cancer [18].

Sclerosing adenosis

A benign proliferative lesion, most common in premenopausal women, sclerosing adenosis can be seen in isolation, as part of a radial scar, or in association with papillary lesions and fibroadenomas. Differentiation from malignancy can be difficult on both imaging and histopathology, while sclerosing adenosis can also coexist with DCIS or invasive cancer, making radiologic–pathologic correlation particularly important. Gill *et al.* reported on imaging appearances in 32 cases where sclerosing adenosis was the dominant pathologic diagnosis [30]. Radiologic lesion types were microcalcification in 15 (60% amorphous, 27% pleomorphic, 13% punctate), and a mass in 17 (circumscribed in 10, indistinctly marginated in 7). Where imaging-guided biopsy shows only sclerosing adenosis in the presence of a stellate lesion or microcalcifications typical for DCIS, the result should be considered discordant and excision advised. Sclerosing adenosis may rarely present as a discrete palpable mass (adenosis tumor), which is associated with an up to 20% upgrade rate to DCIS on excision. There is an estimated 2- to 3-fold generalized increased relative risk of developing breast cancer after a biopsy diagnosis of sclerosing adenosis.

Juvenile papillomatosis

First described by Rosen *et al.* in 1980, juvenile papillomatosis is a condition of young women with a mean age of 23 years (range 12–48 years) [31]. Indeed, it is the combination of clinical and pathologic findings occurring at a young age which defines the condition as a distinct entity. Patients present with a 3–5 cm palpable mass which is often mistaken for a fibroadenoma on clinical examination. Key histopathologic findings are papillary epithelial hyperplasia and extensive cyst formation giving a "Swiss-cheese" appearance [2]. In a series of 180 women fulfilling the criteria for juvenile papillomatosis, a history of breast cancer in either first or second degree relatives was documented in 50 (28%) [31]. As such, these young women, and their close relatives, are probably at substantially increased risk of breast cancer and heightened surveillance is usually recommended [12, 31]. Rosen *et al.* described a related but distinct condition, also in young women, termed *papillary duct hyperplasia* in which the prominent cystic changes seen with juvenile papillomatosis were absent, and in whom the risk of breast cancer is unclear [2, 32].

Atypical ductal hyperplasia, DCIS and lobular neoplasia

ADH and DCIS

In essence, ADH represents a neoplastic intraductal process with cytologic and/or architectural features which approach but do not fulfill the diagnostic criteria for low-grade DCIS. In some cases both the required cytologic and architectural features are present, but the extent of the lesion is too small (less than 2–3 mm or involving only part of 1–2 ducts). From this, it should be clear that ADH and low-grade DCIS are a continuum and that distinction is part-qualitative and part-quantitative. It is then, not surprising that interpretation is to some extent subjective and that even pathologists may disagree over whether ADH or DCIS is present. Although not yet widely accepted, the term *ductal intraepithelial neoplasia* (DIN) has been proposed to include both ADH and DCIS [33].

In the traditional model of breast cancer pathogenesis, it has been considered that there is stepwise progression along a pathway from usual ductal hyperplasia through ADH to DCIS, ultimately giving rise to IDC when abnormal cell growth breaches the basement membrane (Fig. 2.7). This process might also be observed at different stages of development, so that ADH, DCIS and invasive cancer could coexist. Accordingly, if ADH is found on CNB, surgical excision is recommended because there is an approximately 20–50% upgrade rate to DCIS or to invasive cancer when more tissue is obtained for pathologic examination. Similarly, when extensive DCIS is encountered, focal areas of microinvasion may be present in the surgically excised specimen. However, it is now evident from molecular studies that the progression of ADH is only to low-grade DCIS and to low-grade invasive cancer, and that there is no association between ADH and high-grade DCIS [29].

In DCIS then, the proliferation of malignant epithelial cells is confined to the ducts, representing a pre-invasive phase of breast cancer. The rationale for identifying and surgically removing DCIS is based on estimates that, if left untreated, ~50% of DCIS lesions will develop to invasive cancer [34]. However, in many instances DCIS may progress only very slowly over decades rather than years, never reaching the stage of invasion during the patient's lifetime. In such cases, surgical removal and any additional therapy constitute overtreatment.

To be clinically useful then, any classification of DCIS should predict its potential to proliferate and progress to invasion. Histologically, DCIS is divided into low, intermediate or high nuclear grade, using the same features as for grading the nuclear score in invasive cancer. High-grade DCIS is more likely to recur locally if not adequately excised (~80% at 5 years) and has a higher probability of progression to invasive cancer. About 50% of all recurrences after treatment for DCIS are as invasive malignancy.

In addition to grading, comedonecrosis (with or without microcalcification) is noted if present, as this also implies more aggressive disease. When comedonecrosis is absent, the dominant architectural pattern is described (solid and cribriform patterns are more often high grade than papillary and micropapillary). The significance of the micropapillary pattern of DCIS, although usually low grade, is its tendency to ramify extensively through the duct system, making it more difficult to excise with clear margins [29].

However, histologic features of DCIS are overall rather poor predictors of the risks of developing either local recurrence or progression to invasive cancer. As a generalized risk factor, ADH has an approximately 4- to 5-fold increased risk for subsequent invasive cancer, while for DCIS that risk is roughly doubled to 8- to 10-fold [35].

ALH and LCIS

Together, these two entities comprise lobular neoplasia, a term which recognizes that the pathologic process is the same. Similar to DIN, the term *lobular intraepithelial neoplasia* (LIN) has been proposed, but is not universally accepted. Lobular neoplasia or LIN is characterized by a proliferation of loosely cohesive, uniform small cells within the acini of TDLUs. Distinction between ALH and LCIS is purely quantitative and rather subjective, depending only on the extent to which the acini are either partly filled (ALH) or packed and distended (LCIS) by these monomorphic cells. The pathologic process is typically widespread, usually multifocal in the affected breast and often bilateral.

After a diagnosis of lobular neoplasia there is an increase in absolute risk of 15–20% over 15 years, or ~25% over 25 years. Traditionally, it was thought that the increased risk applied equally to both breasts, and that either ductal or lobular cancer could develop, but recent evidence suggests that both assumptions were incorrect. Subsequent invasive cancer arises at least 3-fold more often in the ipsilateral than the opposite breast, adding to evidence that lobular neoplasia is a non-obligate precursor lesion rather than a simple risk factor. Progression of lobular neoplasia is also known to be much more frequently to ILC than it is to IDC [35–37].

Distinction between DCIS and LCIS can be difficult on light microscopy as cancerization of lobules, particularly by solid-pattern DCIS, may closely simulate LCIS. The immunohistochemical stain for the surface adhesion molecule E-cadherin, uniformly absent in LCIS, can facilitate differentiation.

Usually, LCIS is considered to be an incidental finding in CNB samples, although at least in some instances microcalcification may represent a concordant pathologic diagnosis [38, 39]. While it has been argued that there may be little point in proceeding to excision biopsy, because this is likely to only deliver more of the same material, pathologic upgrades often occur in practice. Furthermore, it appears that there are no radiologic findings which help to predict cases in which malignancy is more likely, and even with generous sampling using 11-gauge VAB technique the upgrade rate to DCIS, IDC or ILC is ~20% [39, 40]. Consequently, when LCIS is diagnosed on CNB or VAB, the usual management is to perform surgical excision [36, 39]. Note though that assessment of surgical margins after excision of LCIS does not apply because of the diffuse nature of the condition.

Subsequent options for management of the usual or *classical* form of LCIS are limited to high-risk surveillance with or without chemoprevention (the NSABP P-1 trial demonstrated a >50% reduction in the incidence of invasive breast cancer in women with a history of LCIS who received tamoxifen).

An exception to the usually conservative management of LCIS relates to the clinically aggressive *pleomorphic* subtype, for which treatment implications are similar to high-grade DCIS. Untreated pleomorphic LCIS frequently progresses to pleomorphic invasive lobular carcinoma (see below). Meanwhile, as a generalized risk factor, classical LCIS confers a relative risk of 6- to 10-fold and probably with a lag phase such that >50% of subsequent malignant breast lesions arise more than 15 years after diagnosis [35].

Histopathologic subtypes of invasive breast cancer

The heterogeneity of breast cancer is a significant problem for clinical management. Not only does in situ disease need to be clearly differentiated from invasive

Table 2.8 Histologic subtypes of invasive cancer

Tumor type	%	Key clinical and radiologic features
IDC NOS	70–80%	Most stellate, but high grade can be circumscribed masses
ILC	10–15%	Variable, occult or subtle on XRM, 30% multifocal, 10% bilateral
Tubular	5%	Stellate, long spicules, DD radial scar, good prognosis
Medullary	3%	Circumscribed mass, young age, poorer prognosis
Mucinous	2%	Circumscribed mass, older age, good prognosis
Micropapillary	2%	75% have lymph nodes at presentation, poorer prognosis
Cribriform	1%	Rare, variant of tubular carcinoma, good prognosis
Papillary	1%	Rare, spectrum of papillary lesions (some = DCIS), good prognosis
Mixed	~6–8%	Ductal-lobular ~4%, others tubular-lobular, tubular-cribriform, mucinous

disease, but the variable prognosis of invasive cancer must be recognized. In the following review of the histopathologic classification of invasive cancer, only the most commonly seen subtypes will be discussed, with their corresponding key clinical and radiologic features (Table 2.8). As will be seen, histologic type has implications for predicting tumor behavior, particularly for special types of invasive cancer.

Invasive ductal carcinoma NOS

Some 70–80% of all invasive cancers are designated as IDC "not otherwise specified" or of "no special type." Tumors are variably circumscribed, but often "scirrhous" with a desmoplastic response and spiculated margins. The classic appearance on XRM is the stellate mass but high-grade tumors can be well-circumscribed rounded lesions corresponding to non-infiltrative "pushing margins" on histology. Other variable features include central necrosis and extent of accompanying DCIS, which may be present with or without microcalcification on XRM. Cell membranes stain positive for E-cadherin. As the NOS designation is really a diagnosis of exclusion, and histologic features vary widely, the division into three grades according to differentiation is important to assess prognosis. The clinical biomarkers, ER, PR and HER2 are highly variable among NOS tumors.

Invasive lobular carcinoma

Invasive lobular carcinoma comprises 10–15% of invasive cancers and has increased in incidence in recent decades, with the use of HRT as a possible explanation. The insidious growth pattern, often without a clearly defined mass and with only minimal architectural disturbance, results in ILC being notoriously difficult to detect on XRM, such that ILCs are often large palpable tumors at first presentation. Furthermore, although multifocal or multicentric in >30% and bilateral in 10–20%, ILC tumor extent is often grossly underestimated by conventional imaging.

Histologically, a background of LCIS is present in 70–80% of cases [2]. Some 80–90% of classical ILCs are ER/PR positive and HER2 negative. In cases where histologic appearances are uncertain, negative E-cadherin staining is distinctive, and at the molecular level reflects loss of the gene for production of the protein E-cadherin. This protein is critical for normal cell adhesion, and its loss accounts for the loosely cohesive pattern of these tumors on histology with the typical single-file infiltrative pattern of invasion by linear strands of malignant cells with small nuclei. Importantly, some 10–15% of ILCs do stain positive for E-cadherin, and this feature alone should never be used to suggest ductal lineage in a histologically typical ILC. A key histologic feature of ILC is the lack of desmoplastic host response, which helps explain why many lesions show only low mammographic density and subtle architectural disturbance.

Further evidence that ILC has distinct biologic implications comes from data on clinical outcomes, with a recent large study showing an early survival benefit compared to IDC but a late crossover to reduced overall survival after ~10 years [41]. Metastatic patterns are also different for ILC with fewer lung events, more bone events and a propensity to involve unusual sites including mesenteric nodes, ovaries, peritoneum and meninges. The rare subtype *pleomorphic lobular carcinoma* which usually arises on a background of pleomorphic LCIS has a particularly aggressive clinical course [42].

Tubular carcinoma

The most common subtype after ILC, tubular cancers often present on XRM as small masses with long radiating spicules, making both radial scar/complex sclerosing lesion and sclerosing adenosis important to consider in differential diagnosis. In doubtful cases, stains for myoepithelial cells can be helpful, as this cell layer is consistently absent in a tubular carcinoma. Lesions are uniformly low grade, and named for the characteristic prominent tubule formation. Multifocal tumors are frequent, and there is usually a low-grade DCIS or LCIS component. Overall prognosis is excellent even with nodal metastases, such that tubular cancers are rarely fatal. They are virtually always ER/PR positive and HER2 negative.

Medullary carcinoma

Classical medullary cancers are histologically distinct tumors defined by Ridolfi *et al.* as showing (i) syncytial growth pattern (with solid broad sheets of cells in >75% of the tumor), (ii) microscopic complete circumscription with (iii) pushing margins (non-infiltrating border), (iv) lymphoplasmacytic reaction (inflammatory cell infiltrate), (v) grade 2 or 3 nuclei and (vi) absent glandular structures [43]. The term *atypical medullary* was applied to tumors which lacked one or more of these classical features, e.g., absence of lymphoid stroma or infiltrating rather than pushing margins [44]. Medullary cancers occur in a younger age-group, often under age 40 years, with a relatively good prognosis confined to those cases which fit strict classical medullary criteria, and a significantly poorer prognosis for the remainder. Variable definitions remain problematic and there is significant crossover in reporting of atypical medullary and high-grade ductal NOS cancers with medullary features. Some expert pathologists do not use the term "atypical" at all and classify any tumor which does not fulfill strict medullary criteria as high-grade IDC NOS [2]. Both classical and "atypical" medullary cancers are characteristically triple-negative (ER/PR and HER2 negative) and often overexpress the p53 protein. Central necrosis and cystic degeneration are further recognized features, while associated DCIS is typically absent or only a minor component [2].

Mucinous carcinoma

Also termed colloid or gelatinous carcinomas, these tumors typically show clusters of small uniform cells floating in lakes of extracellular mucin. Tumors are usually well-circumscribed, rounded or lobulated, slow-growing masses occurring in the older age-group (mean age 70 years). The pure form (defined as >90% mucinous pattern) carries a favorable prognosis while variants with a lower mucinous component have a slightly poorer prognosis. There is often DCIS, usually low grade. Tumors are usually ER/PR positive and HER2 negative.

Cribriform carcinoma

Invasive cribriform cancer, with a histologic pattern similar to cribriform DCIS, is a variant related to tubular carcinoma and may show tubular features. The pure pattern has an excellent prognosis, even when nodal metastases are present. Mixed forms between cribriform cancer and IDC have intermediate prognosis. About 80% of tumors have associated DCIS, usually of cribriform type. Tumors are usually ER/PR positive and HER2 negative.

Papillary carcinoma

Literature on papillary lesions reflects the difficulty in drawing distinction between in situ and invasive disease, which may artifactually contribute to the good prognosis reported for papillary carcinoma. Encapsulated (intracystic) papillary carcinoma or intraductal papillary carcinoma have been considered as equivalent to DCIS, often presenting with bloody nipple discharge in the older age-group. Papillary cancers usually remain well circumscribed even when frank invasion is seen histologically, and have a favorable prognosis. Calcifications may be seen within the tumor mass and there is frequently DCIS in the adjacent tissue.

Invasive micropapillary carcinoma

The characteristic histologic appearance of tubular-alveolar or micropapillary structures floating in clear, empty space defines this subtype, a pattern which has the potential for misinterpretation as LVI [2, 12]. It may occur in pure form (<2% of all invasive cancers) or admixed with IDC NOS or mucinous carcinoma, and ~70% are associated with micropapillary or cribriform DCIS [2]. Whether pure or mixed, >90% are grade 2 or 3 and 70–80% have involved axillary nodes at presentation [45]. Overall prognosis is relatively poor, and a high rate of axillary and supraclavicular locoregional recurrence which has particular implications for radiation treatment [45]. About 75% are ER positive and about one-third HER2 positive [2]. On XRM, ~50% of cases present as a mass with microcalcification due to associated DCIS but appearances are not distinctive [12, 46].

Mixed types

Of the estimated 6–8% of "mixed" tumors, some may simply represent adjacent but intermingling cancers of different types, while others are truly indeterminate. Among these, mixed IDC and lobular forms account for 4–5%, while tubular-lobular and other types also occur.

Inflammatory carcinoma

This clinico-pathologic entity is characterized by an erythematous, indurated breast with peau d'orange (skin like an orange), an appearance which correlates with tumor plugging of dermal lymphatics on histopathology. Classified T4d in the TNM system, inflammatory carcinoma is defined as involving at least one-third of the breast skin [33]. The breast may also be diffusely enlarged, warm, tender, edematous and heavy, so that clinical confusion with mastitis can occur. Young women are often affected, and tumors are typically high-grade IDC with an aggressive course and overall poorer prognosis. Mammography shows dermal thickening and a diffusely dense breast within which the primary cancer may be obscured, and is more often identified by US. It should be noted that locally advanced breast cancer invading or ulcerating the skin without the typical clinical changes or tumor emboli in dermal lymphatics does not qualify as inflammatory carcinoma [33].

Combined invasive and in situ disease

Overall, ~80% of all invasive cancers have some degree of associated DCIS on histopathology, although often not evident mammographically. The term *extensive intraductal component* (EIC) has previously been used to describe an IDC with an accompanying prominent DCIS component, and also encompassed extensive predominant DCIS with foci of microinvasion. Although some studies had suggested that an EIC independently predicted increased risk of local recurrence after BCT and overall poorer outcomes, subsequent analyses have indicated that this was more likely a reflection of inadequate surgical excision. Consequently, the concept of an EIC has been largely superseded by greater emphasis on obtaining pathologic clear margins in surgical local excision specimens. Meanwhile, linear measurement of pathologic whole lesion extent, including any DCIS component, has become standard practice, in addition to measurement of the invasive cancer itself (Fig. 2.7). Nevertheless, the term EIC is still used to describe IDC with a large DCIS component.

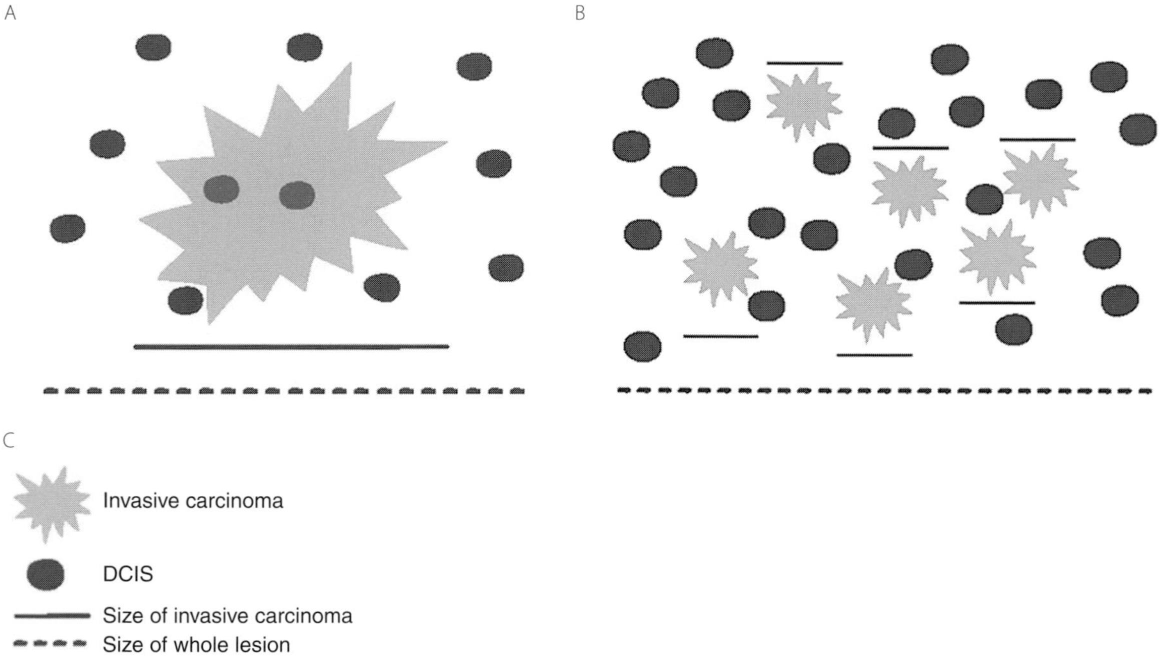

Fig. 2.7 **Measuring IDC and DCIS in combination:** Rather than applying the traditional concept of an EIC, pathologists now tend to simply measure the size of the DCIS component when seen in combination with invasive cancer. Two broad patterns are (A) an invasive cancer with surrounding DCIS and (B) predominant DCIS with foci of microinvasion. See (C) for key to symbols. Used with the permission of NBOCC [104].

Staging and grading of invasive cancer

Traditionally, the three best prognostic indicators for breast cancer are tumor size, nodal status and histologic grade. Breast cancer is staged using the TNM system, which takes into account how far the tumor has progressed in terms of size, extent of local infiltration, nodal status and distant metastatic disease (Appendix 3) [33].

A major division for clinical purposes is into *early-stage breast cancer* (EBC) (corresponding to TNM Stage I and II disease) and *advanced breast cancer* (TNM Stage III and IV disease). An indication of the effect of TNM stage on survival is given in Table 2.9.

With EBC, while it is helpful to know the histologic tumor type, it is more clinically meaningful to think in terms of tumor grade (degree of differentiation) when predicting risk of local recurrence and metastatic potential. It has been shown that histologic grade has prognostic value even for minimal invasive cancers (< 10 mm diameter) [47]. Tumor grade is particularly important as a guide to selection of adjuvant therapy, because it is a measure of tumor aggressiveness.

Histologic grading is recommended for all subtypes of invasive breast cancer, but is particularly important for IDC NOS. A tubular carcinoma, for example, is by definition always grade 1, and in fact has a better prognosis than low-grade IDC [2]. Cribriform cancers are also consistently grade 1, but for ILC and mucinous cancer, grading does appear to add prognostic value [2].

Most widely used is the *Nottingham combined histologic grade* (modified Bloom and Richardson system). This assigns *nuclear*, *mitotic* and *tubular differentiation* scores each from 1 to 3, giving a range of possible combined total scores from 3 to 9. A score of 3–5 is grade 1, 6–7 is grade 2 and the most aggressive grade 3 tumors are defined by a score of 8–9.

Table 2.9 Indicative 5-year survival rates by TNM stage

Stage 0	In situ disease, no invasion	100%
Stage I	Tumor size < 2 cm, no axillary nodes	95%
Stage IIA	Tumor 2–5 cm node negative or < 2 cm with < 3 axillary nodes positive	90%
Stage IIB	Tumor 2–5 cm < 3 axillary nodes or tumor > 5 cm but node negative	80%
Stage III	Chest wall invasion, fixed or > 4 axillary nodes or other regional nodes	60%
Stage IV	Distant metastases	20%

Compared to those with grade 1 lesions, women with grade 3 cancer are more likely to (i) have positive axillary nodes, (ii) develop recurrence and (iii) die from metastatic disease. However, the position of grade 2 lesions is more ambiguous in studies on clinical outcomes, tending to cluster with either grade 1 or 3 lesions rather than having a clearly intermediate prognosis [48].

Hormone receptor and HER2 status

Two further important factors in determining prognosis and for selection of adjuvant treatment, are hormone receptor and HER2 status. Tumors which test positive for ER have a generally better prognosis and are routinely treated with endocrine therapy. Positive HER2 status is an adverse prognostic factor but introduces the therapeutic option of using specific monoclonal antibody therapy (trastuzumab).

Hormone receptors

Estrogen receptor and PR status is usually best determined by IHC staining of paraffin-embedded material from CNB or surgical specimens, but can be performed on cell-block preparations (spun down from cytology fluid and embedded) or even cytologic smears. Both the percentage of nuclei which stain and the intensity of the staining are assessed, although definitions of a positive final result are variable (thresholds of 1%, 10% or even 20% have been used) [49]. Recent guidelines suggest that staining > 1% should be regarded as significant as even low-level ER-positivity may be associated with a clinical benefit from endocrine therapy [2, 50]. Testing is routine for invasive cancer, and can also be performed for DCIS.

HER2 (c-erbB2, HER2/neu)

About 15–20% of EBC overexpress HER2 and there is evidence for poorer outcomes even for node-negative minimal invasive cancers (< 10 mm), up to 30% of which may recur in 5–10 years. Testing is now recommended as a routine for invasive cancers while recent work also suggests a valuable role in predicting biologic behavior of DCIS, with HER2-positive cases being up to 6-fold more likely to be associated with invasion [51]. Assays using IHC are performed on CNB samples or excised specimens to detect overexpression of HER2 protein, augmented by in situ hybridization techniques (FISH or CISH) to score gene amplification. While IHC confirms the presence of the HER2 protein antigen, there is subjectivity in assessing IHC staining. To decide whether trastuzumab therapy is likely to be effective, a high gene amplification score at in situ hybridization is strong evidence for a significant abnormality at the molecular level.

Molecular classification of breast cancer

Since 2000, it has become clear that *gene expression profiling* techniques can be used to classify breast cancer into four major molecular subtypes with important implications for prognosis and treatment [52–56]. Differences in the gene expression profiles of tumors reflect fundamentally distinct cell biology. As such, these molecular subtypes represent distinct diseases in the heterogeneous group of conditions which make up "breast cancer."

Division is first into two broad groups based on ER status (Table 2.10). The ER-positive tumors show a gene expression profile similar to luminal epithelial cells and are therefore termed the luminal group, with distinct subtypes A and B. Luminal A subtype tumors are HER2 negative, although some luminal B type tumors overexpress HER2. As a group, luminal tumors have a generally good prognosis although luminal B tumors are more often high grade. Recently, the Ki-67 proliferation index has been used to differentiate the luminal A and B molecular subtypes, with an index of 15% or greater closely predicting the more aggressive B subtype [57]. Together, luminal subtypes A and B constitute about 60–70% of all breast cancers [2, 58]. The evidence for a possible further luminal subtype C remains controversial.

Among ER-negative tumors, the first group (making up some 15–25% of all breast cancers) is characterized by HER2-positive status although some may show at least weak ER-positivity [2, 58]. The second group express genes characteristic of basal/myoepithelial cells (*basal-like tumors*), and are HER2 negative, constituting 10–15% of breast cancers [2, 52, 59]. Finally, a further proposed subtype of tumors with a gene expression profile resembling normal breast tissue (*normal breast-like tumors*) may be attributable to tissue sampling errors and is not widely accepted.

Table 2.10 Molecular classification of breast cancer

ER-positive tumors
Luminal type A – good prognostic group
Luminal type B – more often high grade, less good prognosis
ER-negative tumors
HER2 positive – poorer prognostic group, but respond to trastuzumab
Basal-like tumors (HER2 negative) – poorer prognostic group, but may respond to PARP inhibitors

Although it would be convenient to assume that luminal tumors originate directly from luminal cells, and that basal-like tumors originate from basal/myoepithelial cells, the process is probably more complex. More likely, multipotential progenitor cells, i.e., stem cells, give rise to these cell lines, with tumors ultimately evolving through pathways yet to be fully elucidated.

Gene expression profiling can help determine which therapeutic options are most appropriate and which patients are most at risk of recurrence. In general, the ER-positive group tumors can be expected to respond well to endocrine therapy and have the best overall prognosis. The ER-negative but HER2-positive tumors are a poorer prognostic group but amenable to trastuzumab (Herceptin) therapy. The basal-like group are a poorer prognostic group and problematic to treat, since neither endocrine therapy nor trastuzumab are suitable. Molecular research could be the key to developing new specific therapies, e.g., recent evidence that basal-like cancers might respond to a class of drugs which inhibit the enzyme poly (ADP-ribose) polymerase (*PARP inhibitors*) [60].

The gene profiles of different tumor types are associated with expression of different cell-surface proteins, allowing correlation with immunohistochemical markers. For example basal-like cancers, which are typically ER, PR and HER2 negative, also stain positively for basal cytokeratins such as CK5/6, CK14 and CK17. Luminal-type tumors stain positive for ER, PR and a different panel of luminal cytokeratins (CK7, CK8/18 and CK19). Stains for hormone receptors and cytokeratins are widely available for use with formalin-fixed and paraffin-embedded sections. For routine clinical work, immunohistochemistry offers a more economic and robust technology than microarray-based gene profiling. A major aim of molecular research is to develop new IHC tumor markers which more closely match with gene expression profiles.

Low- and high-grade pathways model of breast cancer pathogenesis

Initial genomic research showed that where DCIS and IDC coexisted, their gene expression profiles were almost invariably identical, at first seeming to support the classical linear model of neoplasia (Fig. 2.7). However, subsequent array-CGH studies then revealed significant differences in the genetic profiles of different DCIS samples, matched by the synchronous invasive cancer in each case, and it emerged that tumor grade was the key factor consistently reflected in the type of genomic aberration [61, 62]. These findings then called in to question the traditional model of DCIS progression, because it appeared that different grades of DCIS and invasive cancer progressed along multiple parallel pathways.

There is now compelling genetic evidence for the existence of biologically distinct low-grade and high-grade arms in the pathogenesis of DCIS and invasive cancer, representing two entirely separate classes of breast cancer. The gene expression profile of high-grade DCIS and IDC differs markedly from that of low-grade cancers which show much less overall genetic change compared to normal breast tissue. In short, it appears that progression of low-grade DCIS is to low-grade invasive cancer, while high-grade DCIS progresses to high-grade invasive cancer, and crossover between these two major pathways probably occurs only rarely.

What about histologically intermediate-grade DCIS and grade 2 invasive cancers? As observed earlier, while the Nottingham combined score accurately reflects outcome for grade 1 and grade 3 cancers, it has long been known that there is ambiguity in predicting prognosis for grade 2 cancers.

Using genetic indices (such as the 97-gene signature Genomic Grade Index) it appears that the prognosis for histologically grade 2 cancers can be more accurately predicted by stratifying them into either the genomic low- or high-grade pathways [63, 64]. This suggests that the designation of grade 2 cancers may reflect the limitations of histologic grading, and adds further support for the concept of two major high-grade and low-grade pathways [62, 64].

Furthermore, as will be seen, a pathway for the evolution of LCIS to ILC also conveniently fits this model on the low-grade arm.

The "low-grade family" of lesions

Characteristic of the low-grade arm is a group of precursor lesions which includes lobular neoplasia (ALH/LCIS), columnar cell lesions, ADH and low-grade DCIS (Table 2.11). These commonly coexist with low-grade invasive cancers such as grade 1 ductal NOS, tubular and cribriform cancers, classical ILC and mixed types such as tubular-lobular cancer (Table 2.12) [61]. Two distinct pathways within the low-grade arm are the development of (i) classical ILC from lobular neoplasia, and (ii) low-grade ductal cancer types, probably along a pathway which begins with CCLs (columnar cell lesions) before passing through ADH/DCIS [61]. Lesions in the low-grade arm are also frequently ER/PR positive, with evidence suggesting that these represent a "low-grade family" of precursor, in situ and invasive neoplastic lesions belonging to the luminal "A" subtype of breast cancer (Fig. 2.9).

Table 2.11 Low-grade non-obligate precursor lesions

Columnar cell lesions
Atypical ductal hyperplasia
Low-grade DCIS
Atypical lobular hyperplasia
Classical LCIS

Table 2.12 Low-grade invasive cancer subtypes

Tubular
Tubular-cribriform
Tubular-lobular
Invasive lobular carcinoma
Grade 1 ductal NOS

Invasive cancer and DCIS in the high-grade arm

The two most cited molecular abnormalities that predict the biologic potential of DCIS are HER2 status and overexpression of the p53 protein (indicating dysfunction in the p53 tumor-suppressor gene) [65]. The IHC marker of cell proliferation Ki-67 is a further good discriminator between low- and high-grade DCIS. Low-grade DCIS typically shows normal levels of p53, no HER2 amplification and a low Ki-67 index [65].

While over 90% of low-grade DCIS lesions are ER positive and usually HER2 negative, high-grade DCIS lesions are usually ER/PR negative, with about two-thirds overexpressing either HER2 or the p53 protein [66]. Recently it has been shown that DCIS cases which exhibit HER2 overexpression have a more than 6-fold increased risk of progression to invasive breast cancer [51]. Similarly, there appears to be a distinct basal-like DCIS pattern which is characterized by a short "sojourn phase" at the DCIS stage and rapid progression to invasion [67].

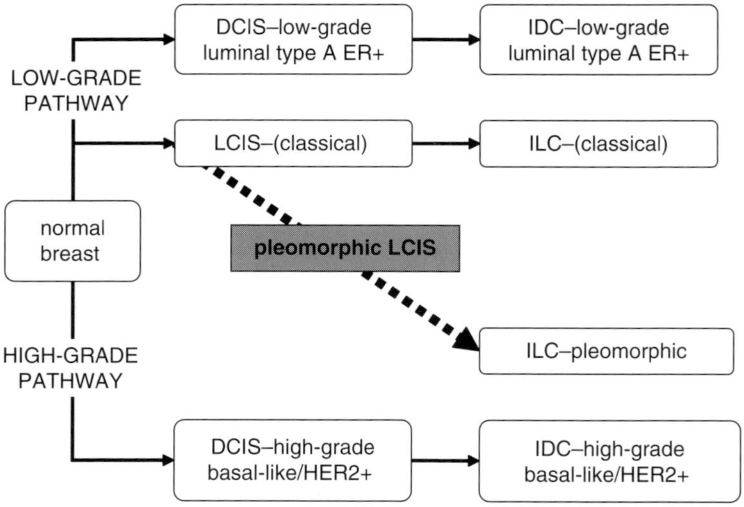

Fig. 2.8 Modern "low- and high-grade pathways" model of breast cancer pathogenesis: Gene expression profiling studies suggest that two distinct parallel pathways of disease progression exist. Molecular research suggests that pleomorphic lobular carcinoma may occupy a unique place in the low- and high-grade pathways model, crossing from low to high in its pathogenesis.

Meanwhile, gene expression profiling of high-grade DCIS samples indicate that most are indeed associated with progression to either HER2-positive or basal-like invasive cancers (Fig. 2.8). From this it follows that DCIS which is most likely to recur or become invasive may be identified by testing for biomarkers like Ki-67, HER2 [51] and those associated with basal-like molecular type [69].

While the low- and high-grade arms are biologically distinct, there are some circumstances where crossover from low-grade to high-grade disease may occur. One such example is the ILC variant, pleomorphic lobular carcinoma, which appears to start off on the low-grade pathway as classical LCIS but then crosses over, via the development of pleomorphic LCIS, to develop into a high-grade invasive cancer (Fig. 2.8) [42, 61] In support of this theory, pleomorphic lobular carcinoma displays overlapping genetic features between classical ILC and grade 3 IDC, [61] and this uncommon tumor is now of considerable research interest in regard to modern models of breast cancer pathogenesis.

Towards a new paradigm for DCIS diagnosis and treatment

A key objective of molecular research is to improve our ability to predict which cases of DCIS are most at risk of recurrence, and more importantly of progression to invasive disease. Identifying those cases may in turn assist in developing more specific adjuvant treatments based on gene expression profiling. That HER2-positivity of DCIS is a major risk factor has raised the possibility that the anti-HER2 monoclonal antibody trastuzumab could have a role in preventing development of invasive disease [34]. The concept of using an anti-HER2/neu vaccine is also under investigation. Similarly, with respect to basal-like cancers, new drugs such as PARP inhibitors might also have a role in slowing the typically rapid progression from DCIS to invasion.

Furthermore, it might be possible to define some subgroups, for example older women with in situ disease in the low-grade arm (DIN or LIN), who were at sufficiently low risk of disease progression that they could be treated solely with chemoprevention. The NSABP P-1 tamoxifen trial showed a 56% risk reduction for women with LCIS, an 86% reduction for those with ADH and an almost 70% reduction in ER-positive invasive cancers overall [69, 70, 71]. Given that the invasive cancers in the "low-grade family" are usually ER positive, taking SERMs or AIs could be a treatment option for their precursor lesions. Trials of tamoxifen as therapy for ER-positive DCIS are currently under way.

BRCA1-related, basal-like and triple-negative cancers

The identification of the BRCA1 gene in 1994 and BRCA2 gene a year later was a breakthrough in familial breast cancer research. Soon after, reports appeared of a high incidence of medullary, atypical medullary and IDC with medullary features in BRCA1-related familial breast cancer [44, 71, 72]. One large study found a 13% incidence of medullary or atypical medullary cancers among BRCA1 carriers compared with only 3% in BRCA2 and 2% among sporadic cancers in a control group [73]. It was also known that medullary-type tumors almost always stained negatively for hormone receptors and were often HER2/neu (c-erbB2) negative as well (triple-negative phenotype), but prior to elucidation of the molecular classification of breast cancer there was no clear basis to separate them from other tumor types.

With the arrival of gene expression profiling techniques, a landmark article by Perou *et al.* in 2000 established for the first time that "estrogen receptor negative breast carcinoma encompasses at least two biologically distinct subtypes of tumors (basal-like and erb B2 positive)" [53]. It was then soon recognized that the features consistently observed in BRCA1-related cancers corresponded closely with the "basal-like" molecular subtype [73]. In one study of 18 cancers found among BRCA1 mutation carriers, all exhibited a basal-like gene expression profile [55].

This strong association is now firmly established, with up to 80–90% of cancers in BRCA1 mutation carriers being triple-negative with a basal phenotype [67]. However, the match-up is not exact, with some sporadic cancers also showing a triple-negative phenotype and basal-like genetic profile [52]. Furthermore, older BRCA1 carriers may present with ER-positive cancers, although whether these are coincidental sporadic cancers or a distinct BRCA1 subgroup is not yet established [74, 75].

Furthermore, while there is strong correlation between triple-negative phenotype (as defined by histology) and basal-like cancers (as defined by gene expression profiling), the overlap here is again incomplete. Based on DNA microarray and IHC comparative analyses, somewhere between 55% and 90% of triple-negative tumors are basal-like [52, 60, 76]. Conversely, not all basal-like cancers are triple-negative, with a certain proportion expressing either ER, PR or HER2 [52, 60, 67]. Therefore it is incorrect to regard triple-negative cancers as synonymous with the basal-like molecular subtype.

A major difficulty is in defining exactly what panel of IHC markers should be used to better define the basal-like genomic profile and improve the degree of overlap. This is necessary because gene expression profiling techniques are not widely available and are unsuitable for routine clinical use. Adding other markers, such as EGFR (HER1) and CK5/6 to the triple-negative phenotype may help to more clearly identify basal-like tumors, which have important implications for prognosis and management [77]. However, markers such as basal cytokeratins, EGFR (HER1), P-cadherin or p53, still do not reliably distinguish between sporadic triple-negative cancers and those who harbor a BRCA1 mutation [78]. Key pathologic features of the basal-like/BRCA1-related subtype of breast cancer are summarized in Table 2.13.

Table 2.13 Features of basal-like/BRCA1-related cancers

Young patient age
High histologic tumor grade
Pushing border of invasion
Stromal lymphocytic response
Geographic or confluent areas of tumor necrosis +/− central fibrotic focus
Small amounts of high-grade DCIS (< 10% of tumor volume)
High Ki-67 index (marker of proliferation)
Extraordinarily rapid clinical growth rates
Triple-negative phenotype (ER, PR and HER2 negative)
Expression of EGFR, p53, P-cadherin, basal cytokeratins 5/6, 14 and 17
Aggressive course, poor prognosis, even when lymph node negative
Propensity for hematogenous spread to brain and lung

It is important to appreciate that while medullary-type cancers are over-represented among BRCA1 mutation carriers, the great majority of BRCA1-related tumors are correctly classified as IDC NOS, usually of high grade (~70% grade 3, 20% grade 2) and often triple-negative. High-grade IDC NOS cancers are also often seen in BRCA2 carriers and in younger women generally [79, 80]. However, in young BRCA1 mutation carriers, cancer growth can be extraordinarily fast, with a mean tumor-volume doubling-time of just 4 weeks reported for women aged < 40 years in a pooled study of three large high-risk screening trials [80].

The distinct biology of BRCA1-related/basal-like cancers

The rationale for breast screening and for surgical management of EBC is based on the premise that there is a predictable progression of disease, with larger tumors being more likely to have positive axillary nodes but still amenable to cure. Among

BRCA1-related cancers, however, the expected relationship between increasing tumor size and the number of positive lymph nodes is disrupted [81]. Interestingly, this is not because small BRCA1-related tumors are more likely to be node positive, but rather that large BRCA1 tumors are more likely to be node negative compared to non-BRCA1-related cancers [81].

Even among node-negative invasive cancers < 10 mm in size, where 10-year survival is ~95%, risk factors for poor outcomes can be defined, including age < 50 years, high tumor grade and ER/PR-negative status [47]. Basal phenotype has itself emerged as an independent and powerful predictor of poor long-term outcome even for small node-negative IDCs [82].

Such findings suggest a significantly different tumor biology, and it now appears that at least some basal-like tumors have a distinct mechanism of early hematogenous spread, with a propensity to metastasize to the brain and lungs, and less often to bone and liver [83, 84]. This combination of rapid growth and aggressive tumor behavior clearly has important implications for screening of known or suspected BRCA1 mutation carriers, and has led to concerns that even using MRI, the potential survival benefit in this group could be less than anticipated [84].

Mammographic correlates of pathologic subtypes

It is clear that correlation exists between features on XRM and histopathologic subtypes of invasive cancer (Table 2.8), so at least to some extent imaging appearances may give an indication of tumor biology. It has been recognized for some time that spiculated masses correlate with low histologic grade, while ill-defined masses and comedocalcification correlate with high histologic grade [85]. Spiculation around low-grade cancers likely reflects slower tumor growth, allowing the host time to develop a desmoplastic response. More than half of all screen-detected small invasive cancers appear as spiculated masses without calcification, a morphologic pattern which has been shown to be a reliable indicator of a good prognosis, independent of tumor grade [86–88]. In fact, Tabar and colleagues have reported 95% survival at 24 years for stellate cancers < 10 mm diameter, and suggested that this may constitute a substantial subgroup where adjuvant therapy adds little benefit [89].

In the Tabar study, however, the XRM finding of a stellate mass with accompanying casting-type microcalcifications due to high-grade DCIS had a dramatically poorer prognosis with 72% and 52% survival for 1–9 mm and 10–14 mm tumors respectively [89]. Similar results have been reported in other series [90, 91] and emphasize the importance of achieving complete surgical excision with clear margins for high-grade DCIS. The combination of a stellate mass and comedocalcification may define a small subgroup of patients with invasive cancer (7% in the Tabar study) who are at risk of a poor outcome, essentially correlating with what has been called an EIC pathologically. However, this remains controversial, with some experts questioning whether this XRM appearance really does constitute an independent risk factor or if it could be due to other confounding effects [92, 93].

Meanwhile, although it is easy to think that circumscribed cancers are usually slow-growing and low grade (e.g., mucinous or papillary types), as earlier illustrated in Fig. 2.6, fast-growing tumors can also result in a circumscribed mass because of rapid concentric expansion. Non-spiculated masses are more difficult to detect on XRM, particularly in dense breast tissue, while the potential for misinterpreting a circumscribed mass as benign has been made clear. These are important limitations of XRM in young women who have generally denser breasts but are also more likely to develop high-grade cancers. It is then unsurprising that a substantial proportion of invasive cancers in premenopausal women escape mammographic detection, often presenting as clinically palpable lumps at a relatively late stage. Basal-like/BRCA1-related cancers with high proliferation rates and rapid growth are a particularly frequent cause of false-negative mammograms [80, 94, 95].

Mammographic correlates of molecular subtypes

So, we have seen that a high proportion of BRCA1-related cancers have a basal-like phenotype and are particularly likely to present as circumscribed masses. In one retrospective study of cancers in known BRCA mutation carriers, 7/21 (33%) were circumscribed non-calcified cancers, all of which were grade 3 tumors in BRCA1 carriers [94]. The presence of DCIS is widely reported as uncommon in BRCA1-related cancers, but it is probably more accurate to say that accompanying high-grade DCIS is often present but limited in extent. In fact, it is likely that a propensity for rapid progression to invasive cancer is the reason why DCIS is often minimal or absent on histopathology with BRCA1-related cancers [96]. If mammographically evident, DCIS with basal phenotype tends to be associated with a comedocalcification pattern, but more often the small DCIS component is non-calcified and occult to XRM.

To appreciate typical imaging features of basal-like cancers, it is equally important to recognize those appearances which correlate with other molecular subtypes. Among 198 premenopausal women with breast cancer, Yang *et al.* found the 38 triple-negative cancers were usually round, oval or lobulated masses. Only 18% had spiculated margins, compared with 50% of HER2-positive and 60% of ER-positive cancers. Only 15% of the triple-negative cancers were associated with calcifications compared with >60% of ER-positive and HER2-positive cancers [97]. In another study, Dogan *et al.* reported that about one-third of triple-negative cancers presenting as mammographic masses had circumscribed margins, while 6/38 (16%) sonographic masses had benign features [98].

In a series of 1944 consecutive screen-detected EBC cases, Luck *et al.* defined basal phenotype as triple-negative plus >10% staining for either CK5/6 or CK14, and found that 12% of cancers fitted this definition [99]. Basal-like cancers were more likely to be ill-defined masses (61% compared with only 24% of non-basal cancers) and showed a low rate of spiculation (20%) which was independent of histologic grade [99]. Meanwhile ~50% of all non-basal cancers appeared as spiculated masses. In that study, however, none of the basal-like cancers were classified as circumscribed masses, and not all studies suggest that a typical basal-like morphology exists [100].

In summary then, basal-like cancers usually manifest mammographically as either circumscribed or ill-defined masses with spiculation a feature in only ~20%. Any DCIS component is usually small but high grade and may exhibit mammographic comedocalcification. In contrast, at least 50% of non-basal (ER- or HER2-positive) cancers present as spiculated masses or show microcalcification.

In contrast to BRCA1 mutation carriers, women with BRCA2 mutations have much less distinctive pathologic features. A study of 157 BRCA2-related tumors showed that although most were high-grade IDC NOS (Table 2.14), often with pushing margins and high proliferative index, usually they were ER-positive and expressed luminal cytokeratins [101]. Associations between BRCA2 mutations and tubular, classical lobular and pleomorphic lobular carcinoma have been suggested by some, [71] while it is noteworthy that up to 20% of male breast cancers may be BRCA2-related [2].

Table 2.14 Grade of BRCA-associated cancers

	Grade 1	Grade 2	Grade 3
BRCA1	10%	20%	70%
BRCA2	10%	30%	60%
non-BRCA	20%	40%	40%

The HER2-positive molecular subtype is also associated with high-grade cancers and an adverse prognosis, although the outlook has substantially improved with the advent of trastuzumab therapy. Comedocalcification is also significantly associated with HER2 overexpression, and patients more frequently present at age < 50 years [102]. This is consistent with evidence that HER2 overexpression in DCIS lesions is associated with more rapid progression to invasive disease [51].

At this point, the reader should have a basic understanding of conventional breast imaging signs and how these relate to traditional histopathologic breast cancer types and to the modern molecular classification. The principles of breast cancer pathogenesis and the importance of early detection of high-grade DCIS and invasive cancers in reducing breast cancer mortality should be appreciated.

MULTIPLE CHOICE QUESTIONS

2.1 Answer true or false to the following statements

- A. Teacup-type calcifications typically represent fibrocystic change and do not require biopsy.
- B. In the Stavros algorithm, at least three malignant criteria should be present to warrant biopsy.
- C. Histologically benign papillary lesions after 14-gauge CNB are never malignant at excision.
- D. The pleomorphic LCIS subtype has treatment implications similar to that for high-grade DCIS.
- E. Molecular studies show that low-grade DCIS progresses to high-grade DCIS and then to IDC.

2.2 Answer true or false to the following statements
   A. A rounded mass lesion in a BRCA1 mutation carrier suggests a possible basal-like cancer.
   B. Cancers seen as spiculated masses without calcification are frequently of luminal type A.
   C. Basal-like cancers most commonly appear as spiculated masses without calcification.
   D. Cancers showing HER2 overexpression may be appropriate for trastuzumab therapy.
   E. Stellate masses with comedocalcification may represent a subgroup with a poor prognosis.

See page 189 for answers.

References

1. Klimberg VS. *Atlas of Breast Surgical Techniques*. Philadelphia, PA, Saunders, Elsevier, 2010.
2. Schnitt SJ, Collins LC. *Biopsy Interpretation of the Breast*. Philadelphia, PA, Lippincott Williams & Wilkins, 2009.
3. Tot T. The theory of the sick breast lobe and the possible consequences. *Int J Surg Pathol* 2007; **15**: 369–75.
4. Sharpe CR. A developmental hypothesis to explain the multicentricity of breast cancer. *CMAJ* 1998; **159**: 55–9.
5. O'Flynn EAM, Morel JC, Gonzalez J, *et al*. Prediction of the presence of invasive disease from the measurement of extent of malignant microcalcification on mammography and ductal carcinoma in situ grade at core biopsy. *Clin Radiol* 2009; **64**: 178–83.
6. Stomper PC, Geradts J, Edge SB, *et al*. Mammographic predictors of the presence and size of invasive carcinomas associated with malignant microcalcification lesions without a mass. *AJR Am J Roentgenol* 2003; **181**: 1679–84.
7. Stavros AT, Thickman D, Rapp CL. Solid breast nodules: use of sonography to distinguish between benign and malignant lesions. *Radiology* 1995; **196**: 123–34.
8. Stavros AT. Ultrasound of solid breast nodules: distinguishing benign from malignant. In: *Breast Ultrasound*. Philadelphia, PA, Lippincott Williams & Wilkins. 2004; 445–527.
9. Camuto PM, Zetrenne E, Ponn T. Diabetic mastopathy. A report of 5 cases and a review of the literature. *Arch Surg* 2000; **135**: 1190–3.
10. Thorncroft K, Forsyth L, Desmond S, *et al*. The diagnosis and management of diabetic mastopathy. *Breast J* 2007; **13**: 607–13.
11. Larsen LH, Peyvandi B, Klipfel N, *et al*. Granulomatous lobular mastitis: imaging, diagnosis, and treatment. *AJR Am J Roentgenol* 2009; **193**: 574–81.
12. Muttarak M, Lerttumnongtum P, Chaiwun B, *et al*. Spectrum of papillary lesions of the breast: clinical, imaging, and pathologic correlation. *AJR Am J Roentgenol* 2008; **191**: 700–7.
13. Brookes MJ, Bourke AG. Radiologic appearances of papillary breast lesions. *Clin Radiol* 2008; **63**: 1265–73.
14. Lam WWM, Chu WCW, Tang AP, *et al*. Role of radiologic features in the management of papillary lesions of the breast. *AJR Am J Roentgenol* 2006; **186**: 1322–7.
15. Liberman L, Tornos C, Huzjan R, *et al*. Is surgical excision warranted after benign, concordant diagnosis of papilloma at percutaneous breast biopsy? *AJR Am J Roentgenol* 2006; **186**: 1328–34.
16. Bernik SF, Troob S, Ying BL, *et al*. Papillary lesions of the breast diagnosed by core needle biopsy: 71 cases with surgical follow-up. *Am J Surg* 2009; **197**: 473–8.
17. Maxwell AJ. Ultrasound-guided vacuum-assisted excision of breast papillomas: review of 6-years experience. *Clin Radiol* 2009; **64**: 801–6.
18. Jacobs TW, Connolly JL, Schnitt SJ. Nonmalignant lesions in breast core needle biopsies. To excise or not to excise? *Am J Surg Pathol* 2002; **26**: 1095–110.
19. Lewis JT, Hartmann LC, Vierkant RA, *et al*. An analysis of breast cancer risk in women with single, multiple, and atypical papilloma. *Am J Surg Pathol* 2006; **30**: 665–72.
20. Tabar L, Dean PB. Stellate lesions. In: *Teaching Atlas of Mammography*, 2nd edn. New York, Georg Thieme Verlag. 1985; 87–136.
21. Cawson JN, Nickson C, Evans J, *et al*. Variation in mammographic appearances between projections of small breast cancers compared with radial scars. *J Med Imaging Radiat Oncol* 2010; **54**: 415–20.
22. Alleva DQ, Smetherman DH, Farr GH, *et al*. Radial scar of the breast: radiologic–pathologic correlation in 22 cases. *RadioGraphics* 1999; **19**: S27–35.
23. Philpotts LE, Shaheen NA, Jain KS, *et al*. Uncommon high-risk lesions of the breast diagnosed at stereotactic core-needle biopsy: clinical importance. *Radiology* 2000; **216**: 831–7.
24. Kennedy M, Masterson AV, Kerin M, *et al*. Pathology and clinical relevance of radial scars: a review. *J Clin Pathol* 2003; **56**: 721–4.
25. Orel SG, Evers K, Yeh I-T, *et al*. Radial scar with

microcalcifications: radiologic–pathologic correlation. *Radiology* 1992; **183**: 479–82.

26. Cawson JN, Malara F, Kavanagh A, *et al.* Fourteen-gauge needle core biopsy of mammographically evident radial scars. Is excision necessary? *Cancer* 2003; **97**: 345–51.
27. Brenner RJ, Jackman RJ, Parker SH, *et al.* Percutaneous core needle biopsy of radial scars of the breast: when is excision necessary? *AJR Am J Roentgenol* 2002; **179**: 1179–84.
28. Linda A, Zuiani C, Furlan A, *et al.* Radial scars without atypia diagnosed at imaging-guided needle biopsy: how often is associated malignancy found at subsequent surgical excision, and do mammography and sonography predict which lesions are malignant? *AJR Am J Roentgenol* 2010; **194**: 1146–51.
29. Sewell CW. Pathology of high-risk breast lesions and ductal carcinoma in situ. *Radiol Clin N Am* 2004; **42**: 821–30.
30. Gill HK, Ioffe OB, Berg WA. When is a diagnosis of sclerosing adenosis acceptable at core biopsy? *Radiology* 2003; **228**: 50–7.
31. Rosen PP, Holmes G, Lesser ML, *et al.* Juvenile papillomatosis and breast carcinoma. *Cancer* 1985; **55**: 1345–52.
32. Rosen PP. Papillary duct hyperplasia of the breast in children and young adults. *Cancer* 1985; **56**: 1611–17.
33. American Joint Committee on Cancer. *AJCC Cancer Staging Manual*, 7th edn. New York, NY, Springer, 2010.
34. Kuerer HM, Albarracin CT, Yang WT, *et al.* Ductal carcinoma in situ: state of the science and roadmap to advance the field. *J Clin Oncol* 2009; **27**: 279–88.
35. Arpino G, Laucirica R, Elledge RM. Premalignant and in situ breast disease: biology and clinical implications. *Ann Intern Med* 2005; **143**: 446–57.
36. Elsheikh TM, Silverman JF. Follow-up surgical excision is indicated when breast core needle biopsies show atypical lobular hyperplasia or lobular carcinoma in situ. *Am J Surg Pathol* 2005; **29**: 534–43.
37. Page DL, Schuyler PA, Dupont WD, *et al.* Atypical lobular hyperplasia as a unilateral predictor of breast cancer risk: a retrospective cohort study. *Lancet* 2003; **361**: 125–9.
38. Georgian-Smith D, Lawton TJ. Calcifications of lobular carcinoma in situ of the breast: radiologic–pathologic correlation. *AJR Am J Roentgenol* 2001; **176**: 1255–9.
39. Mahoney MC, Robinson-Smith TM, Shaughnessy EA. Lobular neoplasia at 11-gauge vacuum-assisted stereotactic biopsy: correlation with surgical excisional biopsy and mammographic follow-up. *AJR Am J Roentgenol* 2006; **187**: 949–54.
40. O'Neil M, Madan R, Tawfik OW, *et al.* Lobular carcinoma in situ/atypical lobular hyperplasia on breast needle biopsies: does it warrant surgical excisional biopsy? A study of 27 cases. *Ann Diagn Pathol* 2010; **14**: 251–5.
41. Pestalozzi BC, Zahrieh D, Mallon E, *et al.* Distinct clinical and prognostic features of infiltrating lobular carcinoma of the breast: combined results of 15 International Breast Cancer Study Group clinical trials. *J Clin Oncol* 2008; **26**: 3006–14.
42. Vargas A, Lakhani SR, Simpson PT. Pleomorphic lobular carcinoma of the breast: molecular pathology and clinical impact. *Future Oncol* 2009; **5**: 233–43.
43. Ridolfi RL, Rosen PP, Port A, *et al.* Medullary carcinoma of the breast. A clinicopathologic study with 10 year follow-up. *Cancer* 1977; **40**: 1365–85.
44. Shousha S. Medullary carcinoma of the breast and BRCA1 mutation. *Histopathology* 2000; **37**: 182–5.
45. Yu JI, Choi DH, Park W, *et al.* Differences in prognostic factors and patterns of failure between invasive micropapillary carcinoma and invasive ductal carcinoma of the breast: matched case-control study. *The Breast* 2010; **19**: 231–7.
46. Adrada B, Arribas E, Gilcrease M, *et al.* Invasive micropapillary carcinoma of the breast: mammographic, sonographic, and MRI features. *AJR Am J Roentgenol* 2009; **193**: W58–63.
47. Hanrahan EO, Gonzalez-Angulo AM, Giordano SH, *et al.* Overall survival and cause-specific mortality of patients with stage T1a, bN0M0 breast carcinoma. *J Clin Oncol* 2007; **25**: 4952–60.
48. Singletary SE, Allred C, Ashley P, *et al.* Revision of the American Joint Committee on Cancer staging system for breast cancer. *J Clin Oncol* 2002; **20**: 3628–36.
49. Oakman C, Viale G, Di Leo A. Management of triple negative breast cancer. *The Breast* 2010; **19**: 312–21.
50. Goldhirsch A, Ingle JN, Gelber RD, *et al.* Thresholds for therapies: highlights of the St Gallen International Expert Consensus on the Primary Therapy of Early Breast Cancer 2009. *Ann Oncol* 2009; **20**: 1319–29.
51. Roses RE, Paulson EC, Sharma A, *et al.* HER-2/neu overexpression as a predictor for the transition from in situ to invasive breast cancer. *Cancer Epidemiol Biomarkers Prev* 2009; **18**: 1386–9.
52. Rakha EA, Reis-Filho JS, Ellis IO. Basal-like breast cancer: a critical review. *J Clin Oncol* 2008; **26**: 2568–81.

53. Perou CM, Sørlie T, Eisen MB, *et al.* Molecular portraits of human breast tumors. *Nature* 2000; **406**: 747–52.
54. Sotiriou C, Pusztai L. Gene-expression signatures in breast cancer. *N Engl J Med* 2009; **360**: 790–800.
55. Sørlie T, Tibshirani R, Parker J, *et al.* Repeated observation of breast tumour subtypes in independent gene expression data sets. *Proc Natl Acad Sci USA* 2003; **100**: 8418–23.
56. Goldhirsch A, Wood WC, Gelber RD, *et al.* Progress and promise: highlights of the international expert consensus on the primary therapy of early breast cancer 2007. *Ann Oncol* 2007; **18**: 1133–44.
57. Cheang MCU, Chia SK, Voduc D, *et al.* Ki67 index, HER2 status, and prognosis of patients with luminal B breast cancer. *J Natl Cancer Inst* 2009; **101**: 736–50.
58. Turner NC, Jones AL. Management of breast cancer–Part II. *BMJ* 2008; **337**: 164–9.
59. Turner NC, Jones AL. Management of breast cancer–Part I. *BMJ* 2008; **337**: 107–10.
60. Elias AD. Triple-negative breast cancer. A short review. *Am J Clin Oncol* 2010; **33**: 637–45.
61. Simpson PT, Reis-Filho JS, Gale T, *et al.* Molecular evolution of breast cancer. *J Pathol* 2005; **205**: 248–54.
62. Moulis S, Sgroi DC. Re-evaluating early breast neoplasia. *Breast Cancer Res* 2008; **10**: 302–5.
63. Sotiriou C, Wirapati P, Loi S, *et al.* Gene expression profiling in breast cancer: understanding the molecular basis of histologic grade to improve prognosis. *J Natl Cancer Inst* 2006; **98**: 262–72.
64. Ivshina AV, George J, Senko O, *et al.* Genetic reclassification of histologic grade delineates new clinical subtypes of breast cancer. *Cancer Res* 2006; **66**: 10292–301.
65. Tsikitis VL, Chung MA. Biology of ductal carcinoma in situ classification based on biologic potential. *Am J Clin Oncol* 2006; **29**: 305–10.
66. Burstein HJ, Polyak K, Wong JS, *et al.* Ductal carcinoma in situ of the breast. *N Engl J Med* 2004; **350**: 430–41.
67. Diaz LK, Cryns VL, Symmans WF, *et al.* Triple negative breast carcinoma and the basal phenotype: from expression profiling to clinical practice. *Adv Anat Pathol* 2007; **14**: 419–30.
68. Gauthier ML, Berman HK, Miller C, *et al.* Abrogated response to cellular stress identifies DCIS associated with subsequent tumor events and defines basal-like breast tumors. *Cancer Cell* 2007; **12**: 479–91.
69. Pruthi S, Brandt KR, Degnim AC, *et al.* A multidisciplinary approach to the management of breast cancer, part 1: prevention and diagnosis. *Mayo Clin Proc* 2007; **82**: 999–1012.
70. Mahoney MC, Bevers T, Linos E, *et al.* Opportunities and strategies for breast cancer prevention through risk reduction. *CA Cancer J Clin* 2008; **58**: 347–71.
71. Armes JE, Egan AJM, Southey MC, *et al.* The histologic phenotypes of breast carcinoma occurring before age 40 years in women with and without BRCA1 or BRCA2 germline mutations. *Cancer* 1998; **83**: 2335–45.
72. Breast Cancer Linkage Consortium. Pathology of familial breast cancer: differences between breast cancers in carriers of BRCA1 or BRCA2 mutations and sporadic cases. *Lancet* 1997; **349**: 1505–10.
73. Foulkes WD, Stefansson IM, Chappuis PO, *et al.* Germline BRCA1 mutations and a basal epithelial phenotype in breast cancer. *J Natl Cancer Inst* 2003; **95**: 1482–5.
74. Lakhani SR, Khanna KK, Chenevix-Trench G. Are estrogen receptor-positive breast cancers in BRCA1 mutation carriers sporadic? *Breast Cancer Res* 2010; **12**: 104.
75. Tung N, Wang Y, Collins LC, *et al.* Estrogen receptor positive breast cancers in BRCA1 mutation carriers: clinical risk factors and pathologic features. *Breast Cancer Res* 2010; **12**: R12.
76. Rakha EA, El-Sayed ME, Green AR, *et al.* Prognostic markers in triple-negative breast cancer. *Cancer* 2007; **109**: 25–32.
77. Cheang MCU, Voduc D, Bajgik C, *et al.* Basal-like breast cancer defined by five biomarkers has superior prognostic value than triple-negative phenotype. *Clin Cancer Res* 2008; **14**: 1368–76.
78. Collins LC, Martyniak A, Kandel MJ, *et al.* Basal cytokeratin and epidermal growth factor receptor expression are not predictive of BRCA1 mutation status in women with triple-negative breast cancers. *Am J Surg Pathol* 2009; **33**: 1093–7.
79. Tilanus-Linthorst M, Verhoog L, Obdeijn I, *et al.* A BRCA1/2 mutation, high breast density and prominent pushing margins of a tumour independently contribute to a frequent false-negative mammography. *Int J Cancer* 2002; **102**: 91–5.
80. Tilanus-Linthorst MMA, Obdeijn I-M, Hop WCJ, *et al.* BRCA1 mutation and young age predict fast breast cancer growth in the Dutch, United Kingdom, and Canadian magnetic resonance imaging screening trials. *Clin Cancer Res* 2007; **13**: 7357–62.
81. Foulkes WD, Metcalfe lK, Hanna W, *et al.* Disruption of the expected positive correlation between breast tumor size and lymph node status in

BRCA1-related breast carcinoma. *Cancer* 2003; **98**: 1569–77.

82. Evans AJ, Rakha EA, Pinder SE, *et al.* Basal phenotype: a powerful prognostic factor in small screen-detected invasive breast cancer with long term follow-up. *J Med Screen* 2007; **14**: 210–14.

83. Luck AA, Evans AJ, Green AR, *et al.* The influence of basal phenotype on the metastatic pattern of breast cancer. *Clin Oncol* 2008; **20**: 40–5.

84. Hamilton LJ, Evans AJ, Cornford EJ, *et al.* Will MRI screening deliver the expected survival advantage in BRCA1 carriers? *Clin Radiol* 2009; **64**: 1045–7.

85. De Nunzio MC, Evans AJ, Pinder SE, *et al.* Correlations between the mammographic features of screen detected invasive breast cancer and pathologic prognostic factors. *The Breast* 1997; **6**: 146–9.

86. Evans AJ, Pinder SE, James JJ, *et al.* Is mammographic spiculation an independent, good prognostic factor in screening-detected invasive breast cancer? *AJR Am J Roentgenol* 2006; **187**: 1377–80.

87. Alexander MC, Yankaskas BC, Biesemier KW. Association of stellate mammographic pattern with survival in small invasive breast tumors. *AJR Am J Roentgenol* 2006; **187**: 29–37.

88. Tabar L, Chen H-H, Duffy SW, *et al.* A novel method for prediction of long-term outcome of women with T1a, T1b, and 10–14mm invasive breast cancers: a prospective study. *Lancet* 2000; **355**: 429–33.

89. Tabar L, Chen TH-H, Yen MFA, *et al.* Mammographic tumor features can predict long-term outcomes reliably in women with 1–14-mm invasive breast carcinoma. Suggestions for the reconsideration of current therapeutic practice and the TNM classification system. *Cancer* 2004; **101**: 1745–59.

90. Thurfjell E, Thurfjell MG, Lindgren A. Mammographic finding as predictor of survival in 1–9 mm invasive breast cancers. Worse prognosis for cases presenting as calcifications alone. *Breast Cancer Res Treat* 2001; **67**: 177–80.

91. Peacock C, Given-Wilson RM, Duffy SW. Mammographic casting-type calcification associated with small screen-detected invasive breast cancers: is this a reliable prognostic indicator? *Clin Radiol* 2004; **59**: 165–70.

92. James JJ, Evans AJ, Pinder SE, *et al.* Is the presence of mammographic comedo-calcification really a prognostic factor for small screen-detected invasive breast cancers? *Clin Radiol* 2003; **58**: 54–62.

93. Evans A, James J, Pinder S. Mammographic casting-type calcification associated with small screen-detected invasive breast cancers: is this a reliable prognostic indicator? *Clin Radiol* 2004; **59**: 163–4.

94. Kaas R, Kroger R, Hendriks JHCL, *et al.* The significance of circumscribed malignant mammographic masses in the surveillance of BRCA 1/2 gene mutation carriers. *Eur Radiol* 2004; **14**: 1647–53.

95. Collett K, Stefansson IM, Eide J, *et al.* A basal epithelial phenotype is more frequent in interval breast cancers compared with screen detected tumors. *Cancer Epidemiol Biomarkers Prev* 2005; **14**: 1108–12.

96. Hwang ES, McLennan JL, Moore DH, *et al.* Ductal carcinoma in situ in BRCA mutation carriers. *J Clin Oncol* 2007; **25**: 642–7.

97. Yang W-T, Dryden M, Broglio K, *et al.* Mammographic features of triple receptor-negative primary breast cancers in young premenopausal women. *Breast Cancer Res Treat* 2008; **111**: 405–10.

98. Dogan BE, Gonzalez-Angulo AM, Gilcrease M, *et al.* Multimodality imaging of triple receptor-negative tumors with mammography, ultrasound, and MRI. *AJR Am J Roentgenol* 2010; **194**: 1160–6.

99. Luck AA, Evans AJ, James JJ, *et al.* Breast carcinoma with basal phenotype: mammographic findings. *AJR Am J Roentgenol* 2008; **191**: 346–51.

100. Gilbert FJ, Warren RM, Kwan-Lim G, *et al.* Cancers in BRCA1 and BRCA2 carriers and in women at high risk for breast cancer: MR imaging and mammographic features. *Radiology* 2009; **252**: 358–68.

101. Bane AL, Beck JC, Bleiweiss I, *et al.* BRCA2 mutation-associated breast cancers exhibit a distinguishing phenotype based on morphology and molecular profiles from tissue microarrays. *Am J Surg Pathol* 2007; **31**: 121–8.

102. Seo BK, Pisano ED, Kuzimak CM, *et al.* Correlation of HER-2/neu overexpression with mammography and age distribution in primary breast carcinomas. *Acad Radiol* 2006; **13**: 1211–18.

103. Love S. Breast cancer: prevention/detection. 2009. http://www.dslrf.org/breastcancer/content.asp?L2=1&L3=1&SID=120 (Accessed August 5, 2009).

104. National Breast and Ovarian Cancer Center and Australian Cancer Network. *The Pathology Reporting of Breast Cancer. A Guide for Pathologists, Surgeons, Radiologists and Oncologists*, 3rd edn. Surry Hills, NSW, Australia, National Breast and Ovarian Cancer Center, 2008.

Chapter 3

Interpreting breast MRI studies

Chapter outline

- Introduction
- Developing a systematic approach
- Analysis of a focus
- Analysis of a mass
- Analysis of non-mass enhancement
- Summary of MRI lesion analysis
- Correlating MRI findings with conventional imaging
- Follow-up of probably benign (BI-RADS 3) lesions

Introduction

When radiologists first learn to read a chest x-ray, a system is adopted to ensure that all important areas are reviewed. Similarly, when they learn how to describe a bone lesion, the best grounding for future development is based on a system which gathers all potentially important findings. Furthermore, understanding of the plain radiographs in both these examples is a vital part of interpretation when further diagnostic techniques such as CT or MRI are required. Breast MRI is really no different – the processes to extract information and give a sensible differential diagnosis are just the same. Mammographic correlation is also an important part of the diagnostic process and the adjunctive role of US is paramount.

Developing a systematic approach

As with technique, there is no absolute right or wrong way to view a breast MRI study. However, adopting a systematic approach to breast MRI interpretation is recommended to minimize errors (Table 3.1). Carefully viewing all sequences helps to build an appreciation of their different strengths and weaknesses while also developing familiarity with the range of normal and pathologic appearances.

Images should be viewed in the same orientation as other cross-sectional imaging (as though looking at the supine patient from the feet), so that the breasts "point" up. For each sequence, window settings should be carefully adjusted so that fat signal, parenchyma and contrast can be distinguished, as areas of complete blackness or saturated white can obscure subtle findings. Any artifacts or positioning errors should be noted, and the location and features of any possible lesions recorded.

Table 3.1 Suggestions for systematic approach to viewing

Workstation review essential, color-mapping and CAD systems optional
Synchronising sequences aids in lesion localization and signal evaluation
Adjust windows carefully as poor image contrast/brightness can obscure lesions
Check for movement, other artifacts and any positioning errors
Check for presence of contrast in breast vessels to confirm adequate injection
Grade background enhancement as minimal, mild, moderate or marked
For each sequence, first compare both sides to observe symmetry
For detailed assessment, pan and zoom to each breast before scrolling through

Both sides should first be compared for symmetry, but scrolling through zoomed images of each breast in turn is best for identifying small lesions. Synchronizing images from different planes is invaluable in lesion localization and for comparing signal characteristics, representing a key advantage of commercial CAD systems.

It is suggested that non-contrast T1- and T2-weighted images are viewed first. These sequences can characterize many benign findings such as duct ectasia, cysts or normal lymph nodes and post-treatment changes such as seroma, fat necrosis or fibrotic scarring (Figs. 3.1–3.5). Any mass, asymmetric density or architectural disturbance on non-contrast images should also be noted, with sagittal

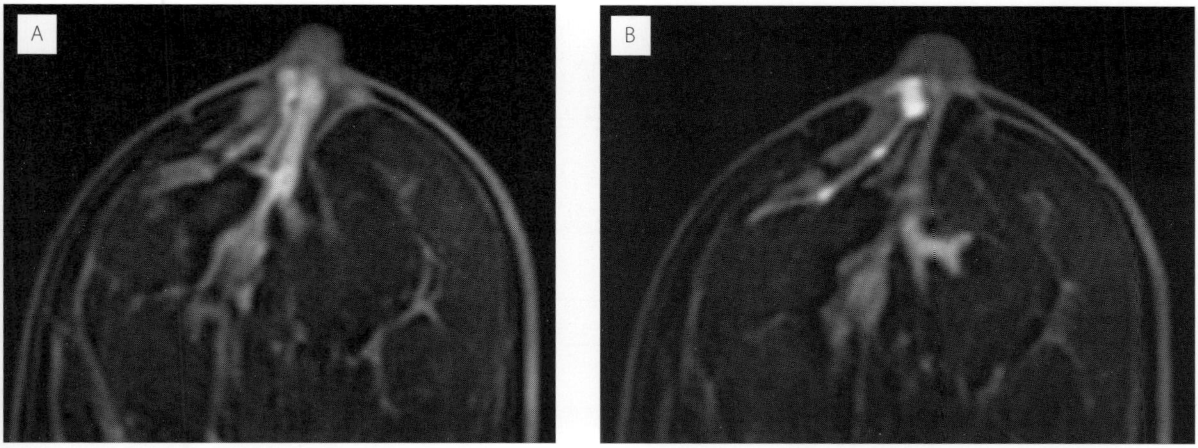

Fig. 3.1 Common benign findings: duct ectasia. Non-contrast axial T1-weighted images (A and B) showing high signal in sub areolar ducts unilaterally consistent with proteinaceous content. Findings must not be confused with ductal enhancement on non-subtracted post-contrast scans.

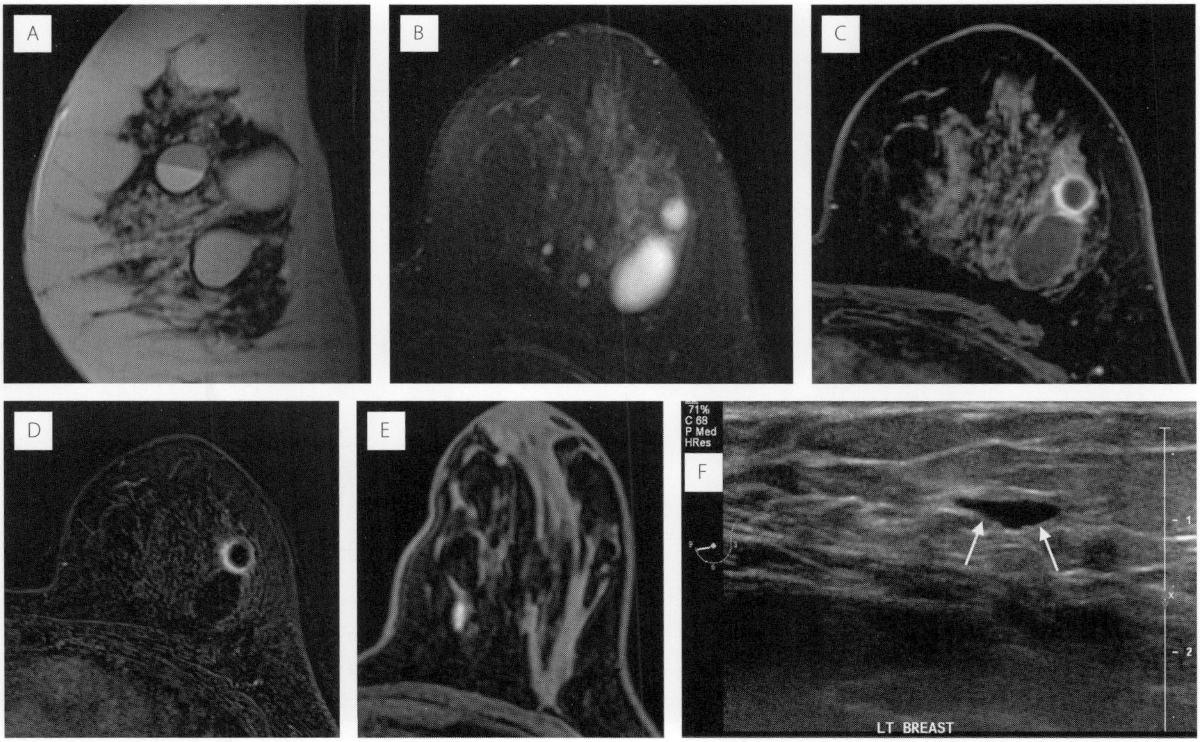

Fig. 3.2 Common benign findings: cysts. Sagittal FSE T2-weighted image (A) showing layering in a cyst, of no pathologic significance. In another case, axial fat-suppressed T2-weighted image (B) shows two cysts, the smaller one with rim enhancement on post-contrast T1-weighted image (C) due to pericystic inflammation, resulting in classic "solar eclipse" sign on subtracted image (D). In a third case, an ovoid mass showing bright signal on non-contrast T1-weighted image (E) was confirmed as a proteinaceous inspissated cyst by TUS (arrows) and FNA (F).

and axial acquisitions ideal to allow easy comparison with standard XRM views. Keep in mind that some malignant lesions show only mild or even absent enhancement. Listing all possible findings on pre-contrast images helps prevent such lesions being overlooked. After completing assessment of the non-contrast scans, the observer can proceed to the contrast-enhanced images.

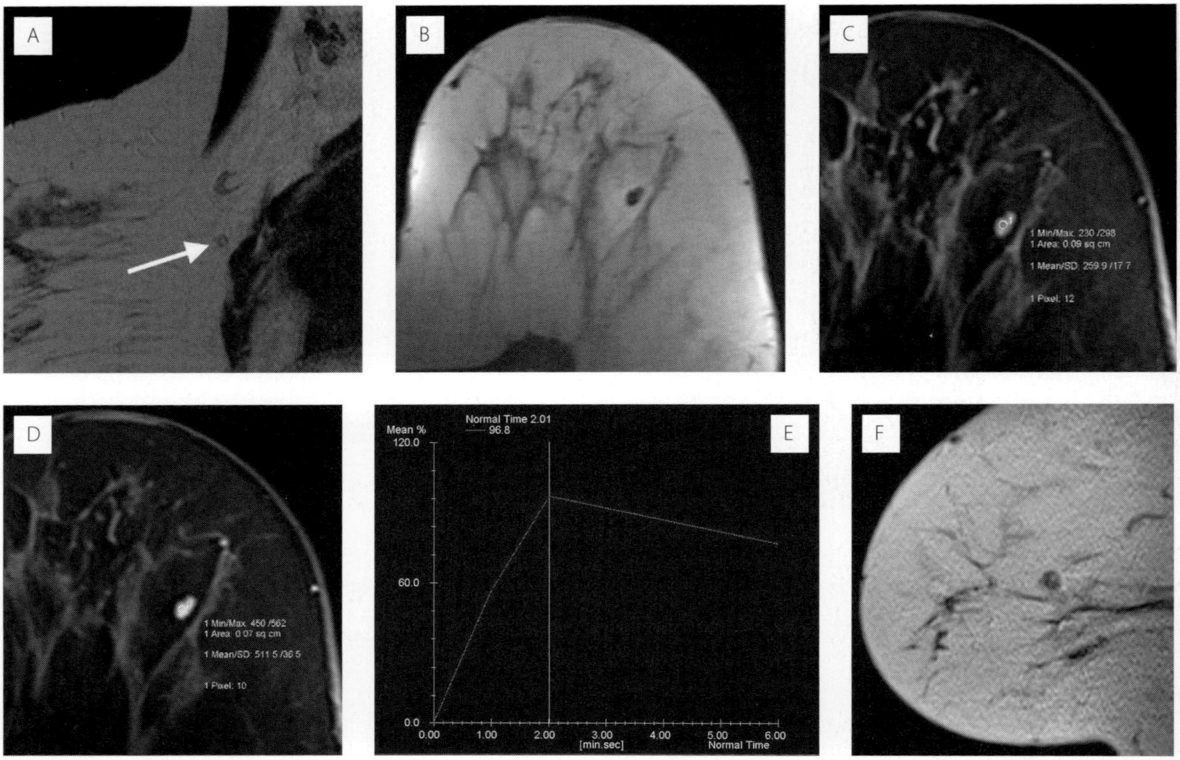

Fig. 3.3 Common benign findings: lymph nodes. (A) Normal C-shaped level I axillary node with fatty hilum on sagittal FSE T2-weighted image and tiny round "donut" node slightly inferiorly (arrow). In another case, a left breast ovoid mass is dark on non-contrast FSE T1-weighted image (B) but bright on non-contrast fat-suppressed T1-weighted image (C) and shows rapid homogeneous enhancement (D) with type 3 curve (E), while reference to sagittal FSE T2-weighted image (F) confirms tiny fatty hilum.

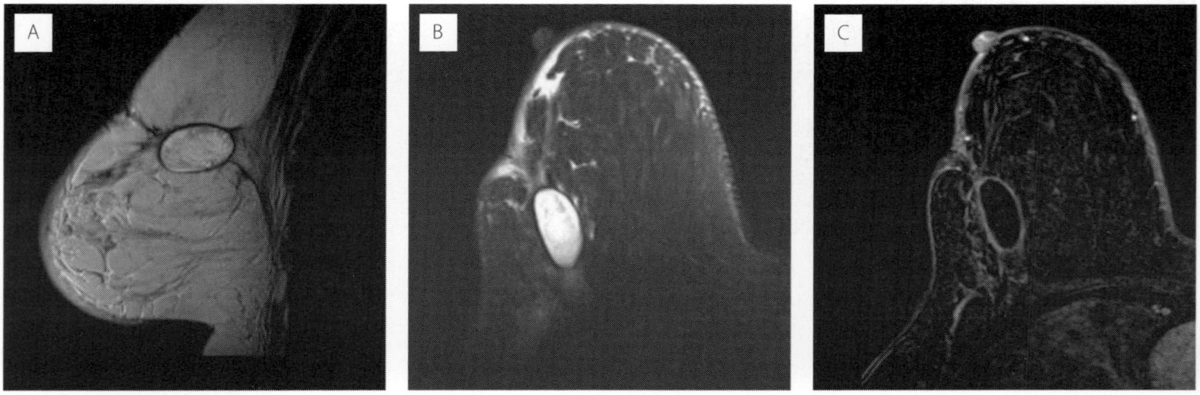

Fig. 3.4 Post-surgical changes: seroma cavity. Sagittal FSE T2-weighted image (A) showing ovoid high-signal cavity with surrounding scarring. Note also skin thickening and edema. Seroma has very high signal on T2 SPAIR image (B). Subtracted image (C) shows normal thin enhancing rim of cavity wall.

In practice, some experienced readers choose to view post-contrast scans first. Because only enhancing lesions are potentially malignant, the argument is that in the absence of abnormal enhancement, there is no significant lesion to further evaluate. Nevertheless, those who adopt this approach must be careful to refer back to the pre-contrast images to extract the important information they contain. Where good contrast opacification of vessels is seen in the breast, this confirms an effective injection. If vascular enhancement is not immediately visible in the breast, it may be that the injection failed. If no contrast is seen in breast

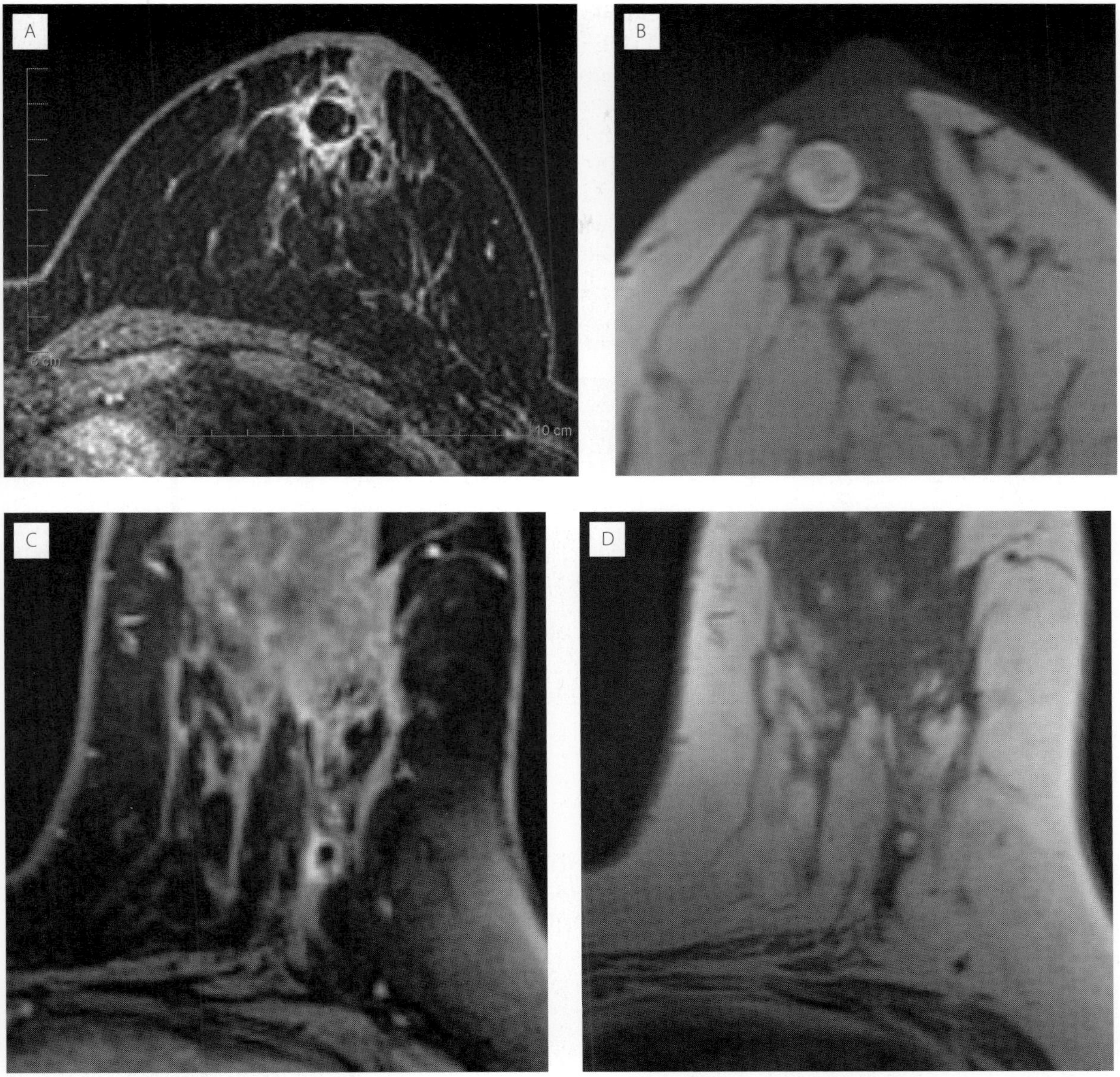

Fig. 3.5 **Post-surgical changes: fat necrosis and oil cysts.** Patient 1 year after breast reduction surgery. (A) Post-contrast fat-suppressed axial T1-weighted image shows marked enhancement surrounding a rounded subareolar lesion with central fat signal. Three years later, non-contrast axial T1-weighted image (B) shows a mature oil cyst which did not enhance. In another patient after lumpectomy, post-contrast fat-suppressed T1-weighted image (C) shows a small rim-enhancing mass, with fat-signal center on (D) non-contrast FSE T1-weighted image, characterizing this as an oil cyst. Note associated post-surgical scarring.

vessels, check if contrast is present in the heart to determine if any gadolinium entered the circulation. Placing a ROI curve on the aorta provides a useful "control" kinetic curve, and should display a classic washout pattern, while a slower rise suggests either an issue with the injection or patient factors (poor cardiac output). Finally, reviewing the "angiogenesis map" provided by MIP images ensures that small vessels in the breast itself have been opacified.

The dynamic scans should be checked for movement causing misregistration on the subtracted images, which in severe cases may render that part of the study uninterpretable. Not only can movement obscure lesions, but it can also produce spurious enhancement, particularly if respiratory motion affects one breast more than the other so that the effect is asymmetric. Blurring of vessels in one breast on MIP images is a clue, while playing a cine-loop of the dynamic series can be helpful for confirmation. Cardiac pulsation artifact is always more marked in the left breast, but is minimized by correct selection of the phase-encoding direction as left to right on axial scans.

If movement is detected, the subtracted scans will need to be interpreted with caution and more emphasis placed on analysis of the fat-suppressed dynamic series. With CAD systems, sophisticated "elastic transformation" software can be used to correct misregistration in all three planes on a pixel-by-pixel basis, and can automatically create a corrected data set as each case is downloaded to the workstation.

After analysis of signal characteristics, morphology and enhancement pattern of any abnormality, information from kinetic curve analysis can be incorporated into the diagnostic algorithm. Finally, it should be remembered that more than just the breasts are demonstrated by MRI. With each study, a mental checklist needs to be applied to ensure that axillary regions, internal mammary nodes, liver, lungs and chest wall have all been carefully evaluated (see Chapter 6).

Grading background enhancement

In ~10% of premenopausal women, a symmetrical diffuse distribution of strong and early enhancement may be seen, even when the study is performed in the optimal second week of the cycle. In these circumstances, a small invasive cancer, or even an extensive region of DCIS, could go undetected in what has been termed the "MRI dense breast," analogous to the reduced sensitivity of XRM in dense parenchyma.

A comment on background enhancement should be routinely included in breast MRI reports. The recent first revision of the BI-RADS MRI Lexicon incorporates a scoring system to grade MRI studies as showing absent or minimal, mild, moderate or marked background enhancement.

Background enhancement reflects not just the range of cyclical hormonal effects within breast tissue, but overlaps with proliferative fibrocystic changes (adenosis and ductal hyperplasia) which are, after all, exaggerated responses to changes in estrogen and progesterone effects. As such, repeating the study at a different phase of the cycle may not alter the appearances. Nevertheless, when marked background enhancement is encountered, the first points to check are whether the study was correctly timed in the menstrual cycle, or if the patient is on HRT.

Kinetic assessment: evaluating time–intensity curves

The concept of the three basic types of kinetic curve was introduced in Chapter 1. To recap, normal parenchyma enhances slowly while most invasive cancers show at least moderate initial phase enhancement. Enhancement rates vary according to the specific MRI system, sequence protocols and local factors such as injection rate and volume. While enhancement rate can be quantified as % signal intensity above baseline at 1 minute from injection, in practice the first post-contrast time point is often used as a convenient reference, and should be kept constant for any given MRI system. The first time point is usually acquired within 60–90 seconds from injection, in order to capture any early enhancement peak, and as a guide, enhancement < 50% above baseline signal intensity is considered slow, 50–100% is moderate and >100% is rapid.

Moderate to rapid enhancement indicates increased vascularity but is relatively non-specific. The "90–90 rule" refers to early enhancement of 90% or more at 90 seconds from injection, and while this is typical for an invasive cancer, ~20% of fibroadenomas and papillomas also show this intense early contrast uptake [1].

Assuming there is significant "wash-in" of at least 50–100%, one of three things can happen after 1–2 minutes, in the late, *post-initial* or *delayed* phase. If the curve continues to rise, albeit at a slower rate, it is a type 1 or *persistent* curve. If it levels off it is a type 2 or *plateau* curve. If it goes down, it is a type 3 or *washout* curve, which is strongly associated with malignancy (Fig. 3.6). Tumor angiogenesis is characterized by

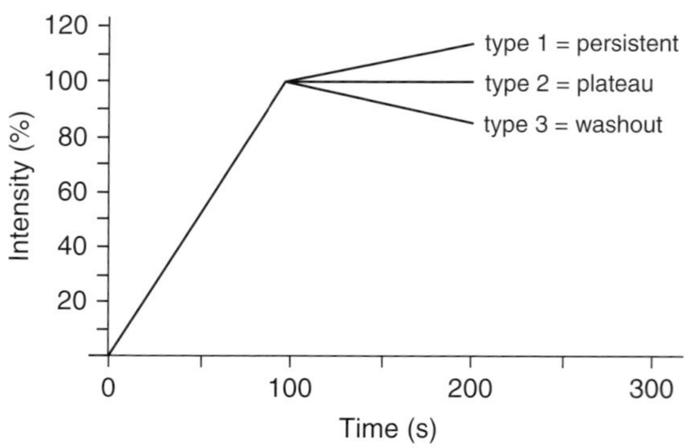

Fig. 3.6 Kinetic curve types: Assuming that at least moderate initial-phase wash-in occurs, three basic late-phase enhancement curve types can be defined. Type 1 is usually benign, type 2 is indeterminate (but often malignant) and type 3 is strongly associated with malignancy.

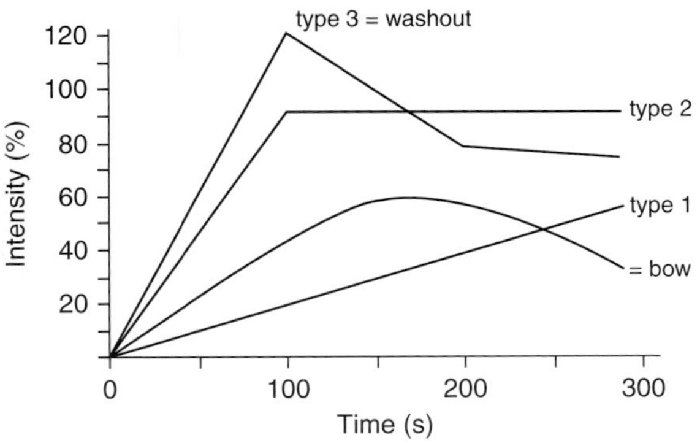

Fig. 3.7 Kinetic curve types: Where initial-phase wash-in is slow, subsequent gradual washout can give a "bow curve" typically seen with ILC and DCIS. Normal parenchyma typically exhibits a very slow and continuously rising type 1 curve.

abnormal "leaky" capillaries which likely accounts for the washout phenomenon being uncommon in benign lesions.

What proportion of invasive cancers show each pattern? Kuhl suggests that ~60% show a type 3 curve, ~30% a type 2 curve and ~10% a type 1 curve [2]. A "bow curve" is also described (type 1B) with "lower and later" peak enhancement and delayed gradual downturn, a pattern reported with ILC and some DCIS (Fig. 3.7).

How much washout must there be to qualify as a type 3 curve? Variation of 10% above or below the horizontal plateau is widely accepted as within the range for a type 2 curve. In practice, kinetic curves are often used as a "tie-breaker" for an otherwise indeterminate circumscribed or slightly irregular mass. A proportion of fibroadenomas will show type 2 curves or even mild washout (usually of no more than ~10%) but specificity of the washout sign increases sharply with percentage drop in peak signal intensity (Fig. 3.8).

What about when there is no significant wash-in? In some lesions, and typically in normal fibroglandular breast parenchyma, there is only very slow enhancement, often well below 50% above baseline in the initial phase. This gradually increases over the duration of the dynamic series, giving a slow persistent type 1 curve (Fig. 3.7). At these very low enhancement levels, attempting to discriminate plateau or washout characteristics is not meaningful. However, invasive cancers with slow enhancement do occur (~10%, often ILC or low-grade IDC) and may be very difficult or even impossible to detect on a background of normal parenchymal enhancement, a phenomenon which accounts for most invasive cancers missed by MRI. Complete absence of enhancement in an invasive cancer is rare, reported at 3% in the IBMC trial [3].

For a morphologically suspicious mass then, type 1 kinetics can never be used to imply benignity. Lesion kinetics are usually also unhelpful in diagnosing DCIS, because many such cases show only slow to moderate enhancement, often with "benign" type 1 kinetic curves.

Using BI-RADS descriptors: the ACR MRI Lexicon

As breast MRI developed, there was a clear need to establish agreed terminology to allow mutual understanding, leading to an MRI section being added to the ACR BI-RADS in 2003 [4]. The ACR MRI Lexicon has since become the accepted worldwide standard and is integral to breast MRI interpretation.

In developing the MRI Lexicon, existing descriptors were retained where possible but with new terms and definitions introduced to describe features unique to MRI, particularly enhancement patterns [5]. The Lexicon was designed to be a "work in progress" so that validated new signs could be added and descriptors found to have no practical value might ultimately be removed in future revisions. Getting familiar with BI-RADS terminology requires some practice, and there is inevitably some subjectivity. Furthermore, BI-RADS terms need not be used exclusively and other descriptors can be included in narrative reports to further clarify meaning.

Following a complete analysis, lesions are placed into BI-RADS final assessment categories. As for XRM and US, a 1–5 grading indicates the level of suspicion of malignancy, plus additional categories 0 and 6 for incomplete imaging and for known cancer respectively (Table 3.2). The BI-RADS 0 category is designed to code a study which is technically unsatisfactory, where further imaging is required such as TUS, or where previous films need to be obtained. The BI-RADS 3 category (probably benign, follow-up recommended) implies a low (<2%) estimated risk of malignancy, so that biopsy is not usually warranted.

Some countries use different scoring systems. A five-point grading system has long been used in Australia, and a similar system has recently been

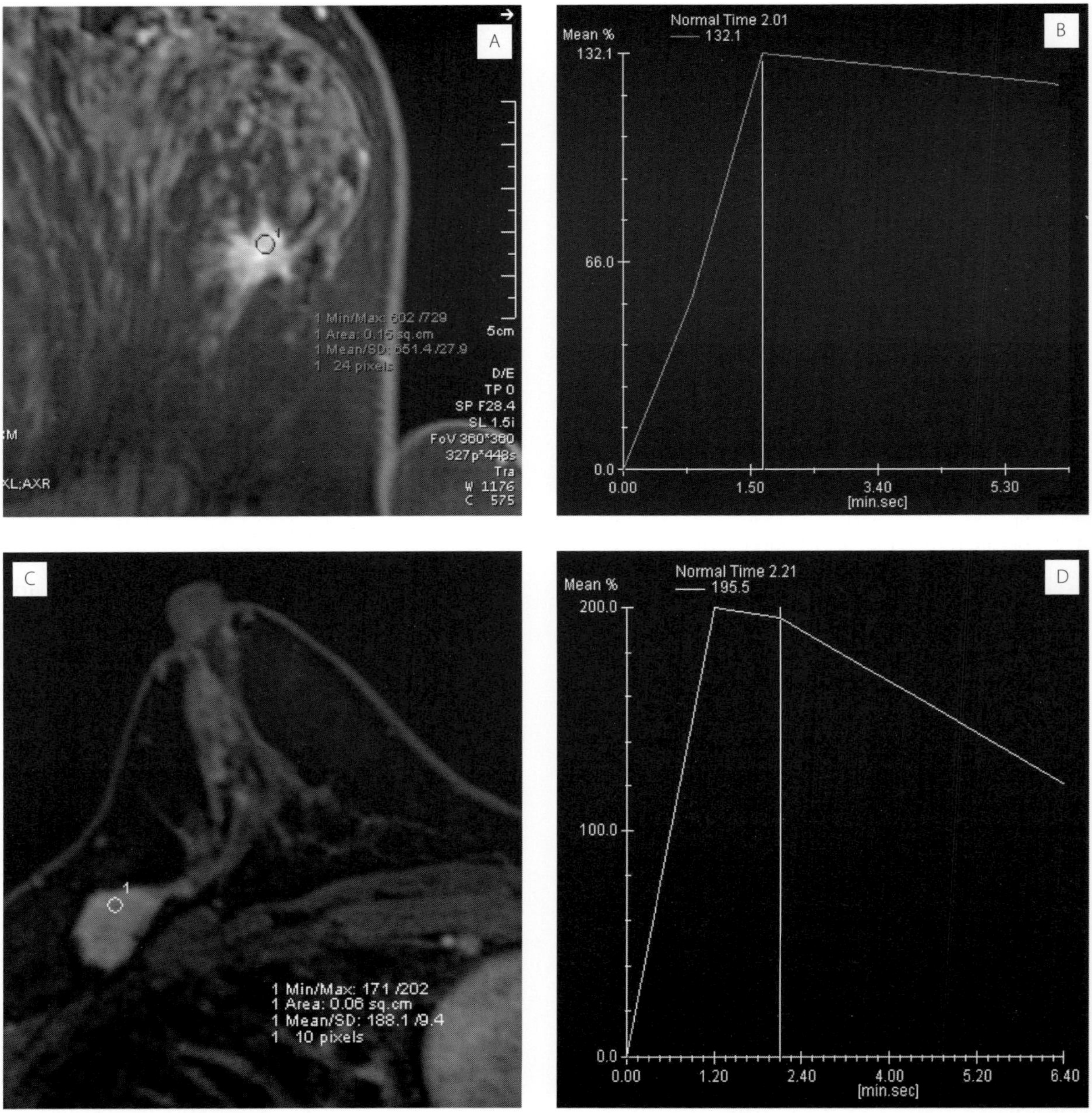

Fig. 3.8 **Semi-quantitative washout analysis:** (A) ROI on stellate IDC shows (B) kinetic curve with rapid initial phase enhancement and ~10% washout, classified as type 2 (plateau). (C) In another case, ROI on slightly irregular mass yields overtly type 3 curve (D) with signal intensity drop from 200% to 120%, or ~40% washout, strongly indicating malignancy (grade 3 IDC).

adopted in the UK [6, 7]. Importantly, both the Australian and UK systems advocate further investigation for lesions in category 3, which are classified as "indeterminate or equivocal." In practice, biopsy is usually performed for such lesions, in contrast to the follow-up recommendation for the ACR BI-RADS 3 category.

BI-RADS definitions for enhancing lesions

When an enhancing lesion is identified on a breast MRI study, the first step in interpretation is to place it in one of three basic groups, classifying it as either a *focus*, a *mass* or as *non-mass enhancement*.

Table 3.2 BI-RADS categories of final assessment after MRI analysis

0 = incomplete assessment – need prior studies, further XRM or TUS
1 = normal – no mass, asymmetry, architectural distortion or suspicious enhancement
2 = benign – abnormal but can return to routine screening
3 = probably benign (98%) short-term follow-up 6 months (1–3 months if thought to be hormonal)
4 = suspicious, possibly malignant, biopsy recommended
5 = probably malignant (95%), biopsy mandatory
6 = known cancer from biopsy

Focus

A spot of enhancement, generally less than 5 mm in diameter, too small to further characterize because its morphology cannot be defined. There should be no correlate visible on non-contrast T1- or T2-weighted images, and if there is, the lesion is displaying characteristics of a mass and enters the next group.

Mass

An enhancing mass is clearly visible as a 3D space-occupying lesion and can therefore be further analyzed in terms of shape and margins. A corresponding lesion is often present on non-contrast T1- and T2-weighted images. To further characterize a mass, its internal architecture and visual enhancement pattern can be assessed.

Non-mass enhancement

Non-mass enhancement implies a lesion larger than a focus, yet which still lacks the features of a mass. There should be no correlate visible on non-contrast T1- or T2-weighted images, with enhancement instead appearing to arise on a background of normal breast tissue. Further analysis is on the basis of distribution and extent of the enhancement, while internal architecture can also be assessed.

A useful concept, popularized by Kuhl, is to think of the distinction between mass and non-mass enhancement as broadly analogous to the distinction between a mass and microcalcification on XRM [2, 8]. The diagnostic implications are similar, because for a mass the major differential is between a benign fibroadenoma and invasive cancer and for non-mass enhancement the major differential is between DCIS or fibrocystic change.

> For an enhancing mass, the major differential diagnosis is between cancer and fibroadenoma. For non-mass enhancement the major differential diagnosis is between DCIS and fibrocystic change.

Analysis of a focus

First, make sure the lesion really is just a focus. The less than 5 mm size guide is only part of the definition of a focus – it must also have no mass-like features. As the resolution of breast MRI improves, more enhancing lesions smaller than 5 mm will have their morphology revealed. If, for example, a 3–4 mm lesion exhibits an enhancing rim or has discernible spiculated margins, it is strictly no longer a focus, and should be redefined as a mass, albeit a small one (Fig. 3.9).

The first step in analyzing a focus is to consider whether other similar lesions are present elsewhere in the same or contralateral breast. Scattered foci are likely to be benign, and symmetry is particularly reassuring. Such changes may be due to cyclical hormonal effects or to focal adenosis (fibrocystic change). A small cluster of foci is termed a *focal area* while widespread scattered foci constitute *stippled* or *punctate* enhancement. These findings place the lesion under the heading of non-mass enhancement and will be considered later.

As Liberman and colleagues have shown, "size does matter" when evaluating the likelihood that an enhancing lesion represents cancer. In a study of 666 lesions, only 1/37 (3%) of lesions < 5 mm was malignant, while the risk increased steadily for lesions >5 mm (Fig. 3.10) [9]. However, in another study, Gutierrez *et al.* reported a higher incidence of malignancy in 5/19 (26%) foci < 5 mm [10]. In both studies the lesions < 5 mm had been selected for excision biopsy because specific morphologic, kinetic or clinical features had increased the level of suspicion. The incidence of malignancy in "non-suspicious" foci is therefore likely to be low, which is usual clinical experience. This forms the empirical basis for what is sometimes called the "Stanford 4 mm rule," which proposes that a lesion of 4 mm or less can be considered to be benign (unless it has features to declare itself as suspicious) while above 4 mm the lesion should be treated as potentially malignant based on its size alone. Other features which redefine a focus as a small mass or which increase suspicion and might lead to a BI-RADS score of 3 or greater are given in Table 3.3.

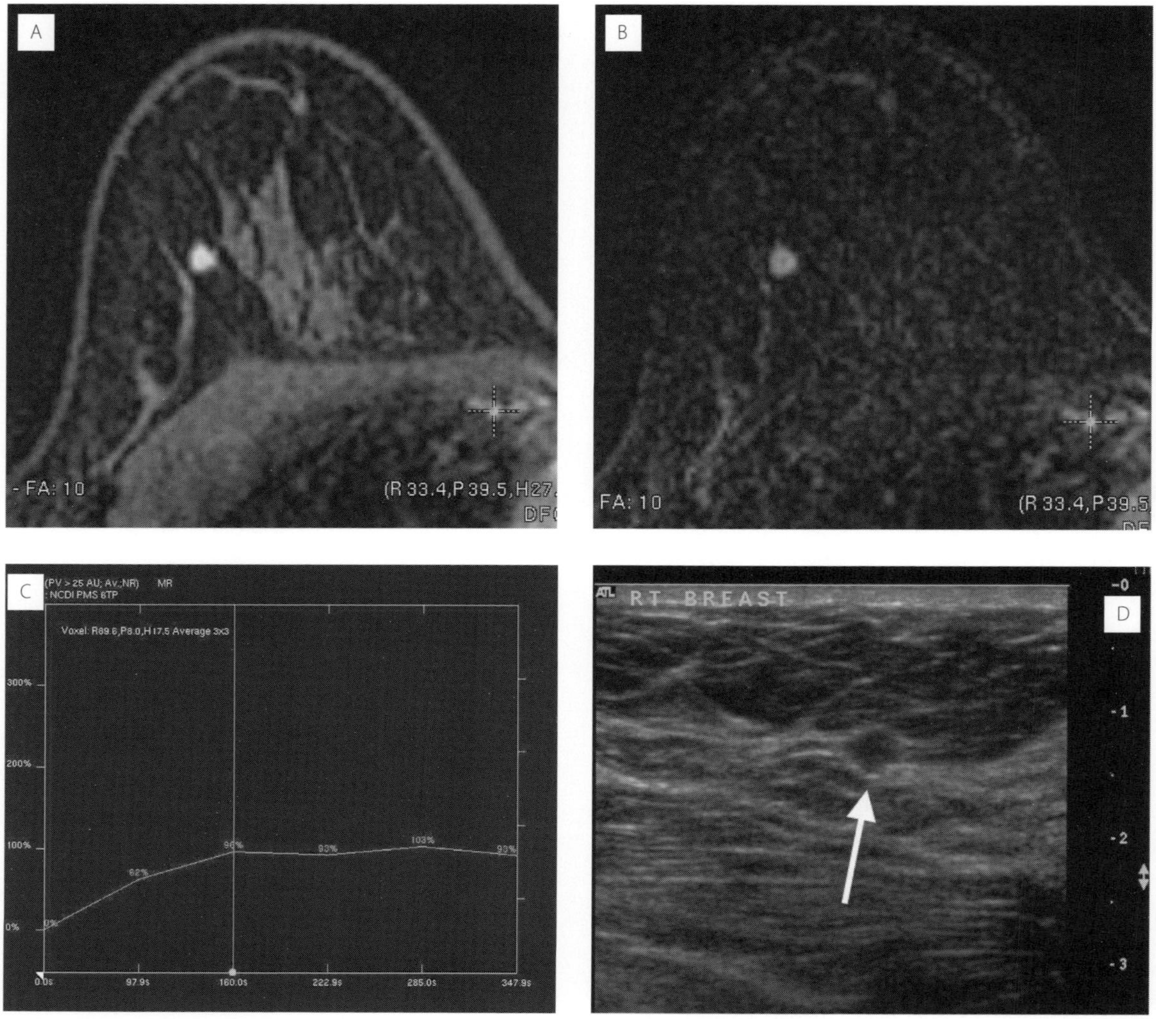

Fig. 3.9 Classifying small lesions: (A) Post-contrast fat-suppressed T1-weighted image shows a 4 mm focus in a patient with ipsilateral index cancer. (B) Subtracted image reveals spiculated margins and rim enhancement, reclassifying the lesion as a mass despite its small size. (C) Kinetic curve shows only moderate initial-phase enhancement of ~60% at 90 seconds from injection with a late-phase plateau. (D) TUS image reveals a 4 mm hypoechoic mass (arrow), grade 3 IDC on 14-gauge CNB.

> The "Stanford 4 mm rule": an enhancing focus under 4 mm usually needs only routine follow-up, while a focus of 4 mm or greater should be regarded as possibly malignant and may require biopsy.

Given that by definition the morphology of a focus cannot be further analyzed, the next question is whether kinetic assessment is of value. Some experts argue that kinetics are unhelpful, as a type 1 curve does not exclude malignancy and benign foci can show a type 3 curve (Table 3.4). Nevertheless, persistent kinetics in a focus reduces the likelihood of malignancy and can reasonably be used to classify it as benign (BI-RADS 2) [11]. Reducing the number of foci subjected to further analysis and particularly biopsy is important in maintaining acceptable specificity. If a type 2 or 3 curve is revealed in a focus > 4 mm in diameter, it is considered equivocal and further assessed (Fig. 3.11), or at least classified as BI-RADS 3, for 6-month MRI follow-up.

Selecting the ROI for kinetic evaluation of a focus

To create a time–intensity curve requires that we first define an ROI. For tiny enhancing foci at only 2–4 mm, this may not be possible, but we know

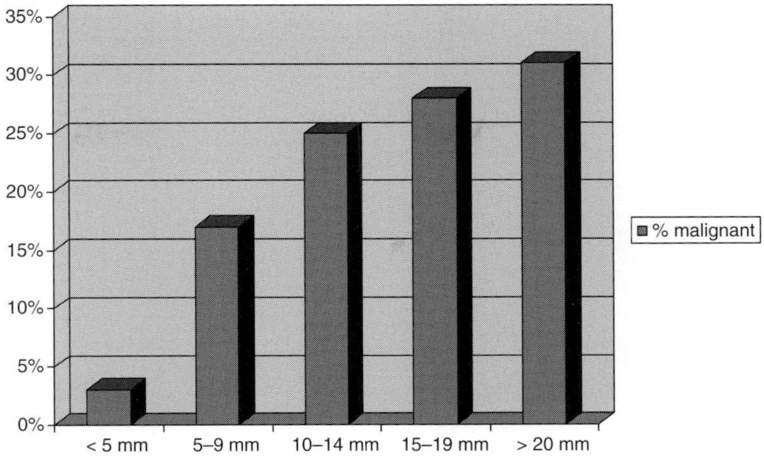

Fig. 3.10 Percentage of malignant lesions by size on MRI: Histogram from data in Liberman *et al.* [9]. In this study, mean lesion size was 10 mm (range 3–70 mm) and over 50% of cancers were DCIS.

Table 3.3 Features in a focus raising suspicion of malignancy

Spiculated margin
Rim enhancement
Correlate on review of pre-contrast T1/T2-weighted images
Solitary lesion, size > 4 mm
Dominant lesion (larger or more intense than other foci)
Type 2 or 3 kinetic curve
Known index cancer in same or contralateral breast
Known BRCA mutation or high-risk history

Table 3.4 Causes of rapidly enhancing focus or small mass +/− washout

Lesion	Rapid wash-in	Washout
Focal adenosis	Frequent	Frequent
Lymph node	Frequent	Frequent
Fibroadenoma	~20%	Rare
Benign papilloma	~20%	Uncommon
Radial scar	Frequent	Occurs

these have an extremely low likelihood of malignancy. Where a focus raises concern, this is often because it exceeds the 4 mm threshold, a size at which an accurate ROI can often be obtained.

Selection of the ROI is usually performed on the first post-contrast image of the fat-suppressed T1-weighted dynamic series. This is particularly appropriate for a focus as only rapid enhancement is likely to be significant. Foci showing only slow persistent enhancement are almost invariably benign. For manual selection, the ROI circle should be adjusted so that it is just large enough to be contained within the focus (Fig. 3.11).

After selection on the first post-contrast image, it is important to ensure that the ROI remains in the focus throughout the dynamic series. If it becomes displaced away from the focus due to patient movement, a bizarre curve or even a spurious type 3 curve can result. To help overcome this, some manual evaluation software allows repositioning of the ROI on images from each time point ("dynamic ROI").

Commercial CAD systems apply color-mapping software to aid in kinetic analysis (Plate 2). Usually CAD software codes the kinetic curve type, assigning blue for persistent (type 1), green for plateau (type 2) and red for washout (type 3). User-defined thresholds can be set for enhancement velocity (for example, only enhancement > 50% above baseline at the first post-contrast time point might be color-coded, as defining curve types has limited value at lower levels). Color-mapping helps locate suspicious lesions, i.e, a solitary red focus seen among several blue ones is singled out for closer inspection.

Most commercial CAD systems have a fixed ROI size set as the default. Dynacad, for example, has a fixed 3 × 3 pixel ROI with the cursor displayed as a cross which represents the central point. A great time-saving advantage of CAD systems is the ability to generate instant kinetic curves "on-the-fly" simply by placing the cursor on the lesion, making

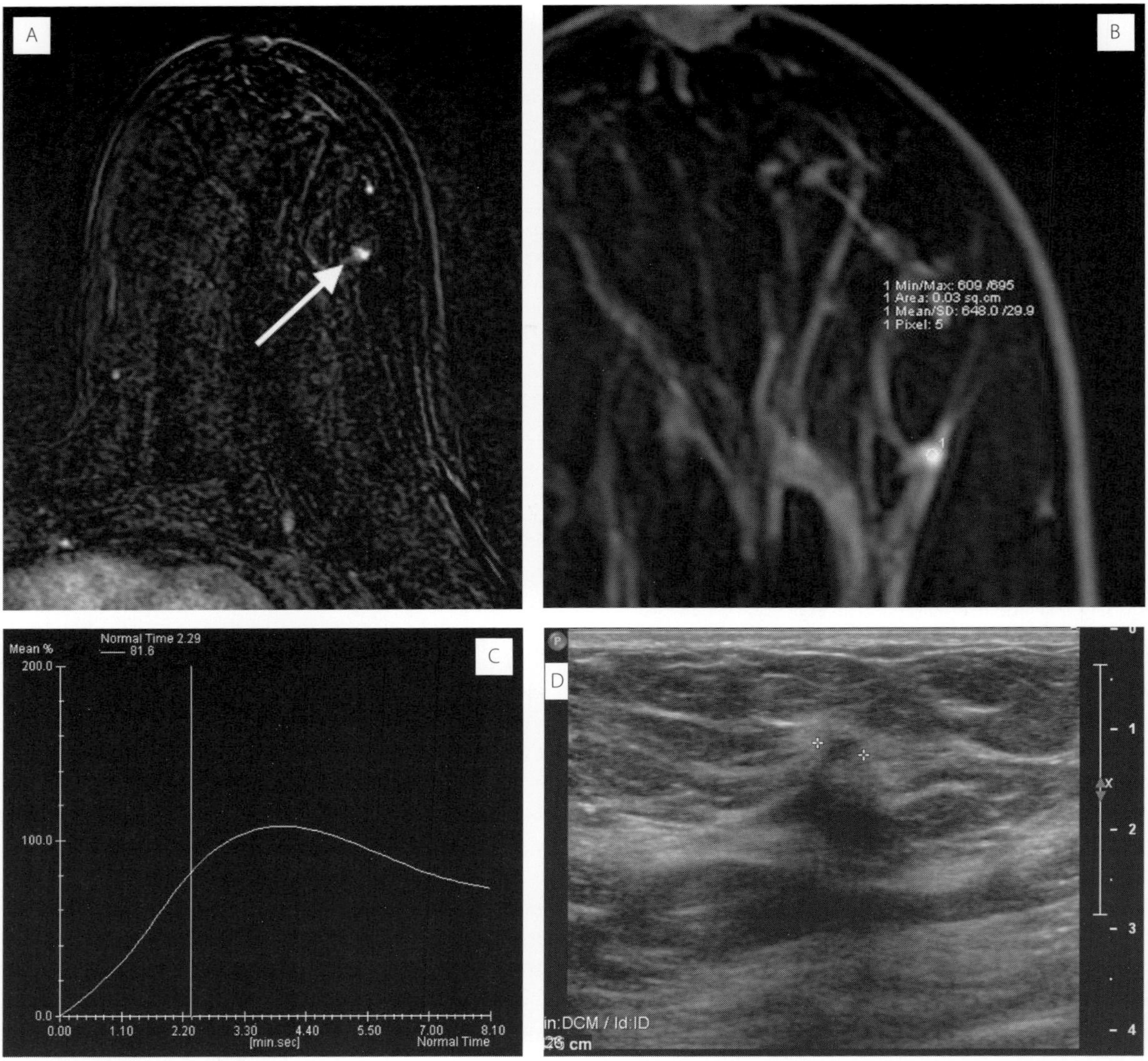

Fig. 3.11 Management of a focus: First screening MRI study in a 43-year-old woman with history of breast cancer in both sisters at ages 38 and 45 years. (A) Subtracted image shows a 4 mm focus in left breast (arrow). The lesion was solitary with no morphologic mass features, no correlate on non-contrast images, and normal XRM. (B) ROI placement and (C) kinetic curve smoothed to show slow early-phase wash-in, delayed peak at ~4 minutes and ~25% late washout ("bow curve"). (D) TUS reveals hypoechoic nidus with echogenic margins, 7 mm ILC on 14-gauge CNB.

the kinetic evaluation very rapid. Routine use of CAD automatic registration software helps minimize issues with patient movement causing spurious colorization.

Table 3.4 lists some common benign lesions presenting as foci or small masses (~5 mm or less) which may be indistinguishable from cancer, because they can exhibit rapid wash-in and in some instances even washout. Such MRI findings often lead to biopsy and a knowledge of potential false positives is important for radiologic–pathologic correlation, further discussed in Chapter 5.

BI-RADS final assessment score for a focus

Given that only a minority of foci are malignant, the object of analysis is to add specificity so that only those lesions with a higher probability of cancer are further assessed. Suggested key steps in the analysis are:

(i) Establishing that the lesion really is a focus and not a small mass.
(ii) Applying a size threshold using the "Stanford 4 mm rule."
(iii) Classifying foci with type 1 kinetics as BI-RADS 1 or 2.

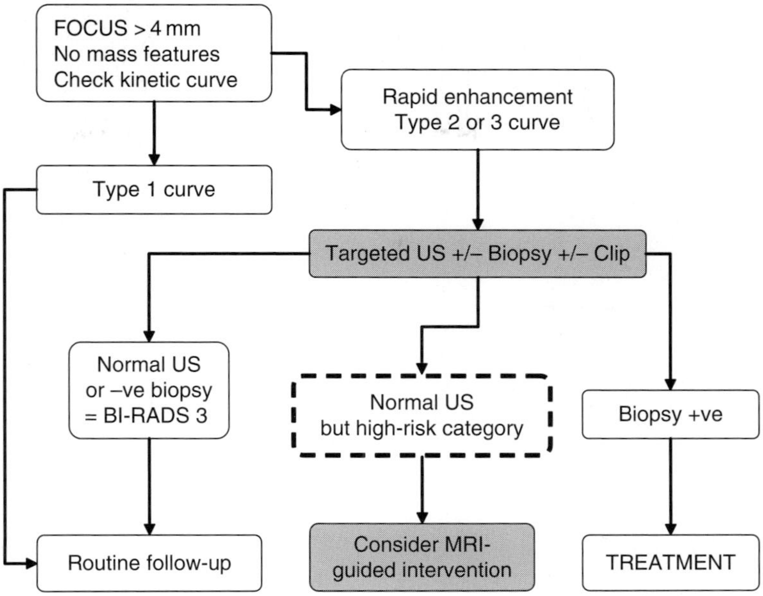

Fig. 3.12 Management flow chart for a focus: Shaded boxes indicate procedural options, broken outlines indicate decision-making. Overall risk of malignancy in a focus is low, and type 1 kinetics help classify most foci as benign. In women with a high-risk profile (known index cancer, BRCA1/2 carrier), MRI-guided intervention is offered at a lower threshold.

So for foci < 4 mm a BI-RADS score of 1 or 2 is usual. For larger or otherwise "suspicious" foci, the individual risk profile is considered, and in some cases will make the difference between a BI-RADS 3 (probably benign) final assessment score and recommending a biopsy (Fig. 3.12).

Analysis of a mass

By definition, a mass is a space-occupying lesion and unlike a focus, a correlate is often seen on non-contrast T1- and T2-weighted images. Analysis of signal on T1- and T2-weighted images then has significant value, and is the suggested first step in the diagnostic algorithm.

Signal characteristics

Whether or not a mass is identified on non-contrast images will depend not only on its size and the nature of its margins, but also on its signal characteristics and those of the surrounding tissue. Most invasive cancers are either isointense or slightly hypointense relative to normal fibroglandular parenchyma on non-contrast FSE T1- and T2-weighted images [1, 12]. This, of course, is precisely why injected contrast is required for diagnosis. On fat-suppressed IR T2-weighted sequences, invasive cancers often show moderately bright signal (similar to parenchyma) but are seldom strongly hyperintense (comparable to water). In one large series, only ~6% of all invasive cancers showed strong high signal on IR T2-weighted images and nearly all of these were special types, e.g., mucinous [13]. Meanwhile, finding even focal high T1 signal in invasive cancers is quite uncommon [14]. The knowledge that a mass which shows significantly bright T1 or T2 signal is unlikely to be malignant can be used to improve specificity.

Non-contrast images are used particularly to help confirm circumscribed masses as benign, including cysts, lymph nodes and fibroadenomas (Figs. 3.2, 3.3 and 3.13–3.15). These all contain fluid, myxoid or highly cellular components which result in bright T2 signal (Table 3.5). However, the "bright T2 mass is benign" rule applies more robustly to non-fat-suppressed FSE T2-weighted images, where signal is compared to normal fibroglandular parenchyma or to pectoral muscle. Kuhl *et al.*, showed that FSE T2-weighted images distinguished fibroadenomas from invasive cancers with an NPV for malignancy of ~90% in women under age 50 years [12]. However, about an equal number of cancers and fibroadenomas were hyperintense on IR T2-weighted images, attributed to the scaling effect on signal intensity when fat suppression is used [12].

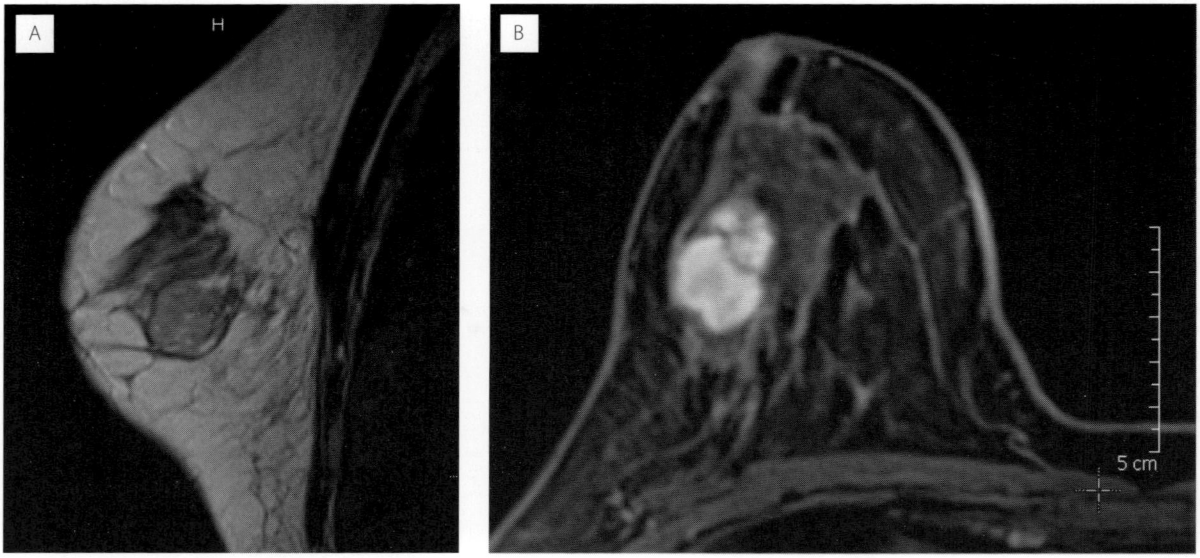

Fig. 3.13 Fibroadenoma: Large circumscribed mass, hyperintense compared to parenchyma on sagittal FSE T2-weighted image (A) with intense enhancement and classic dark internal septations on early post-contrast fat-suppressed T1-weighted image (B). Fibroadenoma confirmed on 14-gauge CNB. See also Plate 2.

"Bright T2 mass is benign rule": a circumscribed or slightly irregular mass showing homogeneous bright signal on non-fat-suppressed FSE T2-weighted images relative to normal fibroglandular breast tissue is usually benign.

Despite this, many centers (particularly in North America) do not include FSE T2-weighted sequences and use only fat-suppressed T2-weighted images, essentially for the identification of cysts. On fat-suppressed T2-weighted images, using an incidental cyst as a visual reference standard can be helpful, as if a lesion shows uniform T2 signal of comparable brightness, this supports a benign diagnosis. Use of pectoral muscle as a reference standard has been validated for IR T2-weighted images, with a lesion to muscle signal intensity ratio value of >5.6 suggested as the threshold for benign lesions (cancers with clearly visible necrosis excluded) [15].

Important exceptions which may show very bright signal on T2-weighted images are mucinous cancers (due to gelatinous matrix) and circumscribed triple-negative or basal-like cancers (due to tumor necrosis) [12, 16, 17]. Some other uncommon invasive cancer types also appear bright on T2-weighted images reflecting various histologic features including high cellularity/abundant cytoplasm, proteinaceous matrix, tumor hemorrhage and edematous non-fibrotic stroma (Table 3.6) [13].

It is also true that circumscribed lesions which show uniform high signal relative to normal fibroglandular

Table 3.5 Benign circumscribed lesions showing bright signal on T2

Cystic – simple, hemorrhagic, galactocoele, oil cyst
Intramammary lymph node
Myxoid fibroadenoma
Papilloma (solid component usually isointense or hypointense, may enhance)
Tubular adenoma/lactating adenoma (rare)
Phyllodes tumor (rare, often large at presentation or show rapid growth)
Juvenile, cellular ("giant") fibroadenoma (rare, large/rapid growth)

Table 3.6 Invasive cancers which may show bright T2 signal

Mucinous (mucoid matrix)
Triple-negative / basal-like cancers (necrosis)
Intracystic (encapsulated) papillary carcinoma
Invasive micropapillary carcinoma
Invasive cribriform carcinoma
Apocrine carcinoma

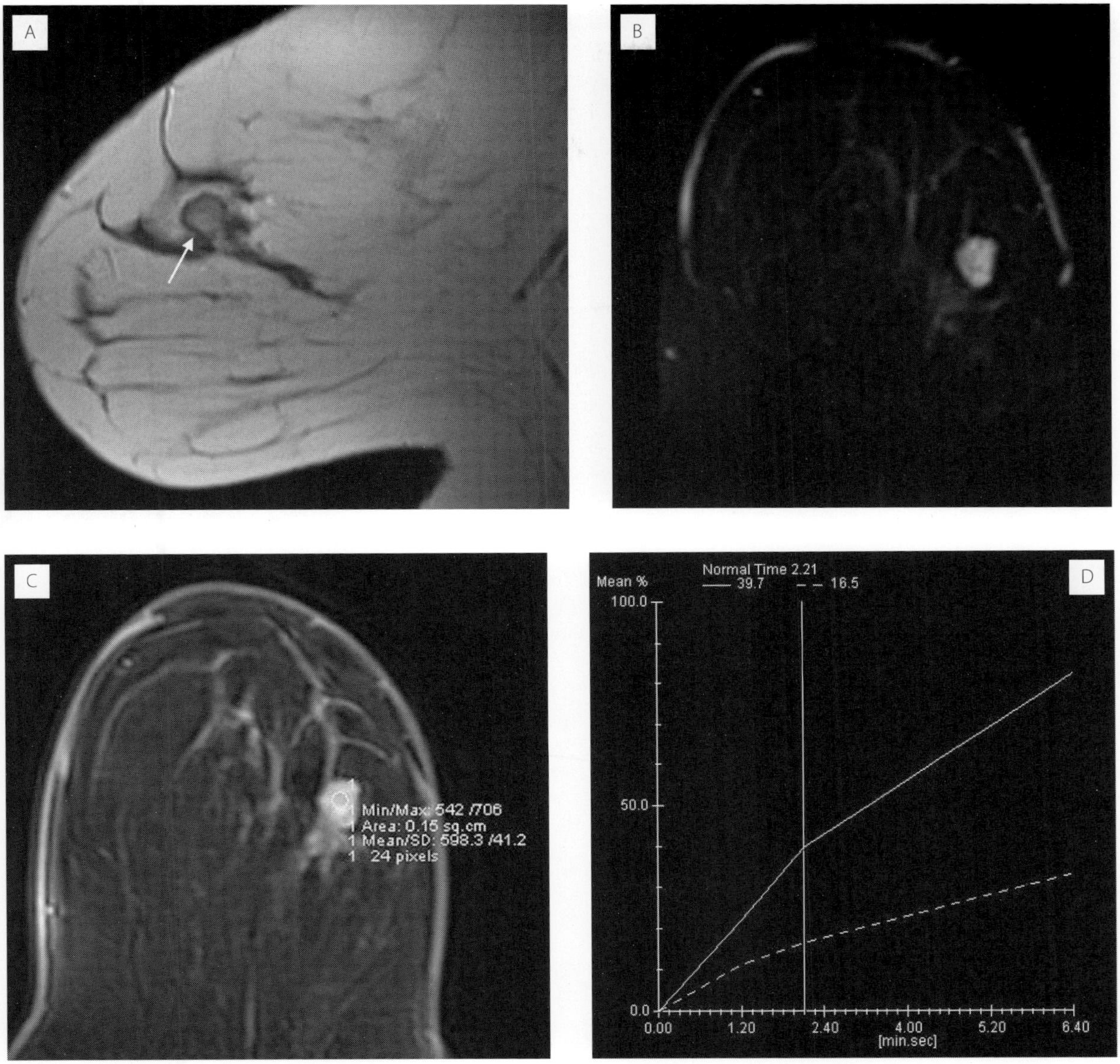

Fig. 3.14 Fibroadenoma: (A) Sagittal FSE T2-weighted image shows mass hyperintense to parenchyma which is also markedly hyperintense on fat-suppressed IR T2-weighted image (B) with subtle dark internal septations on suitably adjusted windows. Post-contrast fat-suppressed T1-weighted image (C) and kinetic curve (D) show slow type 1 pattern (upper solid line with 40% relative enhancement at 2 minutes). Note also the very slow persistent curve (lower broken line) from ROI placed on normal parenchyma for comparison. Despite slightly irregular margins, the presence of non-enhancing internal septations, bright T2 signal and slow persistent kinetics characterize this lesion as a fibroadenoma (no biopsy, stable at > 2 years).

breast parenchyma on non-contrast T1-weighted images are generally benign. This includes proteinaceous cysts and most solid lesions, particularly normal lymph nodes (Figs. 3.2, 3.3 and Table 3.7) and intracystic papillomas with associated blood. Among metastases to the breast, melanoma is often the primary, and a rare exception to the "bright T1 mass is benign" rule [18].

In summary then, on FSE T2-weighted images, signal brighter than fibroglandular tissue in a circumscribed mass favors benignity. This is only true for very bright signal (comparable to water) on fat-suppressed IR T2-weighted images. However, triple-negative/basal-like cancers (common in BRCA1 mutation carriers) and also mucinous cancers are important pitfalls, and biopsy is essential in doubtful cases.

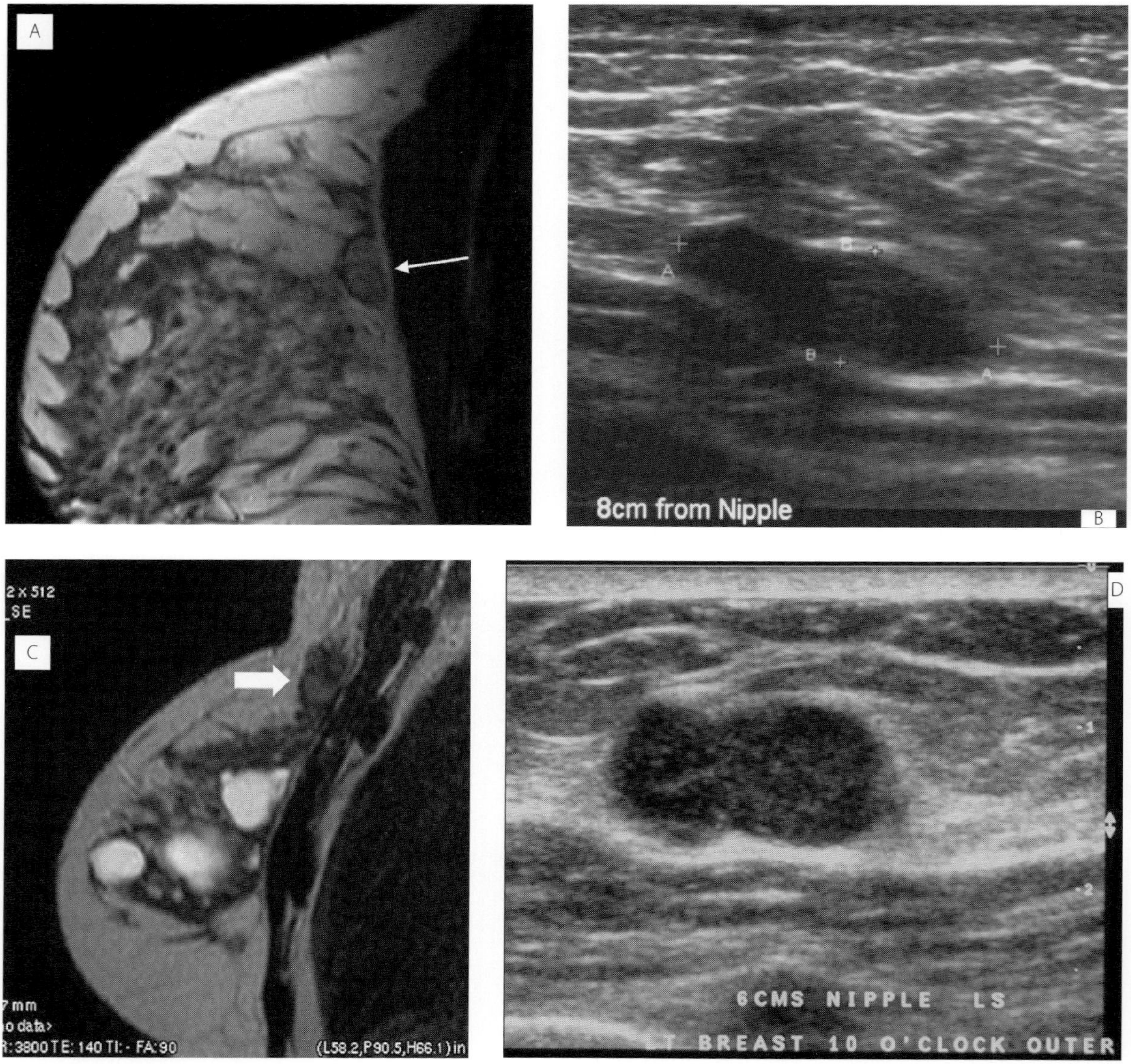

Fig. 3.15 **Differential diagnosis of fibroadenoma:** (A) Circumscribed mass hyperintense to parenchyma with bright T2 signal on sagittal FSE T2-weighted image. Note preserved retroglandular fat layer sign (arrow), typical of a benign lesion. (B) Corresponding US showing hypoechoic gently lobulated, ovoid, wider-than-tall mass typical of a fibroadenoma, which was unchanged over several years. In a different patient sagittal FSE T2-weighted image (C) shows a similar lobulated circumscribed mass hyperintense to parenchyma (arrow) with preserved retroglandular fat layer suggesting a fibroadenoma. However, this was a new finding in a postmenopausal woman and enhancement was heterogeneous with washout kinetics (see also Plate 2). Targeted US (D) confirmed lobulated circumscribed mass suggestive of a benign fibroadenoma. Histopathology showed 25 mm grade 3 IDC, node-negative, triple-negative phenotype.

Nevertheless, in a premenopausal woman with a circumscribed mass, finding very bright T2 signal suggests benignity, and is particularly valuable when used in conjunction with other benign signs discussed later. Circumscribed lesions with bright T1 signal are usually also benign. Finally, a circumscribed mass which shows very marked hypointensity on FSE T1- and T2-weighted images is much more likely to be a sclerosed fibroadenoma or papilloma than an invasive cancer.

Mass morphology

The first two groups of BI-RADS descriptors for mass lesions relate to *shape* and *margins*, although in practice these features can be difficult to separate. Margin analysis is of far greater diagnostic significance and the single best discriminator for benign verus malignant mass lesions.

In the UK MARIBS study, a simplified scoring system was used to combine shape and margins in three categories: (i) lobulated or well-defined, (ii) poorly defined, (iii) spiculated [19–21]. Such a system is easier to apply consistently, and does not preclude the use of shape descriptors if desired. The term "circumscribed" is also in common usage:

(i) circumscribed mass (rounded, ovoid or lobulated shape with smooth margins)
(ii) irregular mass (irregular shape and/or margins)
(iii) spiculated mass (any shape with spiculated margins).

Using this system, most circumscribed masses are benign while lesions in the second group are considered indeterminate. In the third group, regardless of shape, a mass with a spiculated margin has a PPV for malignancy of > 90% [22].

Visual pattern of mass enhancement

The remaining BI-RADS mass descriptors relate to the visual pattern of *mass enhancement* and *internal architecture* and can be conveniently thought of as comprising three pairs of "opposites":

(i) homogeneous versus heterogeneous enhancement
(ii) rim versus central enhancement
(iii) dark non-enhancing versus enhancing internal septations.

Homogeneous versus heterogeneous enhancement

Making this distinction is unreliable in small lesions (< 10 mm), but for larger masses heterogeneous enhancement is a strong malignant predictor, particularly when combined with morphology. In one study, heterogeneous enhancement with irregular or spiculated margins had a 68% probability of malignancy versus only 3% for homogeneous enhancement with smooth margins [10].

Rim versus central enhancement

The finding of *rim enhancement* is a reliable sign of malignancy which can be observed even in very small invasive cancers and has a reported PPV of ~85% [3]. The list of benign conditions which can mimic rim enhancement is limited to an inflammatory cyst (*solar eclipse sign*), an oil cyst in post-traumatic fat necrosis, and normal cortical enhancement of a lymph node, all of which can usually be easily distinguished (Table 3.8 and Figs. 3.2–3.5). Rim enhancement of invasive cancers usually reflects neovascularity at the infiltrating margin and is best evaluated on early post-contrast scans. In the late phase the rim often fades due to peripheral washout and central filling-in of hypovascular areas (centripetal enhancement).

> A rim-enhancing mass which is not either a normal benign lymph node or a cyst with inflammation (solar eclipse sign) has a PPV for malignancy of ~80%, while a spiculated mass has a PPV of ~90%.

In addition to the familiar early-phase pattern (thick rim around spiculated IDC due to central necrosis or fibrosis), a delayed pattern is also reported (thin rim around circumscribed IDC with pushing margins and inflammatory change) [23].

Central enhancement is an uncommon malignant sign, and can be thought of as a variant of heterogeneous internal enhancement. This can occur in

Table 3.7 MRI diagnosis of benign lymph node

Circumscribed mass (smooth margins)
Round, oval, reniform or C-shaped (may need to view multiple planes)
Location in axilla (level I) or lateral half of breast when intramammary
Cortex shows high signal on T2 and often on pre-contrast fat-suppressed T1-weighted images
Short-axis diameter < 5 mm
Fat-signal intensity of hilum (bright on FSE T1/T2, dark on fat-suppressed T1/T2)
Variable – absent or slow enhancement through to rapid with washout kinetics
Uniformly thin cortex (< 2–3 mm) with "donut" or C-shape around fatty hilum

Table 3.8 Rim-enhancing lesions

Invasive cancer (pattern 1) – early phase, thick rim at infiltrating margin
Circumscribed IDC (pattern 2) – delayed phase, thin rim at pushing margin
Inflammatory cyst – solar eclipse sign
Oil cyst – post-traumatic fat necrosis, contents of cyst show fat signal
Intramammary lymph node – cortex enhances around fatty hilus

combination with rim enhancement, giving a "target" appearance.

Dark non-enhancing versus enhancing internal septation

On MRI, *non-enhancing dark internal septations* are reported in 40–65% of enhancing fibroadenomas, and have been considered a strong specific benign sign with an NPV of 95% (Figs. 3.13 and 3.14). However, dark septations are convincingly present in a rather low percentage of small fibroadenomas with Malich and coworkers reporting that only 20% of all benign mass lesions showed this feature [24]. Furthermore, in the IBMC 6883 study, this sign was "not highly correlated with a benign outcome" [3].

To reliably display septations requires high-resolution images and needs careful adjustment of windowing. Early post-contrast T1-weighted dynamic scans show septations best, because although designated as "non-enhancing," in actuality they often slowly enhance and may become obscured on delayed images. Sometimes septations in fibroadenomas are better seen on FSE T2-weighted or T2-weighted fat-suppressed images (Fig. 3.14). They are generally uniformly thin (< 1 mm) and extend to the margins of the lesion, but a variant with thicker swirled internal septations is described [25]. However, it should be kept in mind that necrotic or fibrotic bands in an invasive cancer can also mimic dark septations [26]. Caution is needed to avoid over-interpreting vague curvilinear internal low signal in a mass, and if there is doubt, biopsy should be performed.

The appearance of *enhancing internal septations* relates to areas of necrosis in a cancer with intervening bands of viable tumor tissue. Such bands are typically of variable thickness and enhance strongly, in contradistinction to non-enhancing septations in a fibroadenoma [24]. Enhancing septations are essentially a further variant of heterogeneous internal enhancement in invasive cancers. According to Kaiser, enhancing septa are not common in IDC NOS, and are more characteristic of medullary cancer, ILC or lymphoma, while also occurring in metastases to the breast and in loculated abscesses [1].

Other morphologic signs for masses

As well as BI-RADS mass descriptors, the MRI Lexicon details additional features which should be included in the report when identified (Tables 3.9 and 3.10), while other recognized breast MRI signs are potentially useful discriminators for benign versus malignant masses (Tables 3.11 and 3.12). The more important are discussed here, with many others comprehensively cataloged by Kaiser [1].

Table 3.9 BI-RADS mass descriptors

Shape
Round
Oval
Lobulated
Irregular
Margins
Smooth
Irregular
Spiculated
Mass enhancement
Homogeneous – benign predictor in larger lesions, unreliable in small masses
Heterogeneous – typically malignant, but also in partly sclerosed fibroadenoma
Rim – strong malignant predictor with exception of "solar eclipse sign" and lymph nodes
Central – occasional sign of invasive cancer, may occur with rim enhancement
Dark internal septations – virtually pathognomonic of fibroadenoma
Enhancing internal septations – typically malignant enhancing bands

Table 3.10 Associated findings listed in BI-RADS

Nipple retraction or inversion
Skin retraction
Skin thickening
Skin invasion
Edema on T2-weighted images
Lymphadenopathy
Pectoral muscle invasion
Chest wall invasion
Pre-contrast high T1 duct signal
Hematoma/blood with bright T1 signal
Signal void from clip artifact
Cysts

MRI halo sign

A benign rounded mass lesion may show a thin rim of normal compressed fat around its margins. Although

Table 3.11 Additional benign morphologic signs for masses

Solar eclipse sign (enhancing rim around inflammatory cyst)
Blooming fibroadenoma (centrifugal enhancement pattern)
MRI halo sign (preserved fat plane around lesion)
Marked homogeneous T1 or T2 hyperintensity in circumscribed lesion
Marked T1 and T2 hypointensity in circumscribed lesion (sclerosed or calcified)
If heterogeneous, enhancing parts of lesion are T2 hyperintense (fibroadenoma)

Table 3.12 Additional malignant morphologic signs for masses

Blooming sign ("dissolving aspirin sign") – fuzzy borders in late phase making lesion larger
Perilesional edema (best seen on fat-suppressed T2-weighted sequences)
Vessel sign – unilateral increased vascularity +/– vessel leading to the lesion
Hook sign – long thin strands extending from lesion to the pectoral muscle
Tumor bridges – desmoplastic reaction +/– DCIS or lymphatic infiltration
Disrupted nipple line – loss of normal clear line of demarcation at base of nipple

it has a quite different basis to the mammographic halo sign, this MRI counterpart has a similar high predictive value for benignity, because an invasive cancer will usually infiltrate the adjacent fat [1]. A variant of this sign is the observation of an *intact retroglandular fat layer* where a deep zone lesion abuts the pectoral fascia (Fig. 3.15) [1].

Solar eclipse sign

This description of an enhancing rim due to inflammatory change surrounding a cyst is particularly apt for subtracted images where a round black signal void is seen inside the rim (Fig. 3.2). Oil cysts from post-traumatic fat necrosis (relating to previous surgery) may also show rim enhancement, typically with surrounding edema which gradually subsides over many months (Fig. 3.5).

Blooming sign

This characteristic "fuzziness" of the margins of an invasive cancer develops progressively through the dynamic contrast-enhanced series, resulting in apparent enlargement of the mass. The blooming sign is attributed to enhancement of the peripheral rim of neovascularization, where the tumor is actively infiltrating the surrounding tissues. Fischer *et al.* found a blooming sign present in 324/514 (63%) malignant lesions and in only 41/279 (15%) of benign lesions, giving a PPV of almost 90% [27]. This phenomenon has also been dubbed the *dissolving aspirin sign*, which aptly captures the progressive loss of clarity of the lesion margins. The same sign can be reversed as the *constant sharpness* sign, i.e., a circumscribed mass which remains sharp throughout the dynamic series is probably benign [1]. Recently, an automated CAD method for assessing "morphologic blooming" between images at 1 and 7 minutes from injection has been described with ~90% sensitivity in combination with kinetic interpretation [28].

Blooming fibroadenoma

Confusingly, the term "blooming" has also been applied to describe the *centrifugal* pattern of enhancement (from center to periphery) exhibited by some larger fibroadenomas during the dynamic series [29]. This is a strong benign sign, since invasive cancers typically show peripheral rim enhancement with *centripetal* filling-in towards the center [1]. This should not be confused with the central enhancement seen in a minority of cancers without the subsequent progression to the periphery seen in "blooming" fibroadenomas.

Hook sign

A long thin, usually non-enhancing, hook-like strand of tissue extending from a mass lesion to the pectoral muscle which strongly predicts malignancy [24]. Kaiser has suggested that if the strand does enhance, this usually correlates with lymphatic involvement histologically, whereas a non-enhancing strand probably represents an isolated spicule of desmoplastic reaction, with the specific location perhaps relating to infiltration of Cooper's ligaments [1]. As such, the hook sign may be similar in etiology to the *tumor bridges* sometimes seen between multifocal invasive cancers. Post-surgical or post-inflammatory fibrotic change can also mimic the hook sign [1, 24].

Perilesional edema

This refers to a small area of bright T2 signal around an enhancing lesion, often only visible on fat-suppressed T2-weighted images. This is reportedly a reasonably strong malignant sign, particularly frequently around high-grade invasive or medullary carcinomas [1]. As such, this may correspond to reactive inflammatory change seen with these cancer types.

Nipple line

The *nipple line* is a normal boundary across the base of the nipple, best seen on non-contrast T1-weighted images. This line subsequently shows only low-level enhancement while the nipple surface often enhances intensely. Disruption of the normal intact nipple line with enhancement crossing into the nipple is indicative of malignant infiltration [1, 24]. Usually, there is other direct evidence of a malignant process extending to the nipple, i.e., subareolar mass or non-mass enhancement, often with unilateral nipple retraction.

Vessel sign

The *vessel sign* recognizes that blood vessels are both more prominent and more numerous in the presence of cancer, and may be directly related to the tumor mass [30]. One study using 3D MIP images reported sensitivity of 88% and PPV of 94% for ipsilateral hypervascularity as a sign of invasive cancer (Fig. 3.16) [31]. The vessels seen are prominent early-filling veins, consistent with arteriovenous shunting occurring in the tumor circulation. According to Kaiser, pronounced unilateral increased vascularity may even be observed up to 2 years before cancer is detected [1]. Diffuse increase in breast vascularity is also seen in acute mastitis.

Selecting the ROI for kinetic assessment of a mass

For mass lesions, it is recommended that the ROI is kept small and placed on the most avidly enhancing area of a lesion, often the rim of a suspected cancer. Using a larger ROI around the entire lesion, including the non-enhancing necrotic center, may falsely downgrade the kinetic curve, making the lesion appear less suspicious. The converse is also true, so that a small ROI placed on the most vascular part of a benign lesion could upgrade the kinetic curve to appear more suspicious. Therefore, using a smaller ROI will tend to raise sensitivity but reduce specificity and vice versa [32]. Consequently, experts differ regarding the merits of fixed or variable, smaller or larger ROIs, and there is no published evidence-based consensus [32]. The ACR has stipulated that ROI size should be a minimum of 3 × 3 pixels, but in practice smaller ROIs of between 4 and 9 pixels are often used [32].

The use of color-mapping software aids kinetic analysis by guiding ROI selection. Commercial CAD systems usually allow 3D volumetric analysis, in which a VOI is constructed around a mass. The CAD software can then automatically locate the most suspicious area in the defined volume to display the "worst curve." It is an important point to check that the CAD has not selected an arteriolar blood vessel at the edge of the mass, which invariably yields a spurious type 3 curve.

It is, of course, possible to generate multiple kinetic curves from different ROIs within the same

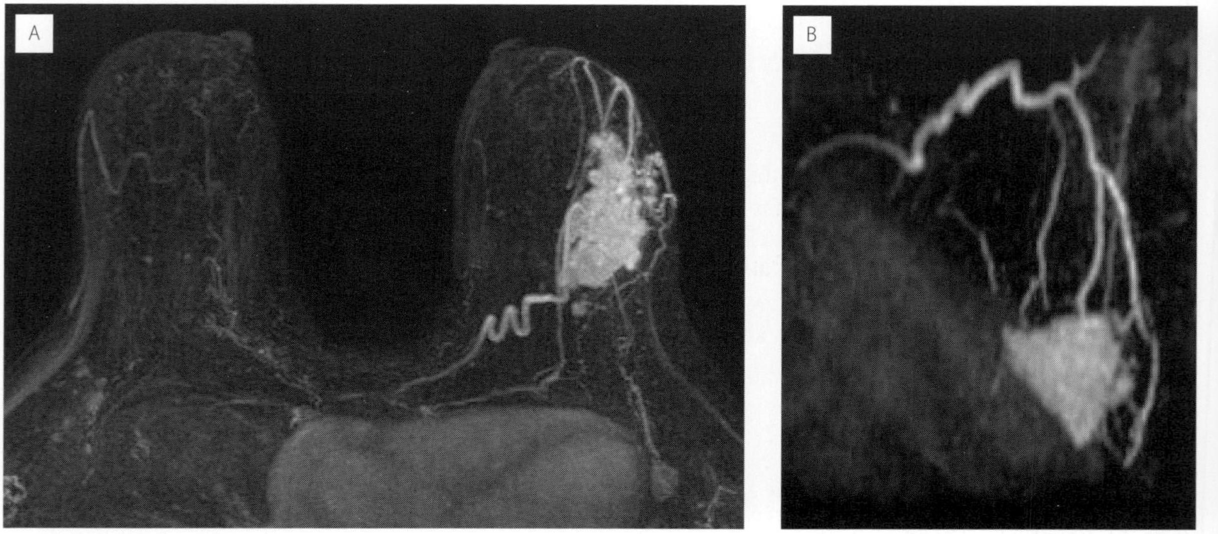

Fig. 3.16 Vessel sign: (A) Axial bilateral MIP image shows increased vascularity around large left breast IDC with (B) coronal subtracted MIP image of left breast showing prominent feeding vessels leading directly to the tumor mass, which was a grade 2 IDC, ER/PR +ve, HER2 –ve.

lesion. This exercise will often show considerable variation even in benign lesions which may appear visually homogeneous. Most CAD systems summarize the kinetics of all voxels in a defined VOI by displaying percentages for each of the three curve types.

An important question then is whether the most predominant curve type (kinetic behavior of the whole lesion) or the "worst curve" is more reliable for identifying cancer. Using CADstream for kinetic evaluation of 125 lesions on MRI, Wang *et al.* found the "worst curve" to be an effective benign versus malignant discriminator, while predominant curve type was not [33]. Therefore, even if only a small part of a lesion shows a type 3 curve, it should be classified as showing washout. Lesions showing purely type 1 kinetics had only a 13% likelihood of malignancy.

The IBMC 6833 trial found that in mass analysis, after lesion margins, rapid early-phase enhancement and kinetic curve type were the best malignant predictors. In that study, a mass with a washout curve, as compared to a persistent curve, had a 5-fold increased risk of malignancy [3].

Combining morphologic and kinetic features in mass analysis

In summary, four key observations contribute to differential diagnosis of masses:

(i) signal characteristics on non-contrast T1- and T2-weighted sequences
(ii) morphology, particularly margins – circumscribed, irregular, spiculated
(ii) visual enhancement – rapidity, heterogeneity, rim pattern, septations
(iii) assessment of the kinetic curve type – persistent, plateau or washout.

Additional BI-RADS findings and MRI signs may further improve specificity, but the golden rule for managing a mass is "if in doubt, biopsy."

Characteristics of specific mass lesions

Cystic lesions

Simple cysts show low signal on T1-weighting and are bright on T2-weighted images. With proteinaceous content, cysts appear bright on T1-weighting with lower signal on T2. Cysts with a fluid level due to layering of the contents are common and do not require biopsy (Fig. 3.2). With a suspected hemorrhagic cyst (high T1 signal) an enhancing mural nodule strongly indicates an intracystic papillary lesion. Inflammation around a cyst is a common incidental finding, giving the classic solar eclipse sign (Fig. 3.2). Fat-signal oil cysts may be observed in the context of post-surgical fat necrosis (Fig. 3.5). The differential diagnosis for cystic lesions is given in Table 3.13.

Papilloma

A solitary intraduct papilloma is suggested by finding an enhancing circumscribed mass near the NAC, while an associated ectatic duct makes the diagnosis almost certain (Fig. 3.17), particularly with very high T1 signal or a history of bloody nipple discharge. However, duct fluid may only be bright on T2-weighted images and discharge may be absent with incidental MRI-detected papillomas (Fig. 3.17) [34]. When a papilloma occludes the duct, the ectatic portion is typically between the lesion and the nipple, with peripheral duct dilation less frequent. Lesions are often ovoid or fusiform and aligned towards the nipple, reflecting their soft friable nature with growth along the duct.

Most solitary small central papillomas (within 1–2 cm of the NAC) are benign, but histology should always be obtained. Most benign papillomas exhibit moderate wash-in, while about 20% show rapid initial enhancement with a post-initial persistent or sometimes plateau curve [1, 29]. Washout occurs occasionally and perhaps relates to the characteristic fibrovascular core (Fig. 3.17). Sclerosed papillomas may not enhance at all.

Intramammary lymph nodes

The morphology of lymph nodes on MRI parallels other imaging modalities. Thus normal benign

Table 3.13 MRI differential diagnosis of cystic lesions

Margins – smooth
Shape – round, oval or lobulated (septated cluster, can mimic fibroadenoma)
Layering effect common on T2-weighted images and does not signify pathology
Hyperintense on T2-weighted images with no internal enhancement = simple cyst
Hyperintense on T1, lower on T2 = proteinaceous or hemorrhagic cyst
Hyperintense on both FSE T1 and T2, dark on fat suppression = oil cyst
Solar eclipse sign of rim enhancement on subtracted images
Look for enhancing mural nodule indicating intracystic papillary lesion

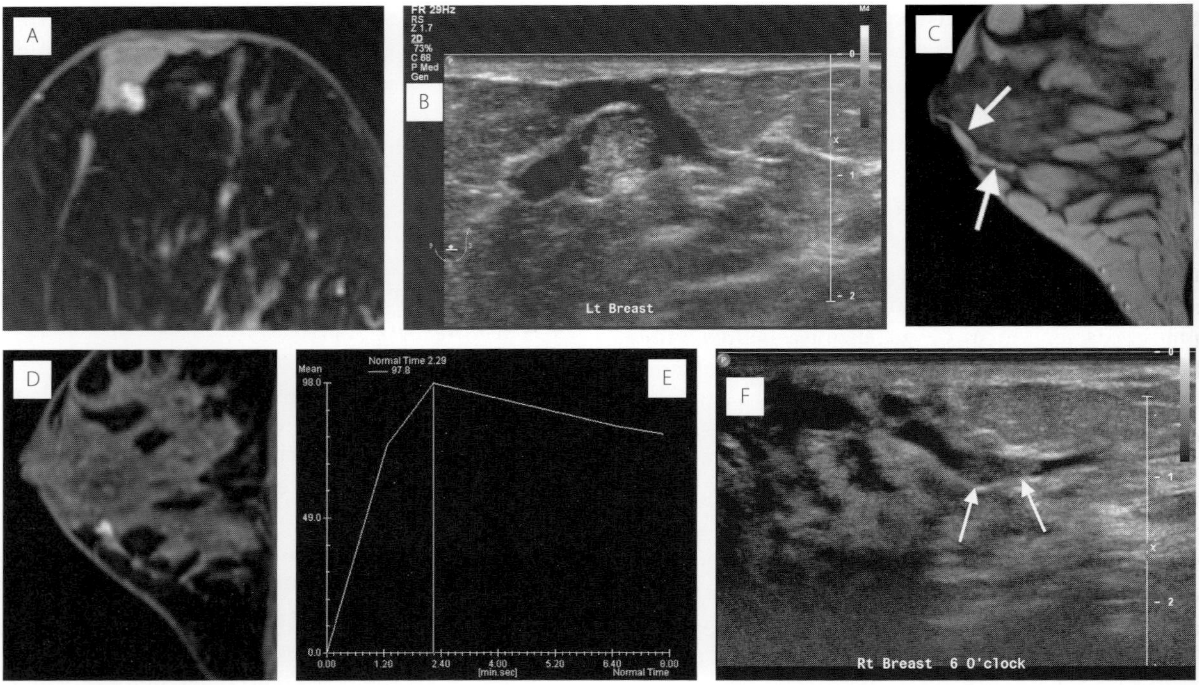

Fig. 3.17 Papillomas: (A) Post-contrast T1-weighted image shows 6 mm rapidly enhancing slightly irregular subareolar mass, a new finding since previous MRI screening round in a BRCA2 mutation carrier. Lesion lies close to the nipple and is associated with an ectatic subareolar duct but the patient had no nipple discharge. (B) TUS image reveals a corresponding intraductal fronded mass with benign papilloma confirmed on excision. In another high-risk woman without nipple discharge sagittal FSE T2-weighted image (C) shows solitary ectatic duct at 6:00 (arrows) associated with (D) lobulated 5 mm dominant focus/small mass on post-contrast T1-weighted image. Kinetic curve (E) shows washout kinetics. TUS image (F) shows intraductal mass (arrows) confirmed as a benign papilloma on excision biopsy.

nodes show an ovoid or reniform shape in long-axis views with a uniformly thin cortex and a preserved fatty hilum (Fig. 3.3). In cross-section on MRI these may appear donut-shaped or C-shaped with preserved hilar fat signal seen on all sequences (Table 3.7). A great majority of benign intramammary lymph nodes arise in the lateral quadrants of the breast, usually in the UOQ or axillary tail. Small round lymph nodes which lack a visible hilum may be implied by their signal, sharp margins and typical location.

Benign lymph nodes typically show high cortical signal relative to normal breast parenchyma on FSE and IR T2-weighted images, and are often bright on fat-suppressed non-contrast T1-weighted images (Fig. 3.3). Enhancement of normal lymph nodes is quite variable, being minimal or absent in some, while others show intense enhancement, often with marked washout (Fig. 3.3). Differentiating features of benign and malignant axillary nodes are discussed in greater detail in Chapter 6.

> Other than a normal lymph node, a mass which shows rapid initial-phase enhancement and late-phase washout >20% has a PPV for malignancy of ~90%, regardless of signal and morphology.

Fibroadenomas

Much like people, the appearance of fibroadenomas depends on their time of life. Young actively growing fibroadenomas (more "adeno" than "fibro") have a myxoid matrix with high water content giving rise to very bright T2 signal, and display a round, oval or gently lobulated shape. About 70% of fibroadenomas show signal brighter than normal parenchyma on FSE T2-weighted images, and below age 50 years the NPV of this finding is ~90% [12]. Enhancement of myxoid fibroadenomas is often rapid and intense, with the late phase showing a persistent (~80%) or plateau curve (Figs. 3.13 and 3.14). Significant washout is rare, reported in < 1% of fibroadenomas [29]. When definite dark internal septations are seen in combination with a T2-hyperintense circumscribed mass and type 1 kinetics, a fibroadenoma can be confidently diagnosed.

At the other end of the spectrum, mature and often almost completely sclerotic fibroadenomas (more “fibro” than “adeno”) may appear dark on T2-weighting, are often irregular in outline and show minimal or absent enhancement. Occasionally, dark non-enhancing spots, profoundly hypointense on all sequences, may be seen in fibroadenomas containing typical coarse “popcorn” calcifications and can readily be correlated with XRM.

Between the myxoid and sclerotic phases, “middle-aged” fibroadenomas may show heterogeneous T2 signal and variable enhancement patterns. This may be related to the structure of fibroadenomas, which are divided into distinct lobules by the fibrous septa. Some lobules then become sclerosed while others remain myxoid. In general, it is the viable adenomatous lobules in a fibroadenoma (bright on T2-weighting) which enhance, while fibrotic parts (with low T2 signal) do not.

In a malignant mass, on the other hand, necrotic areas (bright on T2-weighting) do not enhance while viable tumor areas (with low T2 signal) typically enhance avidly, i.e., opposite to fibroadenoma. This may be a useful benign/malignant discriminator with Malich *et al.* finding that enhancing areas were T2 hyperintense in only 2% of malignant compared with 20% of benign masses [24]. Table 3.14 summarizes the range of MRI appearances of fibroadenomas.

In the absence of dark internal septations, the most likely diagnosis for a circumscribed mass with

Table 3.14 MRI features of fibroadenoma

Circumscribed mass (myxoid), may be slightly irregular (sclerosing)
Homogeneous bright T2 signal (myxoid), may be low T2 (sclerosing)
Internal dark septations in 40–60% – high specificity for fibroadenoma
Rapid type 1 or 2 ~20% (myxoid) slower type 1 ~80% (sclerosing)
Homogeneous enhancement (myxoid), heterogeneous (sclerosing)
Centrifugal enhancement on dynamic scans (“blooming fibroadenoma”)
When heterogeneous T2 signal (sclerosing) – bright T2 parts enhance
Occasional profoundly hypointense parts due to “popcorn” calcifications

bright T2 signal, homogeneous enhancement and a type 1 curve is still fibroadenoma. However, cancers which appear bright on T2-weighting are an important pitfall (Table 3.6). Yuen *et al.* observed that ~90% of such cancers are of special pathologic types [13]. Among these, mucinous carcinomas and triple-negative (basal-like) cancers are the most important considerations (Fig. 3.15).

Mucinous carcinoma

These typically circumscribed cancers usually arise in older women (mean age > 70 years) and have a good prognosis. Lobulated shape and smooth margins are typical, often with prominent thin, dark internal septations which may be non-enhancing on early-phase images [35]. Mucinous composition results in consistently very bright signal on T2-weighted images, while T1 signal is variable, depending on protein content [36]. Peripheral rim enhancement is seen in ~50%, with a heterogeneous pattern in the remainder [16, 35, 37]. A great majority show slow to moderate persistent enhancement kinetics, [13, 16, 33, 36], although with rapid initial enhancement reported in hypercellular pure mucinous tumors and also in mixed lesions [35]. There is the potential for misdiagnosis as fibroadenoma given the bright T2 signal, type 1 kinetics and presence of dark internal septations, although patient age is helpful in differential diagnosis.

Triple-negative/basal-like cancer

This important group of often circumscribed cancers commonly arise in younger women and particularly in BRCA1 mutation carriers. The round, ovoid or lobulated shape reflects rapid growth of these high-grade cancers which mimic fibroadenomas or even cysts on imaging (Fig. 3.15).

In a series of 59 triple-negative cancers, Uematsu *et al.* observed that 40% were smooth masses, and among this group, 95% showed rim enhancement [17]. One-third exhibited very bright signal (comparable to water) on fat-suppressed T2-weighted images which correlated with intratumoral necrosis, and half showed washout kinetics.

In a review of 44 triple-negative cancers by Dogan *et al.*, MRI identified all lesions as malignant. Among 34 masses in that series, MRI features with high PPV were washout kinetics (90%) and rim enhancement (77%), while almost 50% showed bright signal on fat-suppressed T2-weighted images and 30% showed enhancing internal septa [38].

In a cohort of high-risk women, Schrading and Kuhl found 15/64 (23%) invasive cancers had "fibroadenoma-like" morphology, but were distinguishable on MRI by absent non-enhancing internal septations and the presence of rim enhancement or washout kinetics [39]. However, one-third of all cancers in that study showed benign kinetics, with slow or moderate early-phase and persistent delayed-phase enhancement. Most circumscribed cancers (80%) occurred in women who were either proven BRCA1 mutation carriers or at high familial risk (suggesting basal-like molecular subtype). A further observation in that study was that two-thirds of cancers in the high-risk cohort were located in the retromammary zone [39].

So, particularly in the setting of high-risk screening, circumscribed masses on MRI must be regarded with some caution. Of cancers missed by MRI in the MRISC trial, 6/21 were smooth round or lobulated masses < 10 mm diameter, of which three were grade 3 IDC in BRCA1 carriers [40]. Rim enhancement, washout and location in the retromammary zone are clues to identify triple-negative cancers.

Invasive ductal carcinoma NOS

With the exception of low-grade cancers, which may enhance very slowly, and high-grade cancers, which may be circumscribed as discussed above, a majority of invasive cancers appear as irregular or spiculated rapidly enhancing masses. Partly sclerosed fibroadenoma or papilloma are in the differential diagnosis for an irregular mass, with sclerosing adenosis/radial scar and fat necrosis as uncommon benign possibilities for stellate masses (Figs. 3.18 and 3.19).

Inflammatory cancer is essentially a clinical diagnosis based on the finding of an erythematous, indurated and edematous breast with *peau d'orange* (seen as skin thickening on imaging). Although the underlying tumor mass may be difficult to assess on conventional imaging, MRI usually depicts lesion extent and may help direct biopsy. Diffuse edema, typical of inflammatory carcinomas, may manifest on MRI as *prepectoral edema*, although this is also an expected finding following RT (Fig. 3.20) [1]. Differentiation of inflammatory cancer from an acute mastitis may also be possible by MRI, with rim-enhancing fluid-signal collections reliably indicating abscess formation.

Invasive lobular carcinoma

About 10–15% of all invasive cancers are of the ILC subtype, one that is notorious for being subtle or occult on XRM, often leading to delayed diagnosis and large tumor size at presentation. Around 50% of patients diagnosed with ILC present with a palpable abnormality. The incidence of multifocal, multicentric and contralateral tumors is about double that seen with IDC, and disease extent is frequently underestimated by conventional imaging. Difficulty with XRM diagnosis reflects the infiltrative nature of ILC, with minimal desmoplastic reaction and often only subtle architectural distortion. Furthermore, the density of ILC on XRM may be similar to, or even less than, that of normal fibroglandular breast tissue [41, 42]. This pattern of a low-density infiltrating lesion with only subtle architectural distortion on XRM has been likened to a spider's web. Ultrasound is a potentially valuable tool with reported sensitivity of 80–95% in series using high-resolution probes (> 10 MHz) or automated 3D technology [42, 43].

Even on MRI, the diagnosis of ILC can be challenging, with a range of possible morphologic patterns and sometimes only mild persistent enhancement, making lesions difficult to differentiate from surrounding

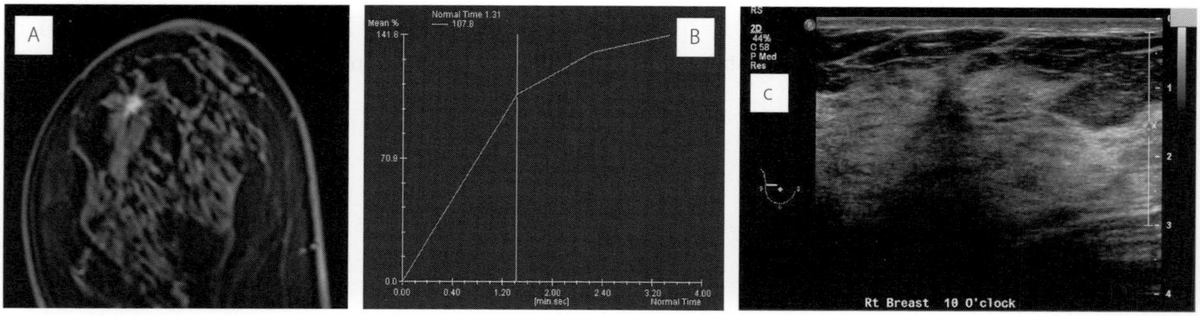

Fig. 3.18 Radial scar: (A) Post-contrast image shows 10 mm enhancing stellate mass, with (B) rapid initial-phase and persistent delayed-phase kinetics (type 1 curve). (C) Image from TUS showing hypoechoic lesion in glandular zone with mild acoustic shadowing found to be radial scar with DCIS on 14-gauge CNB. Lesion was excised, confirming DCIS in association with radial scar but no invasive malignancy.

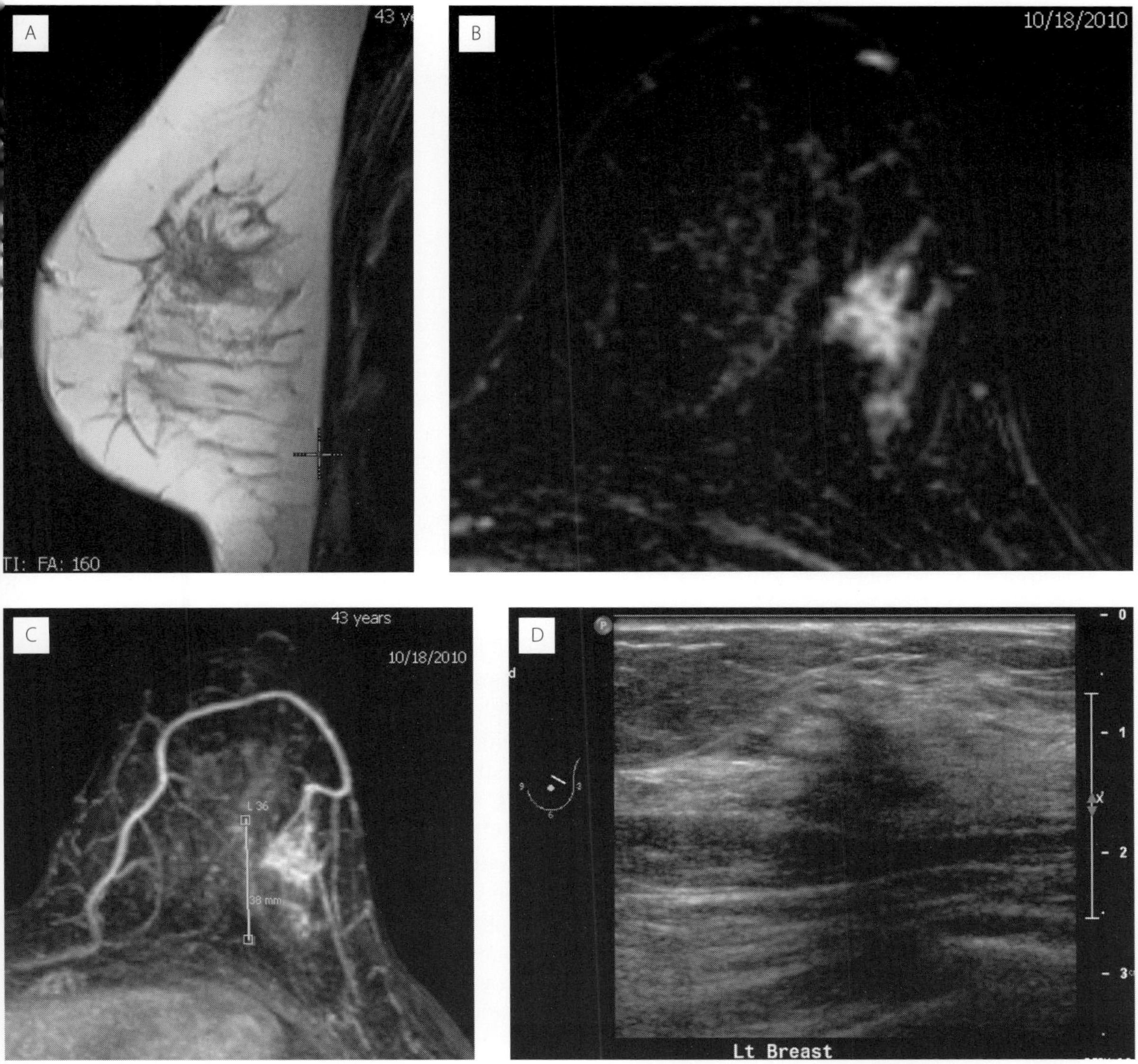

Fig. 3.19 Radial scar: (A) Sagittal FSE T2-weighted image shows stellate architectural distortion with linear enhancement on (B) subtracted post-contrast image, interpreted as probable invasive cancer with DCIS together estimated at 38 mm in size. MIP image (C) shows positive vessel sign. Lesion was identified on TUS (D) with 14-gauge CNB showing complex sclerosing lesion. Surrounding proliferative fibrocystic change was found in the surgically excised specimen but no DCIS or invasive cancer was identified.

parenchyma. Not surprisingly, invasive lobular cancers are over-represented among those missed by MRI due to lack of enhancement.

A problem in gaining accurate data on the performance of MRI with ILC has been that some series have included mixed IDC/ILC tumor types. Recently though, a comprehensive review of data on histologically pure ILC established the sensitivity of MRI at 93% [42]. The study confirmed the superiority of MRI over conventional imaging in delineating tumor extent, with MRI showing excellent histopathologic correlation. Additional ipsilateral disease was shown only by MRI in over 30% of patients, with contralateral cancer occult to conventional imaging revealed in 7%.

Among six studies analyzed in relation to the morphologic appearances of ILC, of a total of 133 pure ILC tumors, 65% were classified as masses and 35% as non-mass enhancement. Of mass lesions, a great majority were either spiculated or irregular (85%), and ILC presenting as a circumscribed mass appears to be very rare [42]. While there is undoubtedly overlap in descriptions by different observers,

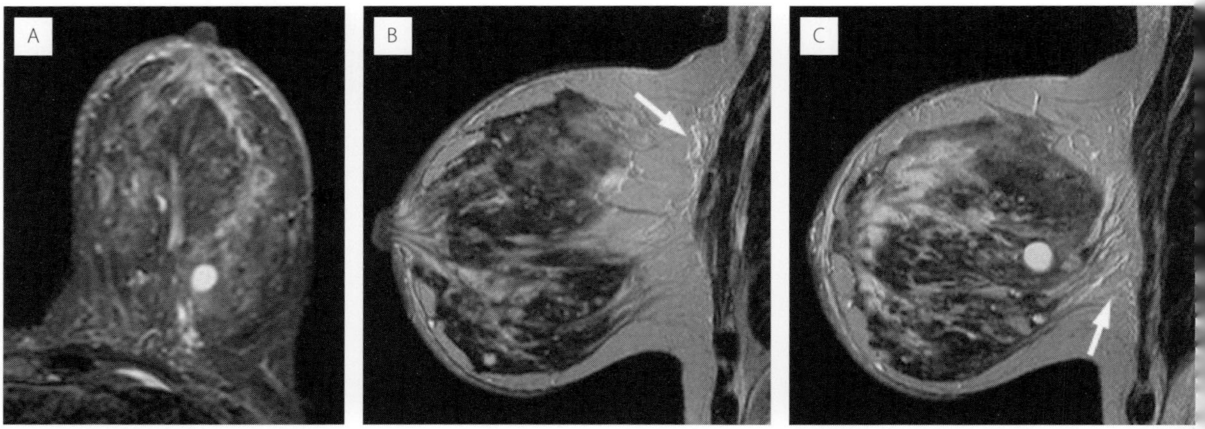

Fig. 3.20 Inflammatory carcinoma: (A) Axial fat-suppressed T2-weighted image shows marked skin thickening and edema in left breast. Sagittal FSE T2-weighted images (B) and (C) show prepectoral edema (arrows).

it is clear that a substantial number of cases present as non-mass enhancement.

Schelfout *et al.* described four dominant patterns in their series of 26 patients with pure ILC [44]. After a solitary spiculated or irregular mass (~50%), the next most common was a dominant lesion surrounded by multiple enhancing foci (30%), while interconnecting enhancing strands between foci (~10%) and architectural distortion alone (~10%) were also observed. Qayyum *et al.* similarly described an appearance of interconnecting strands correlating histologically with the single-file invasion pattern of ILC, seen in one case without any mass or dominant focus [45]. This description corresponds well with the mammographic "spider's web" pattern. Table 3.15 summarizes morphologic appearances of ILC.

Data on the kinetics of ILC indicate that initial-phase enhancement is typically less rapid than with IDC, so that peak enhancement can be delayed beyond 2 minutes. True washout is less common, although a bow-shaped kinetic curve may be seen (Fig. 3.11). The "lower and later" enhancement with ILC has implications for study interpretation, as images at 1–2 minutes after injection may not optimally demonstrate the abnormality [42]. Furthermore, distinguishing such a lesion from marked background enhancement can be problematic.

Table 3.15 Spectrum of MRI morphologic patterns of ILC

Solitary spiculated or irregular mass (~50%)
Dominant enhancing lesion with satellite foci
Multiple enhancing foci with interconnecting strands
Regional enhancement with architectural distortion
Missed due to inadequate enhancement (~7%)
Solitary circumscribed mass (rare)

BI-RADS final assessment categories for masses

Following analysis of signal characteristics and morphology, most benign masses will have been confidently identified and placed in the BI-RADS 2 final assessment category. This group will include cysts, normal lymph nodes and non-enhancing sclerotic fibroadenomas. Other benign mass enhancement is limited to that seen around an inflammatory cyst or an oil cyst in post-traumatic fat necrosis. Normal lymph nodes are an exception where even a type 3 kinetic curve may be present in a lesion given a BI-RADS 2 final assessment score.

Where lesion morphology is suspicious or malignant, kinetics do not influence the final BI-RADS assessment. If the kinetic curve evaluation shows a type 3 curve, this might upgrade a lesion to BI-RADS 5 rather than 4 in the final assessment. However, a type 1 curve should never be used to imply absence of malignancy if morphology is suspicious.

The main role of kinetics is in evaluation of circumscribed masses. With a mass showing typically benign features (dark, non-enhancing internal septations, bright signal on FSE T2-weighted images), a type 1 or 2 curve is considered definitely benign. However, as a type 3 curve in a fibroadenoma is rare, while the PPV of a type 3 curve for malignancy is about 90%, this kinetic finding would generally override the morphologic features and upgrade the lesion to BI-RADS 4.

For a slightly irregular mass with no other malignant features, a type 1 curve may allow a BI-RADS 3 final score to be given, depending on the patient's risk factors. However, a plateau curve would upgrade the analysis to suspicious (BI-RADS 4), while washout of more than 20% would be classified as malignant (BI-RADS 5).

Therefore, where morphology is probably benign, kinetics can be used to decide between early follow-up and biopsy. However, the individual patient risk profile and personal choice play a part in deciding how much uncertainty is acceptable. Presented with the option of biopsy, many women (and particularly those with an elevated risk profile) prefer proof of benignity to "watchful waiting." Correlation with XRM and TUS are further important steps before deciding whether to perform biopsy. A flow chart guide to management of masses is given in Fig. 3.21.

Analysis of non-mass enhancement

Non-mass enhancement occurs on a background of normal parenchyma with fat or fibroglandular tissue usually still visible within it. There are two elements to analysis. First, the distribution of enhancement is classified and then the internal architecture is assessed (Table 3.16). Non-mass enhancement is the typical MRI presentation of DCIS. Occasionally, invasive cancer can present as non-mass enhancement, particularly with pure ILC or mixed IDC/ILC tumors [14]. Compared to descriptors for mass analysis, BI-RADS descriptors for non-mass enhancement are relatively poor benign versus malignant discriminators [10, 46]. Considerable experience is needed to gain familiarity with the wide range of appearances which can be seen with DCIS [47–51].

Distribution

The first step in considering the distribution of non-mass enhancement is to note whether the findings are symmetrical or not (assuming both breasts are present). Bilaterally symmetric non-mass enhancement is always reassuring, but must be confirmed across the whole dynamic series. In many cases DCIS will enhance more rapidly than normal parenchyma in the initial phase, allowing distinction from slower

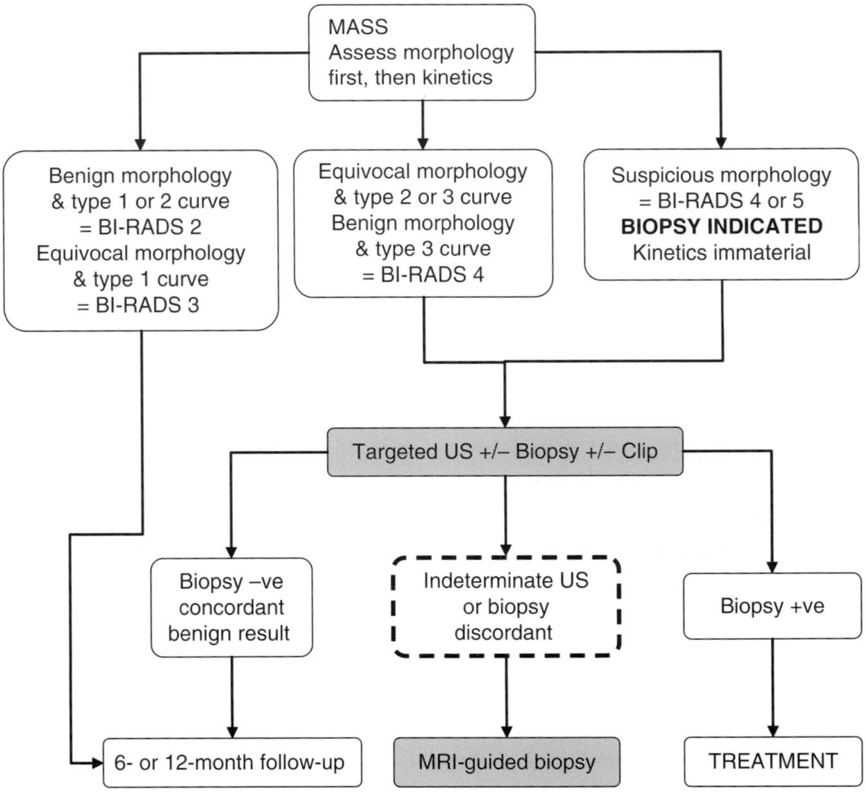

Fig. 3.21 Management flow chart for a mass: Shaded boxes indicate biopsy procedures, broken outlines indicate decision-making. Even with benign mass morphology, a type 3 curve in a lesion which is not a lymph node would prompt TUS with biopsy to exclude high-grade IDC. Normal TUS cannot be used to imply that a mass is benign. If TUS is indeterminate, or a discordant biopsy is obtained, MRI-guided biopsy is performed.

Table 3.16 BI-RADS descriptors for non-mass enhancement

Distribution	
	Symmetric or asymmetric = symmetrical usually benign
	Linear = linear non-specific versus "linear-ductal"
	Ductal = conforms to a duct distribution, high PPV for DCIS
	Segmental = conforming to a segment, high PPV for DCIS
	Focal area = less than 25% of a quadrant
	Regional = a geographic area not conforming to a segment
	Multiple regions = less suspicious, but consider multifocal DCIS/ILC
	Diffuse = whole breast involved, usually benign
Non-mass internal architecture	
	Homogeneous = uniform
	Heterogeneous = non-uniform, irregular or patchy
	Stippled/punctate = multiple scattered foci, usually benign
	Reticular/dendritic = network pattern in fatty breast tissue, often malignant
	Clumped = cluster of foci with confluence as "cobblestone" pattern – high PPV for DCIS

background enhancement, and kinetic assessment or color-mapping may then be helpful. Evaluating the symmetry of non-mass enhancement is also a compelling argument for routinely performing bilateral dynamic breast MRI in the axial plane [52].

In considering the distribution within the affected breast, six BI-RADS descriptors are used, with the volume of tissue involved varying from part of a single duct to the entire breast.

1. *Linear (ductal or non-ductal):* This should be immediately qualified as to whether linear enhancement may be oriented such that it conforms to a duct, in which case it enters the ductal distribution category (Fig. 3.22). If non-ductal, the finding is non-specific and may be a post-surgical scar, inflammatory or related to fibrocystic change.
2. *Ductal:* For the distribution to be ductal, enhancement must be both linear and oriented towards the nipple. Analogous to casting-type microcalcification on XRM, ductal enhancement is suspicious for DCIS (Fig. 3.22). If branching is visible, suspicion of DCIS is even stronger, with a PPV of 38% compared with 11% for a linear-ductal distribution in one study [53]. However, a ductal distribution can also be seen with ADH, LCIS, ductal hyperplasia and fibrocystic change [49].
3. *Segmental:* A segmental distribution is classically described as triangular or conical with the apex at the nipple (Figs. 3.23–3.25). However, keep in mind that anatomic segments are quite variable in shape when deciding if a distribution could conform to a duct system. Segmental distribution is always suspicious for DCIS (analogous to XRM microcalcification) with estimates of the PPV for this MRI finding varying widely, from 25–30% up to as high as 70–80%.
4. *Focal area:* An area is a "small region" of non-mass enhancement defined as occupying less than 25% of a quadrant. This may be too small

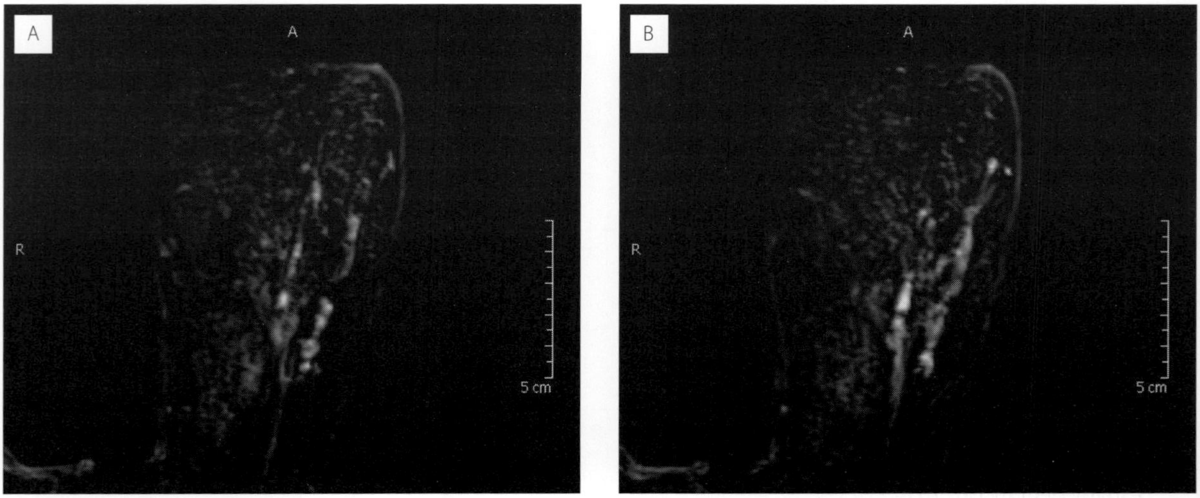

Fig. 3.22 Linear-ductal distribution, clumped architecture: Post-contrast subtracted images (A and B) showing linear distribution conforming to ducts with typical clumped architecture. Pathology confirmed high-grade DCIS which had not been evident on XRM.

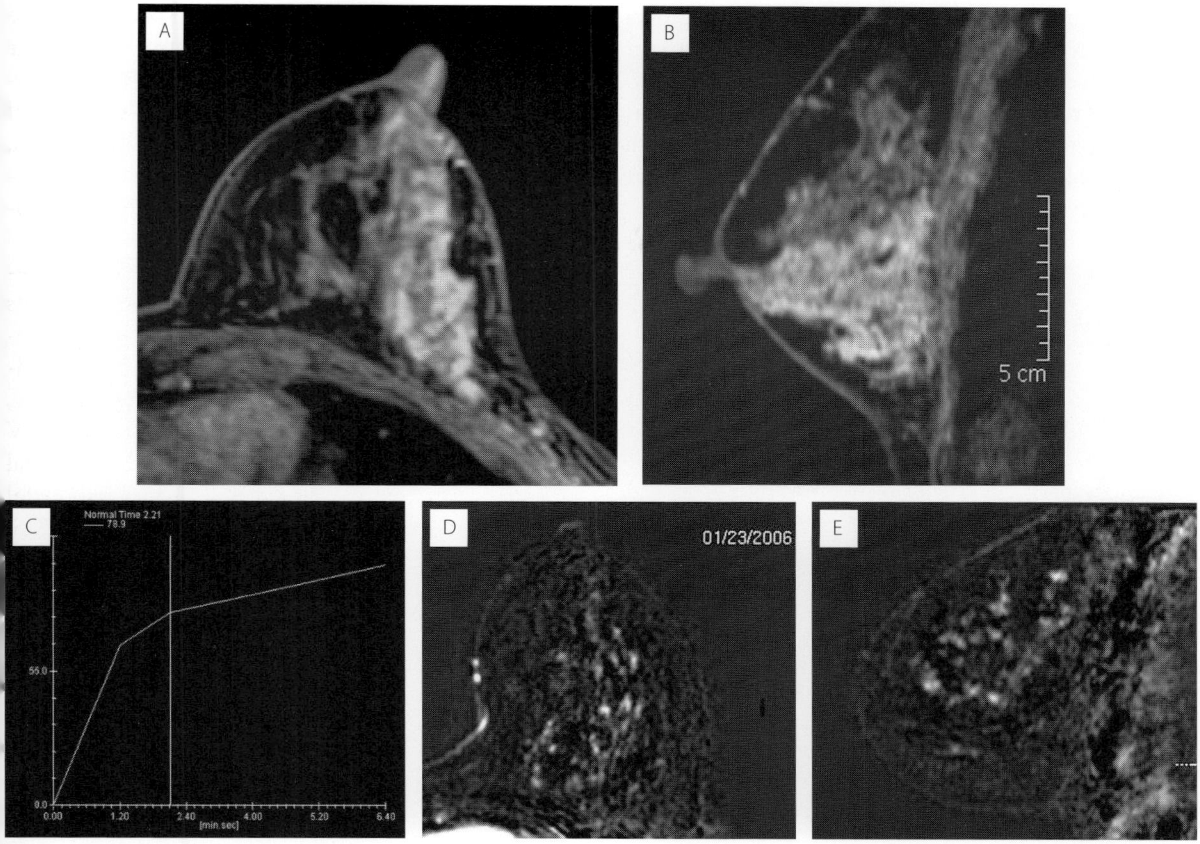

Fig. 3.23 Segmental distribution, clumped architecture: A 61-year-old woman with bloody nipple discharge and positive cytology, normal XRM and US. (A) Axial post-contrast T1-weighted image showing triangular distribution of non-mass enhancement laterally with clumped architecture. Sagittal image (B) confirms conical shape with nipple at apex. (C) Kinetic curve shows only moderate early enhancement rate with persistent late phase (type 1). Pathology showed high-grade DCIS. In another case (second round screening MRI in a 51-year-old woman with history of breast cancer in mother and three sisters), (D) axial and (E) sagittal subtracted post-contrast T1-weighted images show segmental non-mass enhancement (triangular shape with nipple at apex). Internal architecture appears clumped and reticular/dendritic. Both XRM and TUS were normal. Biopsy showed pleomorphic LCIS (equivalent to high-grade DCIS) with foci of microinvasion on final pathology. Subsequent genetic testing revealed BRCA2 mutation.

to determine if it is segmental or not, but internal architecture can still be assessed and may help to add specificity (Fig. 3.26).

5. *Regional (and multiple regions):* A larger volume of tissue than a focal area which is geographic, and not segmental. The likelihood that regional enhancement is due to DCIS is much lower than for a segmental distribution. The IBMC trial showed a PPV of 78% for segmental versus only 21% for regional distribution [3]. The presence of multiple regions further favors benign disease, although multifocal DCIS and ILC should still be considered in differential diagnosis. Bilaterally symmetric regions are usually benign, due to normal vascular inflow phenomenon or cyclical hormonal changes.
6. *Diffuse:* Diffuse enhancement implies wide involvement throughout the breast and is usually benign, although whole breast involvement with DCIS occurs rarely. If diffuse enhancement is symmetrical, it is virtually certain to be benign.

Internal architecture

Five descriptors for internal architectural patterns of non-mass enhancement were listed in the 2003 BI-RADS MRI Lexicon [4]. Since then, Tozaki *et al.* also described *clustered ring enhancement* as a sign with a high PPV for DCIS [51, 54].

1. *Homogeneous:* Uniform linear-ductal enhancement may be seen in the context of an elongated intraduct papilloma. A focal area or small region

of homogeneous enhancement favors hormonal or fibrocystic change. However, DCIS can appear confluent and homogeneous, often in a segmental or regional distribution [55, 56]. This confluent type of homogeneous enhancement often shows loss of intervening normal fibroglandular or fatty parenchyma.

2. *Heterogeneous:* Non-uniform, irregular or patchy enhancement separated by areas of normal parenchyma or fat. Ductal enhancement due to DCIS, whether involving a single duct or several, is almost invariably heterogeneous and may even qualify as clumped. A focal area or region of heterogeneous enhancement is non-specific.

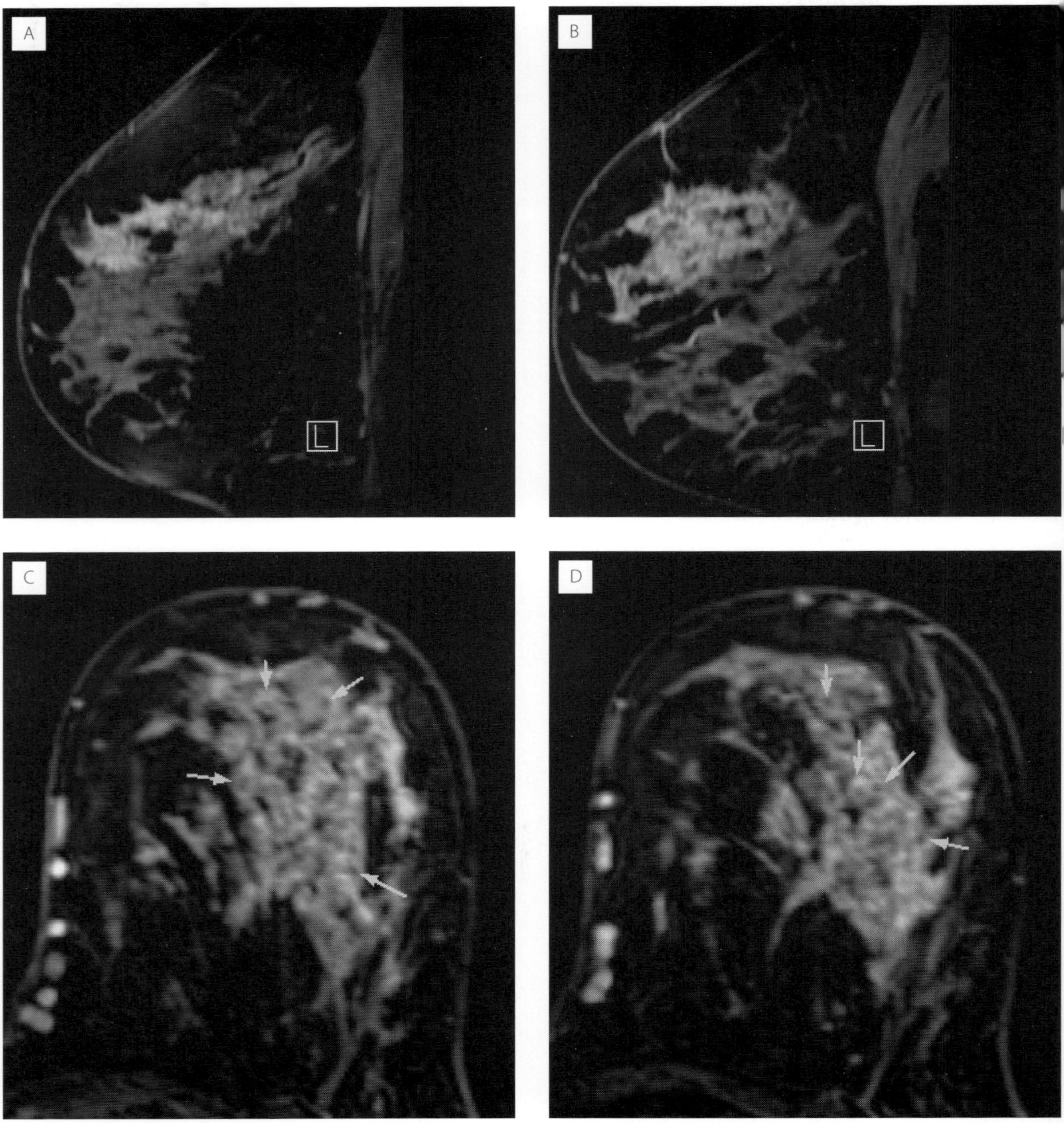

Fig. 3.24 Segmental distribution, clustered ring enhancement: Post-contrast fat-suppressed sagittal T1-weighted images (A and B) show segmental distribution of confluent enhancement throughout parenchyma. Note spared areas of normal fat signal. On axial high-resolution images (C and D) there is a widespread pattern of tiny clustered rings (arrows). Pathology showed micropapillary DCIS of intermediate grade.

Extensive patchy regional or diffuse heterogeneous enhancement usually indicates a benign process.

3. *Stippled/punctate:* Multiple scattered foci are usually benign (hormonal, focal adenosis, fibrocystic change). However, even stippled enhancement is suspicious for DCIS when it occurs in a segmental distribution. When foci are clustered in an asymmetric focal area or region, the finding is non-specific, but usually benign.

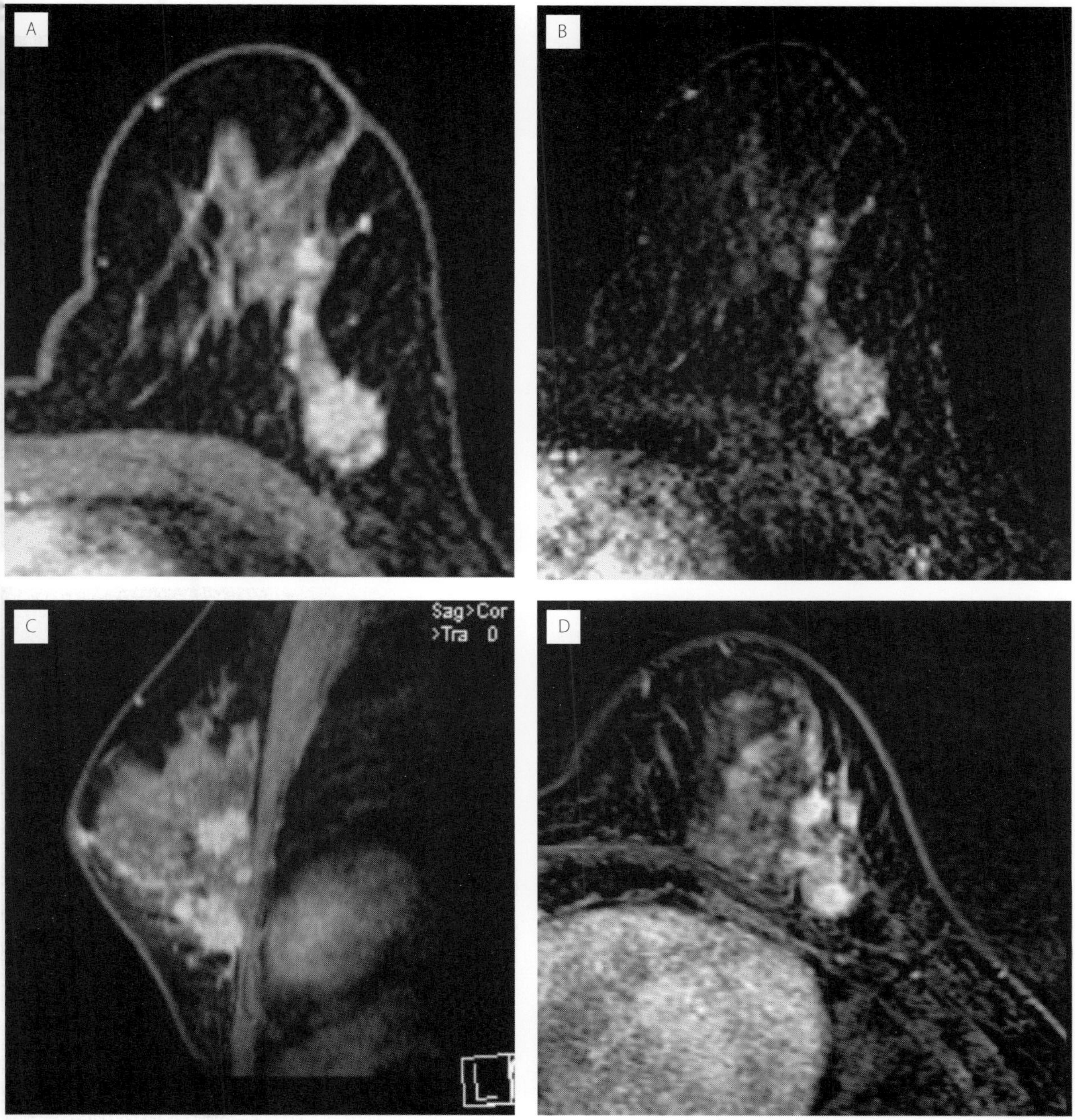

Fig. 3.25 Invasive cancer with EIC: (A) Axial post-contrast T1-weighted and (B) subtracted images show spiculated IDC laterally in left breast, with ~40 mm of irregular linear-ductal clumped enhancement extending anteriorly towards nipple corresponding to EIC. In a different patient with left breast multicentric invasive cancer between 2:00 and 6:00 (C) sagittal post-contrast T1-weighted image shows linear-ductal enhancement typical of DCIS extending to nipple. (D) Axial early post-contrast subtracted image shows confluent low-level enhancement surrounding the invasive foci, also confirmed as EIC on pathology (seven distinct invasive foci up to 25 mm diameter with background of intermediate- and high-grade DCIS).

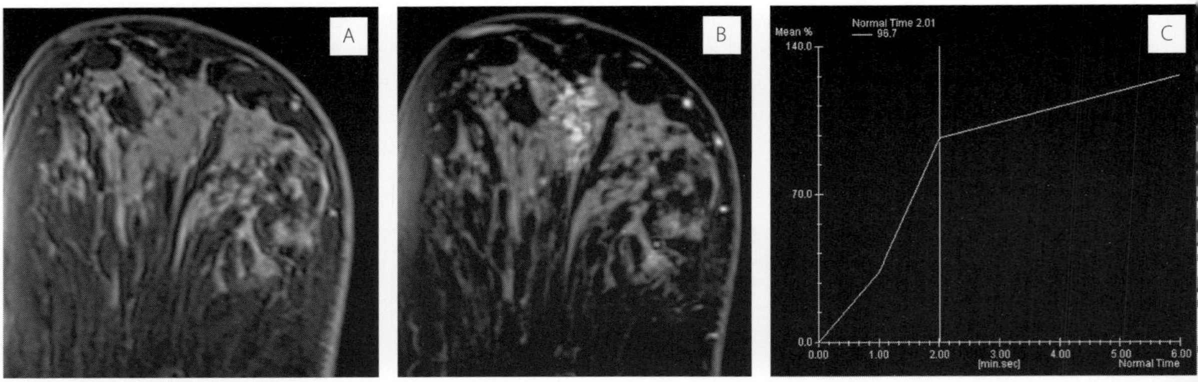

Fig. 3.26 Focal area, clumped architecture: (A) Normal pre-contrast T1-weighted image, with (B) focal area of clumped non-mass enhancement appearing in normal parenchyma. (C) Kinetic curve shows only moderate early-phase enhancement with persistent late-phase enhancement (type 1). Clumped architecture is suspicious despite non-specific distribution (focal area). Benign kinetics do not influence diagnosis. Pathology showed high-grade DCIS.

4. *Reticular/dendritic:* This describes a branching network or thread-like pattern in a fatty involuted breast (Fig. 3.23). Branching or reticular enhancement patterns usually correspond to a ductal pattern of DCIS [1, 51, 57]. In practice, there is significant overlap with the description of ductal distribution with branching.
5. *Clumped:* An aggregate of foci may become confluent in a *cobblestone pattern*, which likely represents heaped-up clumps of intraductal tumor cells expanding the affected ducts [58] sometimes within a fibrous stroma. This pattern is therefore correlated with a ductal distribution, usually with multiple ducts involved, although even a single duct may show a beaded nodular pattern which qualifies as clumped (Figs. 3.22–3.23). Clumped enhancement is considered the most characteristic architectural pattern for DCIS.
6. *Clustered ring enhancement*: In this distinctive pattern, minute enhancing rings with central low-signal intensity are observed in non-mass enhancement due to DCIS (Fig. 3.24) [51, 54]. This has been correlated histologically with expanded and crowded DCIS-filled ducts, suggesting the ring pattern is due to enhancement of the duct wall and periductal stroma. Central necrosis is seen in some cases, but contrast washout from enhancing tumor cells in the duct lumen may also contribute to the clustered ring pattern in others. The clustered ring pattern may be particularly prevalent when DCIS appears as extensive confluent enhancement.

To summarize, a ductal or segmental distribution is always suspicious for DCIS, regardless of architectural pattern, with a PPV of 25–35% [2, 47, 51, 59]. Clumped and clustered ring enhancement, reticular/dendritic and branching are architectural patterns strongly predictive of DCIS, even when seen in a focal area or region. The combination of a segmental distribution with either clumped or clustered ring enhancement has a PPV for DCIS of >90% [51, 54].

On MRI, DCIS most often appears as non-mass enhancement in a ductal or segmental distribution with clumped internal architecture. Kinetic curves are variable, and do not contribute to the diagnosis.

Other morphologic appearances of DCIS

About 70–80% of all DCIS cases appear as non-mass enhancement in a ductal or segmental distribution. In the remaining 20–30% of DCIS, various enhancement patterns are seen, including a focus, mass, focal area or region. Enhancement adjacent to an invasive cancer due to an EIC is often linear-ductal or punctate, and extends towards the nipple (Fig. 3.27) [60–62]. Less commonly, an EIC pattern is seen in which small invasive foci arise on a background of DCIS, identified by MRI in 10/44 (23%) in one study [60]. However, a comprehensive literature review found overall lower sensitivity for EIC (72%), than for pure DCIS (85%) [63].

Kinetic characteristics of DCIS

For pure DCIS it appears that about 70–75% of cases show moderate to rapid initial-phase enhancement (wash-in) while 60–70% show either washout or a plateau in the late phase [64, 65]. Therefore, because up to 30% of DCIS cases show only slow persistent enhancement, kinetics do not help to differentiate DCIS from benign proliferative changes.

Pathologic basis of DCIS enhancement

It was at first considered remarkable that DCIS enhanced on MRI at all, because neovascularity within ducts is not a histologic feature. Instead, intraductal cancer cells are nourished by diffusion from neoangiogenesis induced in the periductal stroma, suggesting this to be the mechanism of MRI enhancement [66]. However, recent work in animal models has shown that gadolinium not only enters the periductal stroma but actually accumulates within DCIS-filled ducts, suggesting that MRI may often directly display the enhancing intraductal cancer [67].

The mechanism by which gadolinium enters the ducts may relate to proteases produced by tumor cells which render the basement membrane leaky. This may even be the first step in development of invasive cancer, enabling intraductal tumor cells to insinuate themselves through the damaged basement membrane.

The importance of this model of DCIS enhancement is that it supports the view that MRI may be a tool for identifying clinically more significant DCIS, i.e., high-grade disease which is likely to rapidly progress to life-threatening high-grade invasive cancer. This is in accord with usual clinical experience that DCIS of high histologic grade is more often shown by MRI than is low-grade disease, with most false-negative findings attributable to weak tumor angiogenesis [63, 64, 68].

> Up to 50% of high-grade DCIS cases are non-calcified and may be shown only by MRI. About 15–25% of all DCIS cases (usually low grade) are not identified by MRI.

Enhancement morphology on MRI appears to show broad correlation with tumor biology [55]. In particular, DCIS seen as extensive confluent segmental or regional enhancement showed biologically aggressive features of ER-negativity, comedonecrosis and high proliferation index (Ki-67). Clumped architecture was also more likely to be high grade than was heterogeneous enhancement.

When DCIS is identified by imaging and confirmed pathologically, good correlation between the radiologic and pathologic disease extent is most important clinically. Overall, MRI is much more accurate than XRM in delineating the margins of both pure DCIS and an EIC associated with invasive cancer [63]. Particularly with low-grade DCIS though, MRI has a tendency to overestimate extent [56].

This usually occurs because low-grade DCIS is often associated with benign non-mass lesions which may also enhance, such as sclerosing adenosis, proliferative fibrocystic change and atypical hyperplasia [55, 56, 63]. Determining the boundary between DCIS and benign changes is difficult when both processes are likely to be seen on MRI as relatively non-specific heterogeneous or stippled enhancement.

Differential diagnosis of non-mass enhancement

Spurious enhancement due to movement artifact

When movement occurs, high signal within small contrast-laden vessels which become displaced relative to the mask may mimic streaky enhancement after subtraction. Usually this is easily recognizable as misregistration artifact, but if one breast moves more than the other, spurious non-mass enhancement with an apparently ductal distribution can suggest DCIS to the unwary beginner if only the subtracted images are viewed.

Color-mapping can also be misleading – because CAD software compares images in the dynamic series with the pre-contrast mask, movement artifact is assigned color on the overlay. Reviewing non-subtracted dynamic scans is most helpful, as if these show no abnormal enhancement, the appearance is probably spurious.

Inflow phenomenon

Symmetrical enhancement localized to the lateral quadrants (particularly the axillary tails) is commonly seen due to normal vascular inflow, reflecting the blood supply from the lateral thoracic branch of the axillary artery. Normal inflow can also be seen at the periphery of the breasts both medially and inferiorly where supply is from intercostal branches of the internal thoracic artery. Enhancement remains symmetrical in appearance throughout the dynamic series, with a "picture-frame" distribution which seldom causes difficulty in interpretation.

Hormonal changes

In premenopausal women, hormonally related enhancement is very common, and should be minimized by booking routine scans between days 5 and 15 of the menstrual cycle. The "three Ps rule" is a helpful reminder of the typical Patchy and Peripheral appearance with Persistent kinetics (usually slow, but can be rapid). Difficulty arises when hormonal enhancement is markedly asymmetric, but a 6- to 12-week follow-up study at a more favorable phase of the cycle usually resolves the issue. Similarly, when confusion arises in postmenopausal women on HRT, short-term follow-up is performed after ceasing HRT, with biopsy only indicated if significant reduction or complete resolution do not occur. Hormonal change should not be diagnosed in postmenopausal women who are not taking HRT.

Selective estrogen receptor modulators (SERMs e.g. tamoxifen and raloxifene) are chemopreventive agents which block ER. They are used for ER-positive cancers in both pre- and postmenopausal women and are taken for up to 5 years. Both the total amount of parenchymal density and the extent to which it enhances become greatly reduced. Consequently, even a focal area or region of non-mass enhancement is viewed as suspicious in these women with biopsy often required.

Fibrocystic change, ADH, LCIS

Fibrocystic change commonly presents as stippled enhancement in a focal area or region with a type 1 curve, although confluent or mass-like lesions also occur and may show rapid initial enhancement with plateau or washout kinetics [69, 70]. Linear-ductal enhancement is uncommon, reported in 2/31 cases of fibrocystic change by Chen *et al.* and in 2/14 by van den Bosch *et al.* (< 10%) [69, 70]. Meanwhile, Liberman and coworkers found 16/88 (18%) of ductal enhancement was due to non-specific fibrocystic change [47]. Fibrocystic change also arises much less frequently in the medical quadrants, where it should be diagnosed with caution.

Intuitively, and based on experience, the association of non-mass enhancement with microcysts on non-contrast T2-weighted images adds support for a diagnosis of fibrocystic change and may allow follow-up rather than biopsy if there are no other features to cause concern (Fig. 3.27). However, clustered microcysts can coexist with DCIS and if the changes are focal and asymmetric, biopsy should be considered even if internal architecture is non-specific.

Unfortunately, MRI is often unable to distinguish between DCIS (particularly low grade) and the range of benign hyperplastic lesions which arise in the breast, some of which reflect "high-risk" tissue [56]. Proliferative fibrocystic change, ductal hyperplasia with or without atypia and lobular neoplasia can all appear as a non-specific focal area or region of non-mass enhancement. As some of these are precursor lesions of DCIS pathologically, it should not surprise that they may also show a ductal or segmental distribution and closely mimic DCIS. This in part accounts for the variable PPV for DCIS based on distribution alone, and highlights the importance of assessing internal architectural features to improve specificity.

Invasive lobular carcinoma

About one-third of ILC cases appear as asymmetric non-mass enhancement which may be ductal, segmental, regional or diffuse, making ILC important to consider in the differential diagnosis of DCIS (Fig. 3.28). Furthermore, the kinetics of ILC are often similar to normal breast tissue with delayed peak enhancement so that classic washout occurs only in a minority of cases [42]. Overestimation of ILC extent can arise where there is a non-mass pattern and a background of diffuse enhancement due to LCIS [71]. The difficulty is identical to that encountered in defining low-grade DCIS extent in a background of benign proliferative changes.

BI-RADS final assessment categories for non-mass enhancement

In many instances, benign non-mass enhancement can be dismissed based on the distribution and absence of malignant features (Table 3.17). For some cases early follow-up may be required for suspected hormone-related enhancement. Alternatively, if it has been resolved to perform MRI-guided biopsy if the enhancement persists, the follow-up study may be scheduled as an intervention. It must be recog-

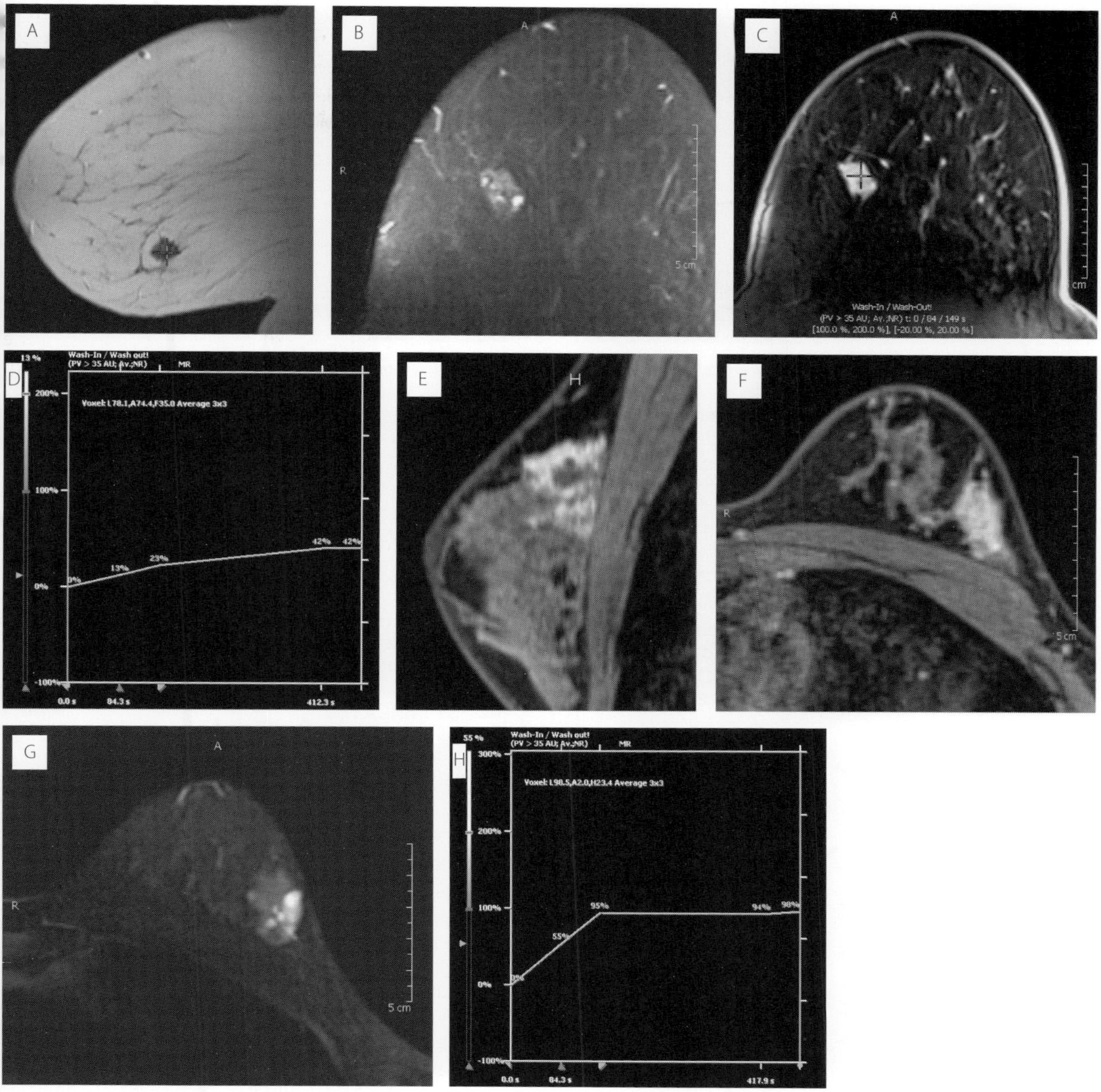

Fig. 3.27 Fibrocystic change: (A) Non-fat-suppressed sagittal T1-weighted image showing 2 cm density in right breast recalled at mammographic screening, with US-guided biopsy showing fibrocystic change (MRI referral was for problem-solving in relation to a different lesion) (B) Axial T2-weighted SPAIR image shows microcysts typical of fibrocystic change. Dynamic post-contrast image (C) with kinetic curve (D) show only slow persistent enhancement, similar to normal parenchyma. In a different patient with BRCA1 mutation, (E) sagittal and (F) axial post-contrast images show segmental distribution of non-mass enhancement. (G) Axial T2-weighted SPAIR image shows microcysts, supporting diagnosis of fibrocystic change. (H) Kinetic curve shows moderate initial-phase enhancement and late-phase plateau (indeterminate). US-guided 14-gauge CNB showed florid proliferative fibrocystic changes.

nized that proliferative fibrocystic changes, ADH and LCIS cannot be distinguished, so that biopsy may be required.

Other causes of non-mass enhancement, often localized as a focal area, include chronic mastitis, PASH, sclerosing adenosis and fibrosis. When these conditions are encountered in biopsy specimens, they can usually be considered to represent concordant benign pathology (Table 3.18). A flow chart guide to management of non-mass enhancement is given in Fig. 3.29.

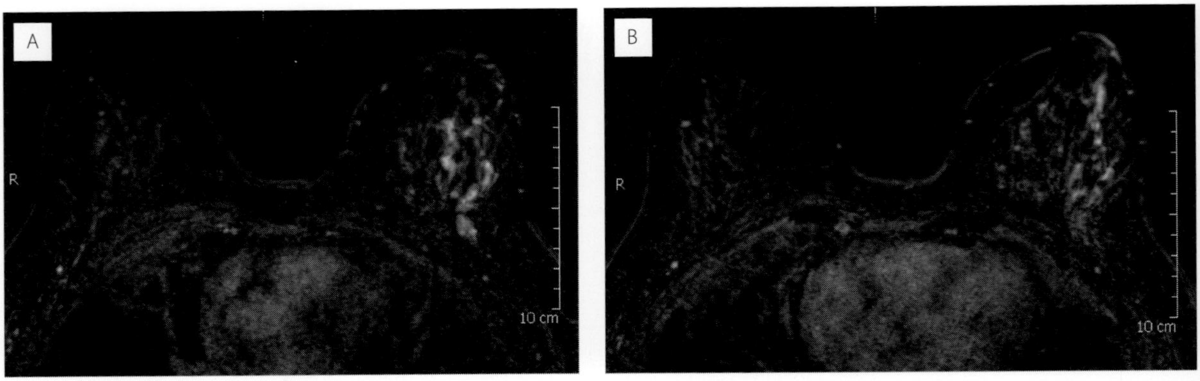

Fig. 3.28 **Invasive lobular cancer as non-mass enhancement:** Axial post-contrast subtracted images (A and B) show extensive segmental non-mass enhancement in the left breast with clumped internal architecture. Pathology showed at least 12 foci of ILC measuring from 0.5 to 10 mm diameter in a background of LCIS. MRI distribution and morphology is indistinguishable from DCIS.

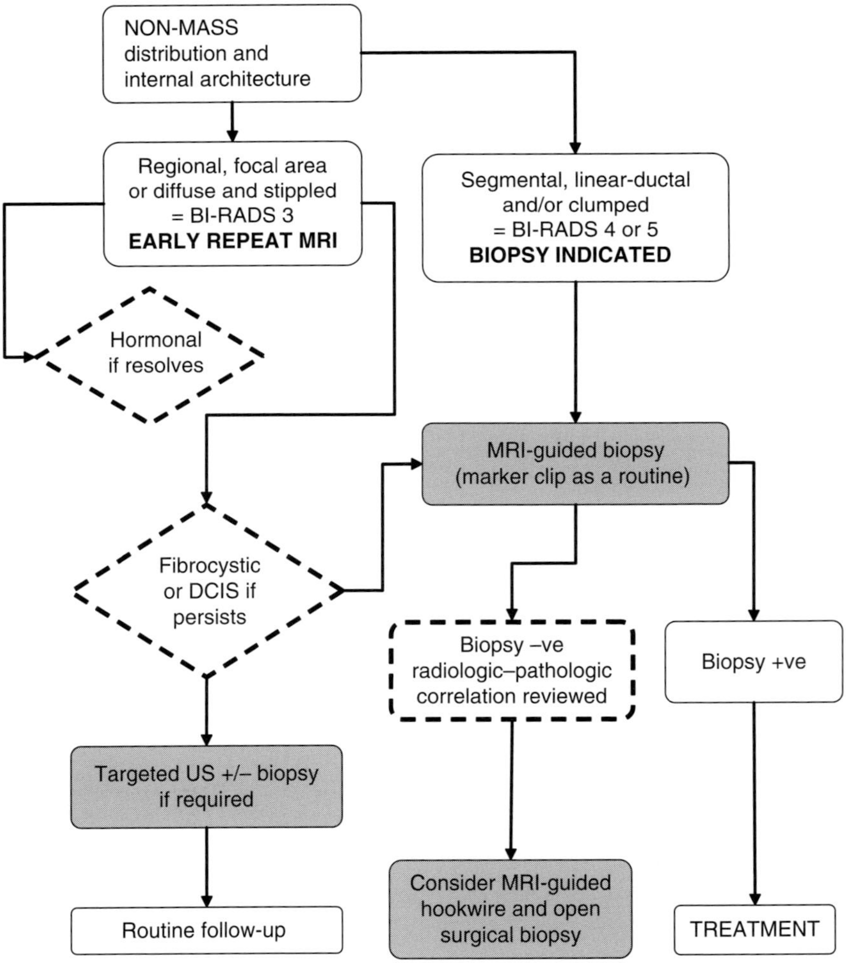

Fig. 3.29 **Management flow chart for non-mass enhancement:** Shaded boxes indicate biopsy procedures, broken outlines indicate decision-making. Diamond-shaped boxes are possible outcomes at 6–12 weeks early follow-up (different phase of cycle if pre menopausal or after suspending HRT). If enhancement persists and features, e.g., microcysts support fibrocystic change, TUS +/– biopsy may be confirmatory, but MRI-guided biopsy is usually preferred for suspected DCIS. Establishing pathology as concordant or discordant is essential following MRI-guided biopsy.

Table 3.17 Features of benign non-mass enhancement

Patchy
Peripheral
Persistent kinetics – usually slow
Presence of microcysts on T2-weighted images
Scattered foci
Single or multiple focal areas or regions
Stippled or punctate diffuse pattern
Symmetrical distribution
Not showing ductal or segmental distribution
Not showing clumped, reticular or clustered ring architecture

Table 3.18 Differential diagnosis of non-mass enhancement

DCIS/ADH/LCIS
Proliferative fibrocystic change (usual duct hyperplasia, sclerosing adenosis)
Focal adenosis especially nodular sclerosing adenosis = stippling/punctate
Cyclical hormonal change (transient, resolves on follow-up scans)
Chronic mastitis (benign pericystic or periductal inflammation/fibrosis)
Fibroadenomatoid hyperplasia
Fibrosis
Fat necrosis (history, fat signal of oil cysts, time course)
Papillomatosis (multiple peripheral papillomas)
PASH (pseudoangiomatous stromal hyperplasia)

Summary of MRI lesion analysis

Table 3.19 summarizes the suggested approach to MRI lesion analysis. Individual patient risk factors and personal choices will play a part in decision-making for all lesion types. Keep in mind that even the clinical indication is a factor to consider – the chance that an unexpected lesion found by MRI is malignant is highest for a patient referred with a known index cancer [9, 72, 73]. Women undergoing high-risk surveillance are also more likely to require biopsy of subtle lesions than those who are having the MRI as a problem-solving study to exclude malignancy in relation to a vague mammographic abnormality. Table 3.20 lists the MRI findings which allow malignancy to be excluded with an NPV of > 95%.

Focus

While the great majority of foci are benign, care should be taken not to dismiss all lesions < 5 mm in size, because small cancers may then be overlooked.

Mass

Margin analysis is the single most important benign versus malignant discriminator. Spiculation, rim enhancement and a type 3 curve (washout) are the best malignant predictors (Table 3.21). The combination of bright T2 signal, internal dark septations and type 1 kinetics has a PPV for fibroadenoma of ~95%. Caution is needed to avoid overlooking circumscribed cancers. Cysts and solid lesions with absent enhancement can be classified BI-RADS 2 (Table 3.22).

Non-mass

Most cases of DCIS appear as clumped enhancement in either a ductal or segmental distribution (Table 3.21). However, DCIS can present a wide range of appearances and distinction from proliferative fibrocystic change and hyperplasia (ADH, ALH, LCIS) is usually impossible without biopsy.

Kinetics

The most common role for kinetic assessment is as a "tie-breaker" for equivocal masses (circumscribed or slightly irregular mass with otherwise benign morphology) where a type 2 or 3 curve may warrant biopsy, but a type 1 curve is sufficiently reassuring to allow follow-up. The high PPV of washout kinetics for invasive cancer (~90%) should always be kept in mind. Slow type 1 curves are seen in ~5% of invasive cancers (often ILC and low-grade IDC) and kinetics can never be used to exclude malignancy. Kinetics have little role in analyzing non-mass enhancement, because at least 30% of DCIS cases show slow enhancement.

Correlating MRI findings with conventional imaging

Mammographic correlation

Whether or not an abnormality has been identified on MRI, a careful review of all previous breast imaging is recommended. An advantage of using the sagittal and axial planes for most MRI sequences is their similarity to the MLO and CC views used in routine XRM. Any possible MRI lesion should be correlated with available

Table 3.19 Summary guide to lesion analysis

Analysis of a focus
Size of lesion ("Stanford 4 mm rule"), solitary or multiple (cluster of foci = non-mass lesion)
Exclude any mass correlate on T1- and T2-weighted images or on enhancement morphology
Kinetics – diagnostic value controversial, omitted by some experts
Review clinical history and prior imaging
Arrange XRM or TUS if required
Assign BI-RADS Score 0–6
Analysis of a mass
Size and location – quadrant and zone (subareolar, glandular, retromammary fat)
Signal on pre-contrast T1- and T2-weighted images (particularly for circumscribed lesions)
Morphology – shape and margins combined as circumscribed, irregular, spiculated
Morphology of enhancement – homo- or heterogeneous, rim enhancement, septations
Additional features, e.g., chest wall involvement, lymphadenopathy
Kinetics – most valuable as "tie-breaker" for circumscribed or slightly irregular lesions
Review clinical history and prior imaging
Arrange XRM or TUS if required
Assign BI-RADS Score 0–6
Analysis of non-mass enhancement
Symmetry – unilateral or bilateral (hormonal/fibrocystic changes often symmetrical)
Size and location – single or multiple quadrants (3D reformatted images useful)
Distribution – ductal, segmental, regional
Pre-contrast T2-weighted images – check for presence of microcysts
Internal architecture – clumped, reticular, dendritic, stippled
Additional features, e.g., suspected area of invasion or lymphadenopathy
Kinetics – diagnostic value limited, omitted by many experts
Review clinical history and prior imaging
Arrange XRM or TUS if required
Assign BI-RADS Score 0–6

XRM images, and additional views (spot compression, microfocus magnification) obtained of any area which may become suspicious in the light of the MRI findings.

Table 3.20 Best benign predictors > 95% NPV

Absent enhancement (or enhancement less than parenchyma)
Cystic lesion by signal characteristics
Circumscribed mass with definite non-enhancing internal septations
Bright T2 signal mass with definite non-enhancing internal septations

Table 3.21 Best malignant predictors

Invasive cancer
Spiculated margin ~90% PPV
Washout kinetics 80–90% PPV
Rim enhancement 80–90% PPV
DCIS
Ductal enhancement 25–60% PPV
Segmental enhancement 25–80% PPV
Clumped architecture 40–90% PPV
Clustered ring enhancement 60–90% PPV

Table 3.22 Benign masses on MRI (BI-RADS 2)

Cyst
Oil cyst
Lymph node
Duct ectasia
Typical myxoid fibroadenoma
Sclerosed fibroadenoma
Sclerosed papilloma
Non-enhancing post-surgical scar
Lipoma
Hamartoma (fibroadenolipoma)

Mass correlation is usually straightforward. An MRI focus has no XRM correlate in the vast majority of cases, but occasionally will be clarified by mammographic review. Correlation with XRM is particularly important for non-mass enhancement, as if a corresponding area of suspicious microcalcification is identified, stereotactic biopsy may be preferred for histologic diagnosis. Table 3.23 gives an overview of the corresponding XRM and MRI features for the most common lesions.

Table 3.23 Typical XRM-MRI correlation for common breast pathology

	XRM	MRI T2 SIGNAL	MRI MORPHOLOGY	MRI KINETICS
Fibroadenoma (myxoid)	Circumscribed mass	Bright T2	Dark internal septations	Rapid wash-in usual Persistent or plateau Washout rare < 1%
Fibroadenoma (sclerosed)	Circumscribed or irregular occasional popcorn Ca^{++}	May be heterogeneous	Circumscribed or irregular Dark internal septations Bright T2 parts enhance	Absent or slow initial Persistent or plateau
High-grade IDC NOS	Circumscribed or irregular Spiculated uncommon	Often bright T2 (necrosis)	Circumscribed or irregular mass May show delayed rim enhancement	Rapid wash-in usual Variable late phase Usually type 2 or 3
Low-grade IDC NOS	Spiculated usual	Low T2 usual	Spiculated mass May show early rim enhancement	Slow initial (absent rare) Persistent or plateau
ILC	Variable mass Often subtle or occult (spider's web pattern)	Similar to parenchyma (some even after contrast)	50% spiculated or irregular mass May be multifocal/multicentric 35% non-mass enhancement	50% rapid initial "Lower and later" peak Bow curve (type 1B)
Fibrocystic change	Classic teacup pattern of layering (milk of calcium)	Bright clustered microcysts	Focal area or region, may be multiple or diffuse, stippled architectural pattern	Variable, often slow initial Persistent late phase usual
Low-grade DCIS	Often punctate or amorphous powderish Ca^{++}	Not applicable	Architecture – often stippled Difficult to distinguish from background Hormonal/fibrocystic change	Often slow initial Persistent late phase usual May be absent
High-grade DCIS	Granular (crushed stones) or linear-casting Ca^{++}	Not applicable	Segmental, ductal distribution Clumped internal architecture Clustered ring enhancement	Rapid initial usual Variable late phase Washout infrequent

The role of targeted ultrasound

In cases where MRI shows a suspicious finding, an US study focused on the area of interest will often reveal the lesion, and may then allow US-guided biopsy. The terms *targeted* or *directed* may be preferable to *second-look ultrasound* since the latter could imply that the "first look" was in some measure inadequate, which is usually not the case. Rather, it is that with the knowledge of an MRI abnormality, findings which could reasonably have been sublimated on a screening US assume greater significance at TUS.

The extent to which TUS is used for MRI correlation is variable, with some using it for all possible MRI lesions while others use it selectively or not at all [74]. Direct MRI-guided biopsy is particularly often favored for non-mass enhancement. One disadvantage of TUS is the dilemma which arises if there is doubt as to whether a sonographic finding really does correlate with the presenting MRI lesion. If US-guided biopsy is attempted and is negative, MRI-guided intervention may still be required, making a case for adopting the principle of performing the biopsy using the same method which first showed the lesion. In a study by Meissnitzer *et al.*, follow-up of 80 benign concordant biopsies at TUS revealed that the sonographic lesion did not actually correspond to the MRI abnormality in 10, with 5 cancers subsequently diagnosed in this group [75].

For a doubtful correlate at TUS then, it may be preferable to defer the biopsy for MRI-guided VAB. However, US-guided biopsy is considerably easier and cheaper, and placement of a marker clip can be used to allow subsequent MRI confirmation of correct lesion sampling in doubtful cases. Personal experience and local factors will determine which option is followed in each individual case.

So how do we optimize the use of TUS? There are a number of questions to be considered: First, how often does TUS identify and allow biopsy of a lesion seen on MRI? Reported rates of lesion identification at TUS vary widely, ranging from 23% to 89% [75–81].

Typically, correlates are found at least twice as frequently for masses as for non-mass lesions [75–77, 81]. As expected, larger lesions are generally more likely to be seen on US, but even for foci/small masses < 5 mm, sonographic correlates were identified in ~50% in two recent studies [75, 81].

Second, what is the risk of malignancy in the absence of a sonographic correlate? While overall cancer detection rates by TUS are typically in the range of 47–57%, among DCIS cases a majority are occult (60–70%) compared to invasive cancers where 60–85% are identified by TUS [75–77, 81]. So, absence of any sonographic correlate, even for a focus, does reduce the risk that invasive cancer is present (but not DCIS). In routine practice, lesions not identified by TUS have probably ~20% risk of malignancy subsequently being found at MRI-guided biopsy [75, 77].

Third, how does the risk profile of the patient population (pre-test probability of cancer) influence outcomes from TUS, particularly in regard to the use of MRI in high-risk screening? Causer *et al.* reported their experience using multimodality screening in a unique cohort of purely BRCA1/2 mutation carriers in which 33/41 cancers were detected solely by MRI in 1015 screening episodes [82]. In total, 15/33 (45%) MRI-only cancers were visible by US (12 IDC, 3 DCIS), similar to other studies. However, among lesions with no TUS correlate, ~40% (13/33 with 8 IDC, 5 DCIS) proved to be malignant at MRI-guided biopsy. The mean size of invasive cancers detected in that study was 11 mm in the prevalent (first) round and 9 mm in incident screening rounds.

So, although useful as an initial approach, TUS fails to identify around half of all malignant lesions, confirming a vital role for MRI-guided biopsy. A normal TUS does not exclude malignancy, even for a mass. Nevertheless, the use of TUS and biopsy successfully resolves a significant proportion of MRI abnormalities from all lesion types. Generally lower rates of successful sonographic correlation though are reported for non-mass enhancement.

An inherent advantage of MRI-guided VAB is the ease with which a large amount of tissue can be obtained from multiple cores of up to 9-gauge after a single insertion of the probe. Until recently, TUS and biopsy has been reliant on CNB, with core sample size limited to 14-gauge. This may be a particularly important consideration when deciding how to approach non-mass lesions, where lesion undersampling is a significant issue. However, the option of US-guided VAB is now becoming more widely available.

Recently, a high success rate for TUS combined with VAB has been reported for non-mass enhancement. Sakamoto *et al.* reviewed 102 consecutive non-palpable, XRM occult, MRI-detected non-mass lesions [53]. Using a 10 MHz probe, TUS was able to identify corresponding hypoechoic nodules or duct-like structures which were successfully biopsied in 93/102 (91%) using US-guided VAB with a yield of 10 cancers (1 IDC, 9 DCIS). The combination of high-resolution TUS and VAB could prove a viable alternative to MRI-guided biopsy for many non-mass lesions.

Practical tips for targeted ultrasound

A high-resolution probe is essential with a machine set-up proven to be effective for breast US. The radiologist who reports the MRI scan should perform the TUS, because it is critical to have a clear idea of the lesion type and location, including size, shape and depth [75, 76, 81]. It can be very helpful to have a simple line diagram to hand showing the target lesion appearance, approximate o'clock position and distance from the nipple. Nevertheless, considerable latitude is needed in estimating lesion location at TUS to allow for geometric differences between MRI (patient positioned prone with the breast dependent and extruded into the coil) and TUS (patient supine oblique with the breast flattened and foreshortened in its anteroposterior dimension). Depth estimation is particularly unreliable, and it is best to limit localization to one of three zones – subareolar (anterior), glandular (middle) or retroglandular (deep).

Key sonographic features for differentiating invasive cancer from fibroadenoma on US, based on Stavros' criteria, are listed in Table 3.24 [83, 84]. However, when correlating a focus or small mass, even a non-specific cyst-like lesion or what appears to be a normal island of fat (surrounded by parenchyma) needs careful assessment and may warrant biopsy. The importance of careful technique and attention to subtle findings cannot be overemphasized, with a recent study observing that one-third of cancers found at TUS did not exhibit any of the typical malignant sonographic signs [81]. Particular caution is advised in younger patients with strong

Table 3.24 Differentiating US features of cancer and fibroadenoma

Feature	Invasive cancer	Fibroadenoma
Shape	Irregular or rounded	Ovoid (elliptical)
Lobulations	Microlobulation	< 4 gentle lobulations
Margins	Spiculated, angular	Smooth
Borders	Thick echogenic halo	Thin echogenic capsule
Orientation of shape	Taller-than-wide	Wider-than-tall
Echogenicity (vs fat)	Hypo- or isoechoic	Hyper/iso or mildly hypo
Shadowing	Frequent	Edge shadowing
Calcification	Fine punctate (DCIS)	Macrocalcification
Ductal/branch pattern	Frequent (DCIS)	Never

family history or known BRCA1/2 mutation, as a high-grade IDC can mimic a fibroadenoma or even appear cyst-like.

Clustered microcysts are typically benign findings which support a diagnosis of fibrocystic change. However, non-calcified DCIS and some invasive cancers may also present as hypoechoic nodules or lobulated masses which could be dismissed as cyst clusters [85]. After TUS evaluation, follow-up of cyst clusters suffices [86], while elastography may have a future role in characterizing some lesions.

Incidental lesions are often encountered at TUS, but if correlation is questionable, it is preferable to defer the case for MRI-guided biopsy where possible. In the event that US-guided biopsy is performed, it is essential to deploy a marker clip to allow subsequent MRI correlation if required [75].

Follow-up of probably benign (BI-RADS 3) lesions

In giving a BI-RADS 3 final assessment score, the estimated risk of malignancy should be < 2% so that biopsy is not warranted. Follow-up MRI is recommended initially at 6 months. If there is no progression on MRI after 2 years, the lesion is considered stable and downgraded to benign (BI-RADS 2). With the increasing availability of MRI-guided biopsy, the trend is to obtain a histologic diagnosis at first presentation.

Short-term follow-up at 6–12 weeks is used for non-mass enhancement suspected to be due to hormonal change. In this circumstance, a unilateral high-resolution sagittal study maximizes diagnostic information in the event that the abnormality persists [82]. Further analysis is then needed to determine if the abnormality may be due to fibrocystic change or if DCIS requires exclusion by MRI-guided biopsy. For foci, where the likelihood of malignancy is generally lower, follow-up is usual.

The reported incidence of malignancy at follow-up for lesions varies from < 1% up to 10% [11, 87]. Liberman *et al.* reviewed outcomes for women undergoing high-risk screening MRI who were given BI-RADS 3 (probably benign) scores [87]. Among 89 such women, 9 (10%) went on to a cancer diagnosis within 2 years, at a location corresponding to the initial MRI lesion. Of the 9 cancers, 4 were IDC (all < 10 mm), and 5 were DCIS, with 6/9 diagnosed from progression on follow-up MRI.

MULTIPLE CHOICE QUESTIONS

3.1 Answer true or false to the following statements

A. Melanoma metastases may show bright signal on fat-suppressed T1-weighted images.
B. Myxoid fibroadenomas may show bright signal on fat-suppressed T2-weighted images.
C. A focal area of non-mass enhancement showing clumped architecture is considered benign.
D. Less than 20% of invasive cancers seen by MRI can be located at TUS.
E. Normal lymph nodes and inflamed cysts may be associated with rim enhancement.

3.2 Answer true or false to the following statements

A. About 30% of all fibroadenomas show strong washout kinetics on MRI.
B. At least 70% of papillomas show intense early-phase enhancement and washout.
C. After rapid wash-in, a type 1 kinetic curve in any lesion virtually excludes malignancy.
D. Most fibroadenomas show type 1 kinetics, while sclerotic lesions may not enhance at all.
E. Up to 5% of invasive cancers show very slow or absent enhancement on MRI.

See page 189 for answers.

References

1. Kaiser WA. *Signs in MR-Mammography*. Berlin Heidelberg, Springer-Verlag, 2009.
2. Kuhl CK. Concepts for differential diagnosis in breast MR imaging. *Magn Reson Imaging Clin N Am* 2006; **14**: 305–28.
3. Schnall MD, Blume J, Bluemke DA, *et al*. Diagnostic architectural and dynamic features at breast MR imaging: multicenter study. *Radiology* 2006; **238**: 42–53.
4. D'Orsi CJ, Bassett LW, Berg WA, *et al*. *BI-RADS Breast Imaging Reporting and Data System, Breast Imaging Atlas*, 4th edn. Reston, VA, American College of Radiology, 2003.
5. Erguvan-Dogan B, Whitman GJ, Kushwaha AC, *et al*. BI-RADS–MRI: a primer. *AJR Am J Roentgenol* 2006; **187**: W152–60.
6. National Breast Cancer Center. *Breast Imaging: A Guide for Practice*. Camperdown, NSW, Australia, National Breast Cancer Center, 2002.
7. Maxwell AJ, Ridley NT, Rubin G, *et al*. The Royal College of Radiologists Breast Group breast imaging classification. *Clin Radiol* 2009; **64**: 624–7.
8. Kuhl C. The current status of breast MR imaging. Part 1. Choice of technique, image interpretation, diagnostic accuracy, and transfer to clinical practice. *Radiology* 2007; **244**: 356–78.
9. Liberman L, Mason G, Morris EA, *et al*. Does size matter? Positive predictive value of MRI-detected breast lesions as a function of lesion size. *AJR Am J Roentgenol* 2006; **186**: 426–30.
10. Gutierrez RL, Demartini WB, Eby PR, *et al*. BI-RADS lesion characteristics predict likelihood of malignancy in breast MRI for masses but not for nonmasslike enhancement. *AJR Am J Roentgenol* 2009; **193**: 994–1000.
11. Eby PR, DeMartini WB, Gutierrez RL, *et al*. Characteristics of probably benign breast MRI lesions. *AJR Am J Roentgenol* 2009; **193**: 861–7.
12. Kuhl CK, Klaschik S, Mielcarek P, *et al*. Do T2-weighted pulse sequences help with the differential diagnosis of enhancing lesions in dynamic breast MRI? *J Magn Reson Imaging* 1999; **9**: 187–96.
13. Yuen S, Uematsu T, Kasami M, *et al*. Breast carcinomas with strong high-signal intensity on T2-weighted MR images: pathologic characteristics and differential diagnosis. *J Magn Reson Imaging* 2007; **25**: 502–10.
14. Bartella L, Liberman L, Morris EA, *et al*. Nonpalpable mammographically occult invasive breast cancers detected by MR. *AJR Am J Roentgenol* 2006; **186**: 865–70.
15. Ballesio L, Savelli S, Angeletti M, *et al*. Breast MRI: are T2 IR sequences useful in the evaluation of breast lesions? *Eur J Radiol* 2009; **71**: 96–101.
16. Kawashima M, Tamaki Y, Nonaka T, *et al*. MR imaging of mucinous carcinoma of the breast. *AJR Am J Roentgenol* 2002; **179**: 179–83.
17. Uematsu T, Kasami M, Yuen S. Triple-negative breast cancer: correlation between MR imaging and pathologic findings. *Radiology* 2009; **250**: 638–47.
18. Ho LWC, Wong KP, Chan JHM, *et al*. MR appearance of metastatic melanotic melanoma in the breast. *Clin Radiol* 2000; **55**: 572–3.
19. Leach MO, Boggis AK, Dixon AK, *et al*. Screening with magnetic resonance imaging and mammography of a UK population at high familial risk of breast cancer: a prospective multicenter cohort study (MARIBS). *Lancet* 2005; **365**: 1769–78.
20. Warren RML, Pointon L, Thompson D, *et al*. Reading protocol for dynamic contrast-enhanced MR images of the breast: sensitivity and specificity analysis. *Radiology* 2005; **236**: 779–88.
21. Warren RM, Thompson D, Pointon LJ, *et al*. Evaluation of a prospective scoring system designed for a multicenter breast MR imaging screening study. *Radiology* 2006; **239**: 677–85.
22. Tozaki M, Igarashi T, Fukuda K. Positive and negative predictive values of BI-RADS-MRI descriptors for focal breast masses. *Magn Reson Med Sci* 2006; **5**: 7–15.
23. Kobayashi M, Kawashima H, Matsui O, *et al*. Two different types of ring-like enhancement on dynamic MR imaging in breast cancer: correlation with the histopathologic findings. *J Magn Reson Imaging* 2008; **28**: 1435–43.
24. Malich A, Fischer DR, Wurdinger S, *et al*. Potential MRI interpretation model: differentiation of benign from malignant breast masses. *AJR Am J Roentgenol* 2005; **185**: 964–70.
25. Nunes LW, Schnall MD, Orel SG, *et al*. Breast MR imaging: interpretation model. *Radiology* 1997; **202**: 833–41.
26. Kurz KD, Roy S, Mödder U, *et al*. Typical atypical findings on dynamic MRI of the breast. *Eur J Radiol* 2010; **76**: 195–210.
27. Fischer DR, Baltzer P, Malich A, *et al*. Is the "blooming sign" a promising additional tool to determine malignancy in MR mammography? *Eur Radiol* 2004; **14**: 394–401.
28. Penn A, Thompson S, Brem R, *et al*. Morphologic blooming in breast MRI as a characterization of margin for discriminating benign from malignant lesions. *Acad Radiol* 2006; **13**: 1344–54.

29. Fischer U. *Practical MR Mammography*. Stuttgart, Thieme Publishing Co, 2004.
30. Fischer DR, Malich A, Wurdinger S, *et al.* The adjacent vessel on dynamic contrast-enhanced breast MRI. *AJR Am J Roentgenol* 2006; **187**: W147–51.
31. Sardanelli F, Iozzelli A, Fausto A, *et al.* Gadobenate dimeglumine-enhanced MR imaging breast vascular maps: association between invasive cancer and ipsilateral increased vascularity. *Radiology* 2005; **235**: 791–7.
32. Kurz KD, Steinhaus D, Klar V, *et al.* Assessment of three different software systems in the evaluation of dynamic MRI of the breast. *Eur J Radiol* 2009; **69**: 300–7.
33. Wang LC, Demartini WB, Partridge SC, *et al.* MRI-detected suspicious breast lesions: predictive values of kinetic features measured by computer-aided evaluation. *AJR Am J Roentgenol* 2009; **193**: 826–31.
34. Daniel BL, Gardner RW, Birdwell RL, *et al.* Magnetic resonance imaging of intraductal papilloma of the breast. *Magn Reson Imaging* 2003; **21**: 887–92.
35. Monzawa S, Yokokawa M, Toshiko S, *et al.* Mucinous carcinoma of the breast: MRI features of pure and mixed forms with histopathologic correlation. *AJR Am J Roentgenol* 2009; **192**: W125–31.
36. Linda A, Zuiani C, Girometti R, *et al.* Unusual malignant tumors of the breast: MRI features and pathologic correlation. *Eur J Radiol* 2010; **75**: 178–84.
37. Okafuji T, Yabuuchi H, Sakai S, *et al.* MR imaging features of pure mucinous carcinoma of the breast. *Eur J Radiol* 2006; **60**: 405–13.
38. Dogan BE, Gonzalez-Angulo AM, Gilcrease M, *et al.* Multimodality imaging of triple receptor-negative tumors with mammography, ultrasound, and MRI. *AJR Am J Roentgenol* 2010; **194**: 1160–6.
39. Schrading S, Kuhl CK. Mammographic, US, and MR imaging phenotypes of familial breast cancer. *Radiology* 2008; **246**: 58–70.
40. Obdeijn IM, Loo CE, Rijnsburger AJ, *et al.* Assessment of false-negative cases of breast MR imaging in women with a familial or genetic predisposition. *Breast Cancer Res Treat* 2010; **119**: 399–407.
41. Boetes C, Veltman J, van Die L, *et al.* The role of MRI in invasive lobular carcinoma. *Breast Cancer Res Treat* 2004; **86**: 31–7.
42. Mann RM, Hoogeveen YL, Blickman JG, *et al.* MRI compared to conventional diagnostic workup in the detection and evaluation of invasive lobular carcinoma of the breast: a review of existing literature. *Breast Cancer Res Treat* 2008; **107**: 1–14.
43. Lander MR, Tabar L. The classic type of invasive lobular carcinoma of the breast is known to be elusive on mammography, but demonstrable when using 3-dimensional automated ultrasound. *Am J Clin Oncol* 2008; **31**: 513.
44. Schelfout K, Van Goethem M, Kersschot E, *et al.* Preoperative breast MRI in patients with invasive lobular breast cancer. *Eur Radiol* 2004; **14**: 1209–16.
45. Qayyum A, Birdwell RL, Daniel BL, *et al.* MR imaging features of infiltrating lobular carcinoma of the breast: histopathologic correlation. *AJR Am J Roentgenol* 2002; **178**: 1227–32.
46. Baltzer PAT, Benndorf M, Dietzel M, *et al.* False-positive findings at contrast-enhanced breast MRI: a BI-RADS descriptor study. *AJR Am J Roentgenol* 2010; **194**: 1658–63.
47. Liberman L, Morris EA, Dershaw DD, *et al.* Ductal enhancement on MR imaging of the breast. *AJR Am J Roentgenol* 2003; **181**: 519–25.
48. Raza S, Vallejo M, Chikarmane SA, *et al.* Pure ductal carcinoma in situ: a range of MRI features. *AJR Am J Roentgenol* 2008; **191**: 689–99.
49. Morris EA. Breast MR imaging lexicon updated. *Magn Reson Imaging Clin N Am* 2006; **14**: 293–303.
50. Menell JH, Morris EA, Dershaw DD, *et al.* Determination of the presence and extent of pure ductal carcinoma in situ by mammography and magnetic resonance imaging. *Breast J* 2005; **11**: 382–90.
51. Tozaki M, Fukuda K. High-spatial-resolution MRI of non-masslike breast lesions: interpretation based on BI-RADS MRI descriptors. *AJR Am J Roentgenol* 2006; **187**: 330–7.
52. Friedman PD, Swaminathan SV, Herman K, *et al.* Breast MRI: the importance of bilateral imaging. *AJR* 2006; **187**: 345–9.
53. Sakamoto N, Tozaki M, Higa K, *et al.* Categorization of non-mass-like breast lesions detected by MRI. *Breast Cancer* 2008; **15**: 241–6.
54. Tozaki M, Igarashi T, Fukuda K. Breast MRI using the VIBE sequence: clustered ring enhancement in the differential diagnosis of lesions showing non-masslike enhancement. *AJR Am J Roentgenol* 2006; **187**: 313–21.
55. Esserman LJ, Kumar AS, Herrera AF, *et al.* Magnetic resonance imaging captures the biology of ductal carcinoma in situ. *J Clin Oncol* 2006; **24**: 4603–10.
56. Kumar AS, Chen DF, Au A, *et al.* Biologic significance of false-positive magnetic resonance imaging enhancement in the setting of ductal carcinoma in situ. *Am J Surg* 2006; **192**: 520–4.

57. Groves AM, Warren RML, Godward S, *et al.* Characterization of pure high-grade DCIS on magnetic resonance imaging using the evolving breast MR lexicon terminology: can it be differentiated from pure invasive disease?*Magn Reson Imaging* 2005; **23**: 733–8.

58. Liberman L, Morris EA, Lee MJY. Breast lesions detected on MR imaging: features and positive predictive value. *AJR Am J Roentgenol* 2002; **179**: 171–8.

59. Morakkabati-Spitz N, Leutner C, Schild H, *et al.* Diagnostic usefulness of segmental and linear enhancement in dynamic breast MRI. *Eur Radiol* 2005; **15**: 2010–17.

60. Shimauchi A, Yamada T, Sato A, *et al.* Comparison of MDCT and MRI for evaluating the intraductal component of breast cancer. *AJR Am J Roentgenol* 2006; **187**: 322–9.

61. van Goethem M, Schelfout K, Kersschot E, *et al.* Enhancing area surrounding breast carcinoma on MR mammography: comparison with pathologic examination. *Eur Radiol* 2004; **14**: 1363–70.

62. Ikeda O, Nishimura R, Miyayama H, *et al.* Magnetic resonance evaluation of the presence of an extensive intraductal component in breast cancer. *Acta Radiol* 2004; **45**: 721–5.

63. Schouten van der Velden AP, Schlooz-Vries MS, Boetes C, *et al.* Magnetic resonance imaging of ductal carcinoma in situ: what is its clinical application? A review. *Am J Surg* 2009; **198**: 262–9.

64. Neubauer H, Li M, Kuehne-Heid R, *et al.* High grade and non-high grade ductal carcinoma in situ on dynamic MR mammography: characteristic findings for signal increase and morphological pattern of enhancement. *Br J Radiol* 2003; **76**: 3–12.

65. Jansen SA, Newstead GM, Abe H, *et al.* Pure ductal carcinoma in situ: kinetic and morphologic MR characteristics compared with mammographic appearance and nuclear grade. *Radiology* 2007; **245**: 684–91.

66. Gilles R, Zafrani B, Guinebretiere J, *et al.* Ductal carcinoma in situ: MR imaging–histopathologic correlation. *Radiology* 1995; **196**: 415–19.

67. Kuhl CK. Science to practice: why do purely intraductal cancers enhance on breast MR images? *Radiology* 2009; **253**: 281–3.

68. Kuhl CK, Schrading S, Bieling HB, *et al.* MRI for diagnosis of pure ductal carcinoma in situ: a prospective observational study. *Lancet* 2007; **370**: 485–92.

69. van den Bosch MAAJ, Daniel BL, Mariano MN, *et al.* Magnetic resonance imaging characteristics of fibrocystic change of the breast. *Invest Radiol* 2005; **40**: 436–41.

70. Chen J-H, Liu H, Baek H-M, *et al.* Magnetic resonance imaging features of fibrocystic change of the breast. *Magn Reson Imaging* 2008; **26**: 1207–14.

71. Mann RM, Veltman J, Barentsz JO, *et al.* The value of MRI compared to mammography in the assessment of tumour extent in invasive lobular carcinoma of the breast. *Eur J Surg Oncol* 2008; **34**: 135–42.

72. Gutierrez RL, DeMartini WB, Eby P, *et al.* Clinical indication and patient age predict likelihood of malignancy in suspicious breast MRI lesions. *Acad Radiol* 2009; **16**: 1282–5.

73. Han B-K, Schnall MD, Orel SG, *et al.* Outcome of MRI-guided breast biopsy. *AJR Am J Roentgenol* 2008; **191**: 1798–804.

74. Bassett LW, Dhaliwal SG, Eradat J, *et al.* National trends and practices in breast MRI. *AJR Am J Roentgenol* 2008; **191**: 332–9.

75. Meissnitzer M, Dershaw DD, Lee CH, *et al.* Targeted ultrasound of the breast in women with abnormal MRI findings for whom biopsy has been recommended. *AJR Am J Roentgenol* 2009; **193**: 1025–9.

76. LaTrenta LR, Menell JH, Morris EA, *et al.* Breast lesions detected with MR imaging: utility and histopathologic importance of identification with US. *Radiology* 2003; **227**: 856–61.

77. DeMartini WB, Eby PR, Peacock S, *et al.* Utility of targeted sonography for breast lesions that were suspicious on MRI. *AJR Am J Roentgenol* 2009; **192**: 1128–34.

78. Sim LSJ, Hendriks JHCL, Bult P, *et al.* US correlation for MRI-detected breast lesions in women with familial risk of breast cancer. *Clin Radiol* 2005; **60**: 801–6.

79. Beran L, Liang W, Nims T, *et al.* Correlation of targeted ultrasound with magnetic resonance imaging abnormalities of the breast. *Am J Surg* 2005; **190**: 592–4.

80. Wiratkapun C, Duke D, Nordmann AS, *et al.* Indeterminate or suspicious breast lesions detected initially with MR imaging: value of MRI-directed breast ultrasound. *Acad Radiol* 2008; **15**: 618–25.

81. Abe H, Schmidt RA, Shah RN, *et al.* MR-directed ("second-look") ultrasound examination for breast lesions detected initially on MRI: MR and sonographic findings. *AJR Am J Roentgenol* 2010; **194**: 370–7.

82. Causer PA, Jong RA, Warner E, *et al.* Breast cancers detected with imaging screening in the BRCA population: emphasis on MR imaging with histopathologic correlation. *RadioGraphics* 2007; **27**: S165–82.

83. Stavros AT, Thickman D, Rapp CL. Solid breast nodules: use of sonography to distinguish between benign and malignant lesions. *Radiology* 1995; **196**: 123–34.

84. Stavros AT. Ultrasound of solid breast nodules: distinguishing benign from malignant. In: *Breast Ultrasound*. Philadelphia, PA, Lippincott Williams & Wilkins. 2004; 445–527.

85. El Khoury M, Khetani K, Kao E, *et al*. Pseudocystic lesions and clustered cysts: radiologists beware. *AJR Am J Roentgenol* 2006; **186**: A79–83.

86. Berg WA. Sonographically depicted breast clustered microcysts: is follow-up appropriate? *AJR Am J Roentgenol* 2005; **185**: 952–9.

87. Liberman L, Morris EA, Benton CL, *et al*. Probably benign lesions at breast magnetic resonance imaging. Preliminary experience in high-risk women. *Cancer* 2003; **98**: 377–88.

Chapter

4 MRI-guided biopsy techniques

Chapter outline

Introduction

The sensitivity of MRI for invasive cancer and DCIS far exceeds that of XRM, and a substantial proportion of these malignant lesions either cannot be seen at all on TUS or cannot be identified with sufficient confidence to allow biopsy. Accordingly, a means of performing MRI-guided tissue sampling is an essential part of any breast MRI service. Frequently, MRI-only lesions (not seen on TUS or XRM) are foci (< 5 mm), small masses (< 10 mm) or focal areas of ductal non-mass enhancement, which can be challenging targets for the relatively small tissue volumes yielded by 14-gauge CNB. Accordingly, the more robust biopsy options of MRI-guided hookwire localization or VAB are preferred.

The dilemma posed by small MRI-only lesions has been historically similar to that once presented by the XRM finding of an indeterminate small cluster of microcalcification. Initially, x-ray stereotactic hookwire localization and open surgical excision biopsy was the only option. The need for a less invasive nonsurgical solution was partly fulfilled by the advent of x-ray stereotactic CNB, while stereotactic VAB subsequently became the method of choice because of the advantages offered by the greater volume of tissue retrieved.

The evolution of MRI-guided biopsy techniques

In the early years of breast MRI, the development of clinical applications was severely hampered by the lack of any generally available equipment for MRI-guided needle localization. The management options for lesions seen by MRI, but with no mammographic or sonographic correlate ("MRI-only" lesions), were extremely limited. Usually, a "watchful waiting" approach had to be adopted with MRI follow-up initially at 6 months and then for at least 2 years, using lesion stability to indirectly exclude malignancy.

The situation was greatly improved with the introduction of MRI-compatible hookwires for localization and surgical excision in the early 1990s. Breast coils with an open-sided design were used to allow lateral access to the breast in the prone position. Systems were developed using combined compression-grid systems or "stereotactic" external needle guides, while others used "freehand" techniques (similar to CT-guided biopsy, requiring no special needle-guidance equipment and allowing any angle of needle entry to be chosen) [1, 2]. Hookwire localization using MRI became established as a relatively simple and reliable technique. With the advent of helical CT, another innovative approach was to circumvent the problem entirely by performing CT-guided hookwire localization after using iodinated contrast to identify the MRI-enhancing lesions [3].

There remained a clear need to develop direct MRI-guided biopsy techniques to avoid the invasive nature and other disadvantages inherent with surgical excision (Table 4.1). Although some series using FNA technique reported good results, the rate of inadequate sampling was often unacceptably high. Developing MRI-compatible biopsy devices with acceptably low artifact required the use of either low-ferrous steel or titanium. Both these materials have reduced mechanical strength, a significant problem

Table 4.1 Advantages of MRI-guided biopsy over hookwire

Outpatient procedure
Avoids risk of wire displacement
Easier to schedule as no surgical coordination needed
No general anesthetic required
Faster, cheaper and less invasive as avoids diagnostic surgery
Avoids scarring and distortion in the breast after benign biopsy

in developing needles suitable for core biopsy. When these manufacturing issues were overcome, MRI-guided CNB became widely preferred to FNA. In initial experience with MRI-compatible 14-gauge large core biopsy technique, Kuhl *et al.* achieved a 98% success rate [4]. Even so, CNB had technical limitations in sampling small lesions (< 10 mm), which were easily obscured by susceptibility artifact from the needle, [4, 5] and could be missed entirely if targeting was imperfect.

Initially used for x-ray stereotactic biopsy, the Mammotome device (Devicor Medical Products, Cincinatti, OH, USA), introduced in 1995, was the first commercially available VAB system. The probe features an integrated co-axial design in which negative pressure can be applied to the lumen. During biopsy, breast tissue is sucked into the central collection chamber of the needle through a side aperture, and the core is taken by advancing a rotating cutter. The side aperture can be adjusted to face toward any o'clock radius by means of a thumbwheel, allowing multiple core samples to be taken from a single probe insertion, although each core has to be retrieved manually.

Used stereotactically, the Mammotome vacuum biopsy system proved to be greatly superior to conventional CNB in sampling microcalcifications, with the larger tissue volumes obtained allowing more accurate pathologic diagnosis. It was clear that the same advantages would directly translate to MRI, if the system could be adapted to get around the massive artifact caused by the large-caliber steel VAB needles. To do this required that some form of MRI-compatible marker be substituted for the VAB needle during targeting in the bore of the magnet, with the patient then being withdrawn from the tunnel for actual lesion sampling by VAB.

Using the Mammotome system, the procedure for MRI-guided VAB was pioneered in Europe by Heywang-Köbrunner and coworkers in the mid to late 1990s. In 2002, a large multicenter study was published in which 11-gauge VAB had been successful in 334/341 (98%) of lesions [6]. All of the seven technical failures were recognized either at post-interventional imaging or on histopathologic correlation, with no missed cancer diagnoses. Hematoma was the main complication, three requiring surgical intervention (< 1%) while six others > 3 cm in size were managed conservatively, and one became infected at 6 weeks. In the European centers, the use of stereotactic needle guides and compression plates with flexible parallel "ribs" allowed an angled lateral approach for MRI-guided VAB [6, 7]. A thin titanium substitute needle was used as the MRI-compatible marker.

Meanwhile, in the USA, prior to VAB becoming available, a similar strategy using an MRI-compatible titanium sheath was developed to allow 14-gauge CNB sampling to be performed outside the bore of the magnet with standard stainless steel needles [8, 9]. Then in 2003, a 9-gauge VAB device developed by Suros Surgical Systems (Hologic, Bedford, MA, USA), featuring a plastic introducer sheath and localizing obturator, was approved for MRI-guided VAB. A number of USA centers then reported on MRI-guided VAB using the Suros ATEC Breast Biopsy System with the *grid method* (allowing horizontal needle entry). These studies confirmed success rates of > 95%, procedure times typically of 30–60 minutes for a single target and malignant yields of 25–60% [10–13]. The European concept that an angled approach provided better access to some lesions (far anterior or posterior) evolved into the alternative *pillar-and-post method.*

The advent of commercially available MRI-guided VAB systems effectively overcame the limitations of CNB, with several advantages stemming from the ability to rapidly acquire large tissue samples (Table 4.2). Accordingly, VAB has become the standard MRI-guided biopsy procedure, and most MRI-only lesions can now be histologically diagnosed without surgical involvement.

Table 4.2 Advantages of MRI-guided VAB over CNB

Larger tissue volume obtained in shorter time
More tolerant of slight targeting inaccuracy
Higher overall rate of successful sampling
Even small lesions (< 10 mm) can be successfully biopsied
Better sampling of high-risk lesions, e.g., papilloma, radial scar
Less likely to underestimate non-mass lesions, e.g., ADH, DCIS

Nevertheless, hookwire localization remains as a versatile procedure with a proven high success rate and is the fallback option for MRI-only lesions which are not amenable to VAB for technical or medical reasons (Table 4.3). As stated in recent European consensus guidelines: "If a lesion is deemed to be not accessible to MR-guided VAB, MR-guided needle localization followed by surgery is recommended" [14]. Therefore, every case should first be carefully assessed, with hookwire localization offered when appropriate, rather than risking an abortive attempt at VAB where there is a limited chance of success. The final choice may depend on several factors, including characteristics of the target lesion, level of experience of the radiologist and preferences of the individual surgeon and patient. With this in mind, we can look in more detail at the practical principles applicable to both forms of MRI-guided intervention.

Principles of MRI-guided interventions

The use of MRI-guided interventions is now well established, with equipment vendors usually offering excellent applications support to allow radiologists to learn the requisite skills. Watching a video demonstration (DVD or internet), featuring the biopsy system you are using, is an excellent way to prepare for a procedure. It is a good idea to keep a non-sterile kit for practicing technique, particularly if interventions arise relatively infrequently (an olive in a chicken fillet wrapped in cling-film makes a reasonable phantom). Rehearsal sessions should ensure that the team of technologist, radiologist and assisting nurse all become familiar with their roles. Nevertheless, live patients are invariably more challenging than chicken fillets! The following points may help to avoid some of the difficulties encountered in the learning phase.

Table 4.3 Circumstances where MRI-guided hookwire localization may be preferred to VAB

Target lesion close to chest wall, especially in the axillary tail
Retroareolar lesions where satisfactory stability may be difficult to achieve
Superficial lesions, particularly in a small thin breast where VAB may be impossible
Target lesion adjacent to a silicone implant
Isolated focus or very small mass lesion (< 6–7 mm) to allow more confident sampling
Solitary linear-ductal morphology where hookwire +/– bracketing allows more confident sampling
Previous failed attempt at VAB, usually due to difficult lesion location
Previous discordant VAB result requiring definitive open surgical biopsy
Anticoagulated patients where suspending treatment is considered clinically too hazardous
Patients with known severe clotting disorder at high risk of significant bleeding from VAB

Heywang-Köbrunner *et al.* [14], Schrading *et al.* [18], Noroozian *et al.* [23]

Patient positioning

Careful positioning prior to the procedure is the key to achieving a high success rate. Innovative methods are sometimes required to access difficult lesions, and technologists with experience in XRM and stereotactic biopsy have invaluable skills in this regard. It is important that the patient is made as comfortable as possible so they keep still for the often lengthy duration of the procedure. Arms should be above the head to keep them clear of the interventional field. Light compression of the breast is used, sufficient to immobilize and support the breast without compromising blood flow. As a general principle of breast biopsy (with any guidance method), a line of approach roughly parallel to the chest wall is chosen to avoid pain from entering the pectoral muscle, and to minimize the risk of pneumothorax.

Describing anatomic relations

For breast MRI interventional procedures, it is strongly recommended that only the unambiguous terms *head, feet, nipple* and *chest* should be used to describe anatomic relations. Otherwise, with the patient in the prone position and a different orientation of displayed images on the console, confusion easily arises using "anterior/posterior" and "superior/inferior."

Fiducial markers

Both the commercially available localization techniques – the grid method and the pillar-and-post – rely on surface fiducial markers to determine the skin entry point over the underlying enhancing target lesion. The fiducial markers contain dilute gadolinium which gradually loses potency over time, so prior to performing a biopsy these must be replenished (using 1 ml of gadolinium in 20 ml of saline) if not recently used. With the grid method, a Vitamin E capsule taped inside one of the squares can be used as an alternative surface marker.

Choice of contrast sequence

To visualize the fiducial markers and the enhancing target, fat-suppressed IR T1-weighted images are widely used for MRI-guided procedures. The use of subtraction has the disadvantages of removing useful topographic landmarks and lengthens image processing time. Nevertheless, running a pre-contrast series is recommended (this avoids the pitfall of mistaking an incidental proteinaceous cyst with high T1 signal for the enhancing target lesion). In general, the aim is to keep sequences as short as possible to minimize procedure time. Use of fast gradient-echo 3D volume acquisitions provides multiple planes (sagittal and axial) from the one sequence.

Target fails to enhance

In up to about 10% of cases scheduled for an MRI-guided intervention, the enhancing target lesion may no longer be apparent [6, 7, 15, 16]. Usually this is because the "lesion" was simply due to a transient hormonal phenomenon, resolving after re-scanning in a different phase of the menstrual cycle or after at least 4 weeks off HRT [7]. However, in some instances breast compression can restrict blood flow and prevent the enhancement of a cancer [6]. In a study of 29 MRI lesions which could not be biopsied due to absent enhancement, four reappeared at short-term follow-up without compression of which two were due to invasive cancers [17]. This probably occurs because the delicate thin-walled capillaries associated with neoangiogenesis are more easily occluded than normal vessels.

Vanishing target

The *vanishing target* phenomenon refers to the problem of enhancing lesions becoming less conspicuous as time elapses after the initial contrast injection. Fading of the target results from a combination of contrast washout from the lesion and overall increase in normal background enhancement. Using visual landmarks in the breast parenchyma often allows the target location to be reidentified even when the contrast fades, but it is important to work as efficiently as possible. One useful strategy is to divide the total maximum gadolinium dose of 3 ml/kg to allow for multiple smaller injections, e.g., 3 × 10 ml doses. Re-injection is more likely to be successful in improving conspicuity of lesions with strong washout kinetics [18].

Targeting lesions without contrast

For any lesions which can be clearly identified on non-contrast (usually T2-weighted) images there is the potential to locate the target without gadolinium. Contrast injection is then reserved for confirming accurate placement of the hookwire tip (or the obturator tip in the case of VAB) next to the target just prior to deployment (or before VAB sampling). If a T2-weighted sequence is used, care should be taken not to obscure the target by excessive use of deep local anesthetic. With steadily improving resolution, it may be possible to target an increasing number of lesions using only topographic landmarks in the breast, a point proposed as a potential advantage for interventional breast MRI at 3T [19].

Grid method

This method employs a compression plate device divided into 2 cm grid squares, into which a *needle block* can be fitted to guide a needle into the breast perpendicular to the compression grid. A range of needle blocks are manufactured for various needle sizes, with arrays of holes which allow the needle to pass through horizontally. The larger the needle of course, the fewer the number of holes in the block. The needle block for a hookwire localization may have an 8 × 8 or 9 × 9 matrix of 64 or 81 holes, while that for a 9-gauge VAB typically has only 9 access holes in a 3 × 3 matrix. An innovative needle block configuration in the SenoRx Encor VAB system allows 13 points of access for the probe (Fig. 4.1).

When an intervention is performed, the localization device may be attached to the side of the biopsy coil, while some systems, e.g., the InVivo 7-channel Breast Biopsy Array Coil (Philips, Best, The Netherlands), have the device fully integrated into the coil design (Plate 3). Recent 16-channel coils have a closed-in design to accommodate the extra elements and are not suitable for performing biopsy, so vendors supply a companion open-design 4- or 7-channel biopsy coil.

The principle of the grid method is that from a series of sagittal images, the target can be localized in two planes (x and y coordinates), while the depth from the skin to the target (z coordinate) can be ascertained by calculating number of slices × slice thickness. Important to note is that the skin surface is only visible because it is indented by the grid from the application of mild compression (the plastic grid itself is completely invisible on MRI). The skin must pillow into the square grid fenestrations when setting up, not only for adequate immobilization but also to make the grid lines visible on MRI.

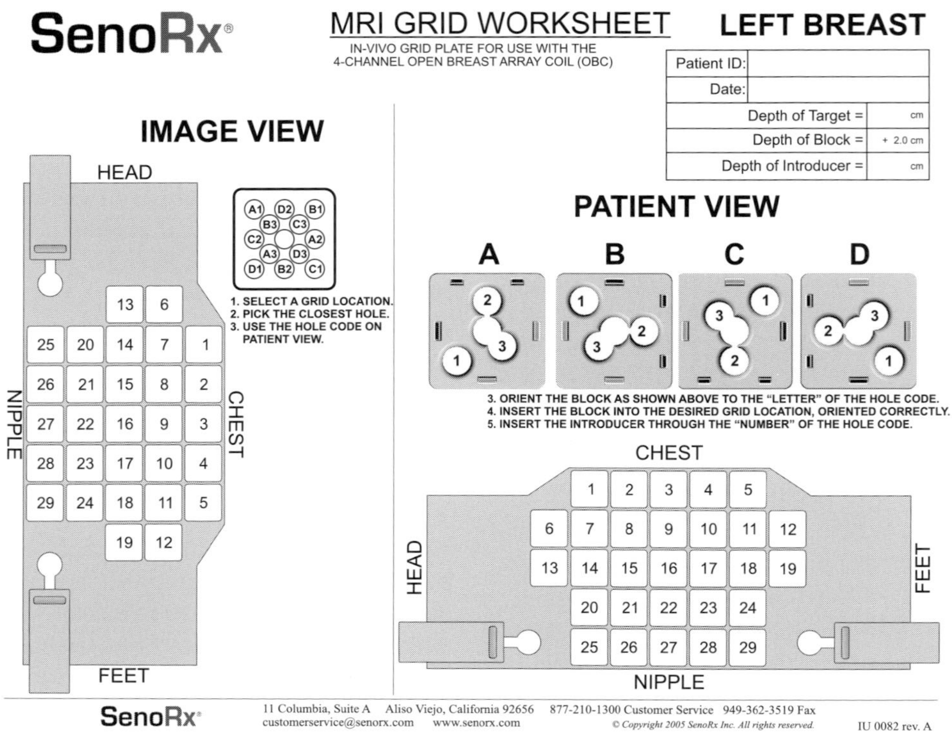

Fig. 4.1 MRI grid worksheet for SenorRx Encor biopsy system used with Noras 4-channel biopsy array coil. Targeting begins by marking fiducial and target on "image view" before transferring to "patient view" for insertion of the trochar. The needle block design allows 13 different entry points. Reproduced with permission.

An advantage of the grid method is its inherent geometric simplicity, wherein the needle entry is horizontal and no angles need to be calculated, making it easy to perform manually. Nevertheless, commercial CAD systems provide interactive software which can potentially make the task quicker and easier to perform, although at the expense of some loss of operator control.

The main disadvantages of the grid method is that it allows only horizontal needle entry, so that lesions far posteriorly in the breast (within 2–4 cm of the pectoral muscle) may be impossible to get within the field of the grid. Anterior (subareolar) lesions can also be problematic because of excessive mobility of this portion of the dependent breast.

Image and patient view

A potential source of confusion and error with the grid method is the need to correlate the different orientations of "image view" (seen on the monitor screen) and "patient view" (as the breast is seen during the biopsy). Accordingly, vendors of biopsy systems supply worksheets to help ensure that grid-positioning details are correctly transcribed (Fig. 4.1). Before starting, it is essential to check that the correct worksheet is selected, e.g., right breast, lateral approach.

Target between holes in needle block

For hookwire localization using the grid method, the large number of holes in the needle block ensures that the needle can be inserted directly over the lesion. However, for larger CNB and VAB needles, with fewer holes in the matrix, it is possible for the target to "hide" between holes in the needle block. While this could be problematic for MRI-guided CNB, an inherent advantage of VAB devices is their ability to compensate for minor errors in needle positioning, because of the vacuum effect. Occasionally the target may "hide" behind one of the intersections of the grid itself, in which case it is advisable to adjust the position of the breast slightly and retarget.

Pillar-and-post method

This alternative method uses a movable pillar in place of the grid compression plate but has the same ability to fix a point of entry over the target. A tubular *needle guide* attached to the pillar allows the appropriate gauge needle (for either hookwire or VAB) to pass through its central lumen. The key difference is that the needle guide allows for an angled aproach, typically at increments of 15 degrees above or below the horizontal (Plate 3). This can be particularly helpful for targeting lesions which are far posterior or anterior in the breast. However, guidance software is needed to calculate the possible combinations of angle and depth needed to access the target, so a purely manual technique is not possible.

Technical innovations continue to emerge, with the Verity™ angled software device (Hologic, Bedford, MA, USA) being a particularly attractive option to add pillar-and-post type functionality to a standard grid system. The device plugs into the grid squares and allows any entry angle to be selected, with accompanying software guiding the appropriate trajectory (Plate 4).

Potentially difficult lesions

Certain locations are particularly challenging to access. In some instances, this may lead to a decision not to attempt VAB, or to modify the technique. Some systems allow alternative medial or even craniocaudal access. If both grid and pillar-and-post methods are available, the latter is chosen where an angled approach would improve accessibility.

Potentially difficult target locations include the following:

(i) Medial lesions – most recent biopsy coils now allow direct medial access (using a plate to blank off the aperture for the contralateral breast), but in practice a lateral approach may still be easier (for a hookwire, check that the long course is acceptable to the surgeon). Using extreme obliquity to place the breast in the contralateral aperture of the coil may be an alternative with some systems (but remember to alert the technologist and to take care with image and patient view chart selection if the grid method is used).

(ii) Posterior lesions – for lesions close to the pectoral muscle, particularly in the axillary tail, the patient should be positioned obliquely to rotate the target as anteriorly as possible, while sacrificing any excess padding from the coil can add a few extra centimeters.

(iii) Retroareolar lesions – because of the mobility of the dependent anterior breast, cushioning may be required for support and stabilization. Generous deep local anesthesia is also recommended.

(iv) Superficial lesions – VAB may be impractical, particularly in small breasts which become thin when compressed. For hookwire localization it is strongly advisable to place the tip of the wire slightly deeper to the lesion than usual to avoid dislocation.

(v) Lesions adjacent to breast implants – hookwire localization is usually the only option to avoid damaging the implant, and in some instances a freehand or semi-freehand technique may be preferred.

MRI-guided hookwire localization

Informed consent

The importance of patient cooperation in preventing wire dislocation or breakage must be emphasized. If the breast contains an implant, the possibility of causing rupture must also be discussed. All other complications such as bleeding and infection are exceedingly rare, and no special precautions are needed. The chance that the target lesion may not be visible should be mentioned.

Technique

In North America, prior to the advent of MRI-guided VAB, the grid method was widely used for hookwire localization [16]. While MRI-guided VAB is now standard procedure for most lesions, hookwire localization is still used for targets which are difficult to access for VAB, or where other medical factors make VAB unattractive (Table 4.3).

Compared to VAB, hookwire insertion using the grid method is both quicker and easier to perform with a reported procedure time of ~30 minutes (range 15–60 minutes) [16]. Ideally, for a small target, the wire should pass through the lesion with the hook lying 5–10 mm distal to it.

For a lesion close to the pectoral muscle, if the wire tip can be placed even within 10–20 mm from the target, it can still be successfully retrieved if the relationship between the target and tip of the wire is clearly conveyed to the surgeon [16]. With larger, usually non-mass targets, two hookwires can be used to "bracket" the abnormal area, particularly where an elongated DCIS lesion is suspected. Both these practices are analogous to XRM stereotactic hookwire localization.

Targets which are a problem for VAB can be challenging even for hookwire localization and often require modifications of technique. In some instances, removal of the needle block and use of a semi-freehand method has been described as a helpful strategy for lesions which are very superficial or close to an implant [20]. For far posterior lesions, outside the grid, it is also feasible to insert the wire through the space between the grid and the biopsy coil to bring it closer to the lesion [20].

Step-by-step instructions for manual placement of a hookwire using the grid method are given in Table 4.4. For lesions which may be difficult to access by the grid method, the pillar-and-post method may be preferred if available. Instructions for the pillar-and-post method given in Table 4.5 relate to the

Table 4.4 MRI-guided hookwire localization using manual grid technique

Finding the target
Gently compress breast between grid plates, with skin pillowing slightly into the squares
Place surface marker in grid square near to expected lesion location
Annotate fiducial location as "F" on "patient view" chart and then transfer to "image view" chart
Scan breast in sagittal plane (usually fat-suppressed T1-weighted) to include grid and show fiducial marker
Ensure expected target location is within grid – if not, reposition patient or modify technique, e.g., freehand
Inject contrast and repeat sagittal fat-suppressed T1-weighted 3D volume acquisition
Determining the target coordinates
Mark target location with cursor on sequential sagittal images to find its surface coordinates
On skin surface slice showing grid indentation, count squares down and across between "F" and target
Annotate "image view" chart with the corresponding main grid square marked "T" for target
Annotate "image view" chart with the closest needle block hole (defines exact x and y coordinates)
Transfer "image view" annotations to the "patient view" chart
Calculate depth (z-axis) from skin surface to target = (number of slices × slice thickness in mm)
Allow additional depth of 20 mm for needle block and 5–10 mm to traverse lesion with hookwire tip
Deploying the hookwire
Prep skin surface in the main grid square, infiltrate superficial local and insert sterile needle block
Set depth-stop and insert hookwire assembly through selected needle block hole to calculated depth
Check needle position with sagittal and axial fat-suppressed T1-weighted images and adjust if necessary
Deploy hookwire and remove co-axial outer needle
Relax compression, repeat axial fat-suppressed T1-weighted images to show relation of wire tip to target
Carefully remove needle block and compression plate over the wire and secure spare wire length to skin
Perform XRM prior to surgery to show hookwire course and tip location

Table 4.5 MRI-guided hookwire localization using pillar-and-post technique

Finding the target
Gently compress breast between immobilization plates, with skin bulging slightly through
Position fiducial marker in needle guide device as appropriate for expected lesion location
Set all three coordinates (x-, y- and z-axes) to zero and position the fiducial at 0 degrees (horizontal)
Scan breast in axial plane (usually fat-suppressed T1-weighted) to include needle guide and fiducial
Ensure expected target location is accessible – if not, reposition patient or modify technique, e.g., freehand
Inject contrast and repeat axial fat-suppressed T1-weighted 3D volume acquisition
Determining the target coordinates
Using guidance software, place one cursor at tip of fiducial marker and another on the target
Software calculates required coordinates for each possible angle of entry (−30, −15, 0, +15, +30)
Select best approach, print worksheet, set x-axis, height on pillar (y-axis) and angle of needle guide
Allow additional depth for needle guide
Deploying the hookwire
Prep skin surface through immobilization plate, infiltrate superficial local at skin entry point
Replace fiducial marker with needle guide of appropriate gauge
Set depth-stop and insert hookwire assembly through selected needle guide to calculated depth
Check needle position with sagittal and axial fat-suppressed T1-weighted images and adjust if necessary
If position acceptable, advance needle to place hookwire tip 5–10 mm beyond target
Deploy hookwire and remove co-axial outer needle
Relax compression, repeat axial fat-suppressed T1-weighted images to show relation of wire tip to target
Carefully remove immobilization plate over the wire and secure spare wire length to skin
Perform XRM prior to surgery to show hookwire course and tip location

Table 4.6 MRI-guided hookwire localization using freehand technique

Localizing the target
No compression or only gentle immobilization or padding can be used
Place surface marker at approximate entry site laterally
Inject contrast and scan in axial plane (usually fat-suppressed T1-weighted) to localize lesion
Determine craniocaudal distance between marker and lesion from slice positions on serial axial scans
Measure on skin surface and adjust surface marker position, then re-scan region to confirm
With the plane of approach thus fixed, measure distance and angle to target
Deploying the hookwire
Prep skin surface, infiltrate superficial local and advance co-axial needle close to lesion
Repeat axial scan series to check correct approach to pass through lesion, adjust angle if necessary
If position acceptable, advance needle to place hookwire tip 5–10 mm beyond target
Deploy hookwire and remove co-axial outer needle
Repeat axial scan series to show relation of wire tip to target
Perform XRM prior to surgery to show hookwire course and tip location

Noras biopsy device (Noras MRI Products, Hochberg, Germany) and the exact procedure may differ slightly for other equipment. A freehand technique, which requires no special equipment, is another option for challenging lesions (Table 4.6) [21]. For very superficial lesions where even hookwire localization may be unsuitable, the freehand technique can also be used to position an MRI skin marker directly over the target prior to surgical excision. Reported success rates using various techniques for MRI-guided hookwire localization are 95–100% [1, 16, 21, 22].

Wire dislocation or breakage

The low-ferrous steel or titanium used in MRI-compatible hookwires results in reduced mechanical strength, and those involved in the procedure must be aware that gentle treatment is needed. Wire dislocation or breakage with a retained fragment are the usual cause of failure to retrieve diagnostic material [16]. Surgeons should be warned that diathermy contact with MRI-compatible hookwires should be avoided as at least anecdotally this may result in breakage [16].

MRI-guided vacuum-assisted biopsy

Although the principles for MRI-guided VAB are similar to those for hookwire localization using either the grid or pillar-and-post methods, the much larger gauge needle used makes the technique more complex and is associated with more significant complications, particularly bleeding. The steps involved in VAB are outlined in Table 4.7 (grid method) and Table 4.8 (pillar-and-post method), based on the Noras device (details may differ for other equipment). The recent European consensus guidelines are summarized in Table 4.9.

Informed consent

The consent process should explain the procedure and the need to insert a metal marker clip. All possible complications should be listed including severe bleeding or hematoma, which is occasionally severe enough to require surgical evacuation (< 1%); exit wound; vasovagal reaction; risk of late infection. It is also important that the patient is aware that biopsy cannot be performed if the target lesion is no longer visible and that VAB may be aborted if the lesion cannot be safely accessed or severe bleeding occurs. The possibility of an equivocal pathology result should also be explained.

Preparation

To minimize risk of bleeding, anticoagulants or aspirin should be discontinued, and if this is not clinically acceptable, hookwire localization substituted. Local anesthetic with epinephrine (adrenaline) is widely used for deep infiltration. Routine oral sedation is recommended with lorazepam 1.0–2.0 mg (Ativan, Wyeth-Ayerst Laboratories). This can be divided into an initial oral dose 20–30 minutes before commencing and supplementary doses given as required during the procedure. Where possible, feet-first entry into the magnet may help to overcome claustrophobia and can improve access to the breast.

Procedure duration

It is essential to allow adequate time. A recent study reported the average time needed in the MRI suite for VAB using a standard grid method was 58 minutes (range 30–109 minutes) even for experienced operators [23]. Realistically, at the beginning of the learning curve for VAB, it is suggested that 90–120 minutes

Table 4.7 MRI-guided VAB using manual grid technique

Finding the target
Gently compress breast between grid plates, with skin pillowing slightly into the squares
Place surface marker in grid square near to expected lesion location
Annotate fiducial location as "F" on "patient view" chart and then transfer to "image view" chart
Scan breast in sagittal plane (usually fat-suppressed T1-weighted) to include grid and show fiducial
Ensure expected target location is within grid – if not, reposition patient or consider alternative method
Inject contrast and repeat sagittal fat-suppressed T1-weighted 3D volume acquisition
Determining the target coordinates
Mark target location with cursor on sequential sagittal images to find its surface coordinates
On skin surface slice showing grid indentation, count squares down and across between "F" and target
Annotate "image view" chart with the corresponding main grid square marked "T" for target
Annotate "image view" chart with the closest needle block hole (defines exact x and y coordinates)
Transfer "image view" annotations to the "patient view" chart
Calculate depth (z-axis) from skin surface to target = (number of slices × slice thickness in mm)
Allow additional depth of 20 mm for needle block, usually plus 5–10 mm to allow for slight tissue shift
Establishing the biopsy track
Prep skin surface in the main grid square and loosely engage the sterile needle block
Place plastic introducer sheath through selected needle block hole to create a circular skin indentation
Remove needle block, infiltrate superficial and deep local anesthetic at marked skin entry point
Make ~5 mm skin nick, sufficient to allow clean entry of trochar assembly without dragging skin
Set depth-stop to calculated depth, firmly reinsert needle block into grid and insert trochar and sheath
Advance trochar and sheath with smooth back and forth rotating action to limit of depth-stop
Carefully remove trochar, leaving introducer sheath in place – the sheath must not move!
Insert plastic obturator, the tip of which will mark the center of the VAB sample collection chamber
Check obturator position with sagittal and axial fat-suppressed T1-weighted images and adjust if required
Use sagittal scans to plan the optimal arc for sampling the lesion
Obtaining the samples
Withdraw patient from magnet, remove obturator and insert probe to commence VAB sampling

Table 4.7 *continued*

Reinsert obturator and repeat sagittal and axial images to confirm adequate lesion sampling
Replace obturator with clip insertion device, deploy clip and then rotate device 180 degrees
Repeat sagittal and axial images to confirm marker placement relative to biopsy cavity
Reinsert obturator and then remove obturator and introducer together
Gently release and remove compression plate and apply pressure to biopsy site
Place specimens in formalin and arrange XRM to show clip location

Table 4.8 MRI-guided VAB using pillar-and-post technique

Finding the target
Gently compress breast between immobilization plates, with skin bulging slightly through
Position fiducial marker in needle guide device as appropriate for expected lesion location
Set all three coordinates (x-, y- and z-axes) to zero and position the fiducial at 0 degrees (horizontal)
Scan breast in axial plane (usually fat-suppressed T1-weighted) to include needle guide and fiducial
Ensure expected target location is accessible – if not, reposition patient or consider option of hookwire
Inject contrast and repeat axial fat-suppressed T1-weighted 3D volume acquisition
Determining the target coordinates
Using guidance software, place one cursor at tip of fiducial marker and another on the target
Software calculates required coordinates for each possible angle of entry (−30, −15, 0, +15, +30)
Select best approach, print worksheet, set x-axis, height on pillar (y-axis) and angle of needle guide
Allow additional depth for needle guide, usually plus 5–10 mm, to allow for slight tissue shift
Establishing the biopsy track
Prep skin surface between the bars of the immobilization plate and remove fiducial marker
Place plastic introducer sheath through selected sterile needle guide to create a circular skin indentation
Infiltrate superficial and deep local anesthetic at marked skin entry point
Make ~5 mm skin nick, sufficient to allow clean entry of trochar assembly without dragging skin
Set depth-stop to calculated depth, then insert trochar and sheath through needle guide and into skin nick
Advance trochar and sheath with smooth back and forth rotating action to limit of depth-stop

Table 4.8 *continued*

Carefully remove trochar, leaving introducer sheath in place – the sheath must not move!
Insert plastic obturator, the tip of which will mark the center of the VAB sample collection chamber
Check obturator position with sagittal and axial fat-suppressed T1-weighted images and adjust if required
Use sagittal scans to plan the optimal arc for sampling the lesion
Obtaining the samples
Withdraw patient from magnet, remove obturator and insert probe to commence VAB sampling
Reinsert obturator and repeat sagittal and axial images to confirm adequate lesion sampling
Replace obturator with clip insertion device, deploy clip and then rotate device 180 degrees
Repeat sagittal and axial images to confirm marker placement relative to biopsy cavity
Reinsert obturator and then remove obturator and introducer together
Gently release and remove compression plate and apply pressure to biopsy site
Place specimens in formalin and arrange XRM to show clip location

Table 4.9 Summary of main recommendations of European consensus on VAB technique

Reserve MRI-guided VAB for MRI-only lesions (use conventional means where possible)
If lesion deemed not accessible to VAB, perform MRI-guided needle localization instead
Ensure that the lesion is clearly and reproducibly visible on MRI
Emphasized that VAB is preferred to CNB because of superior sampling
Routinely obtain 24 cores (11-gauge) to remove small lesions
Perform an immediate post-biopsy scan to assess extent of sampling
Record result as definite sampling, equivocal or inadequate
Undertake multidisciplinary review after obtaining pathology
Undertake appropriate follow-up arrangements
Regularly audit success rates and review outcomes

Heywang-Köbrunner *et al.* [14]

should be set aside for each case. Clearly the patient also needs to be able to tolerate keeping still in the same position for up to about an hour. With appropriate patient selection, the number of image acquisitions (rather than any specific lesion or patient factors) appears to have the most influence on procedure duration, with a minimum of five scan series usually required (Fig. 4.2) [23]:

(i) Pre-contrast – exclude spurious bright T1 signal, e.g., proteinaceous cyst.
(ii) Post-contrast – to show target lesion.
(iii) Confirm obturator position – to check proximity of target to sampling chamber and to plan the sampling arc.
(iv) Immediate post-biopsy scan – to assess adequacy of sampling.
(v) Final scan after clip deployment – to show marker clip location.

Technique

Although design features and functionality vary, all MRI-guided VAB systems have the following basic co-axial arrangement of components:

(i) Sharp MRI-compatible solid metal stylet (the trochar) which needs to be capable of penetrating even very dense breast tissue.
(ii) Outer plastic introducer sheath (inserted with the trochar).
(iii) Blunt plastic localizing obturator which is substituted for the trochar to allow imaging confirmation of accurate targeting (tip of obturator indicates the center of the biopsy probe side collection chamber).
(iv) Biopsy probe device with hollow metal cutting needle and side collection chamber with vacuum attached, inserted through the sheath for final tissue sampling, performed outside the bore of the magnet.

As the actual process of tissue extraction cannot be monitored in real time, accuracy of the biopsy location is based on calculated coordinates, with the potential for failure of sampling if displacement of the target lesion is not recognized. Therefore, a major consideration in MRI-guided VAB is avoiding tissue displacement, which can occur at three possible locations:

(i) At the skin surface, due to dragging of the skin during trochar insertion – to prevent this an adequate skin nick needs to be made at the entry point (use of disposable titanium scalpels is recommended).
(ii) Along the track leading to the target lesion, usually in dense tissue – the tendency for "tissue shift" is minimized by using a very sharp trochar design and careful technique, discussed in more detail below.

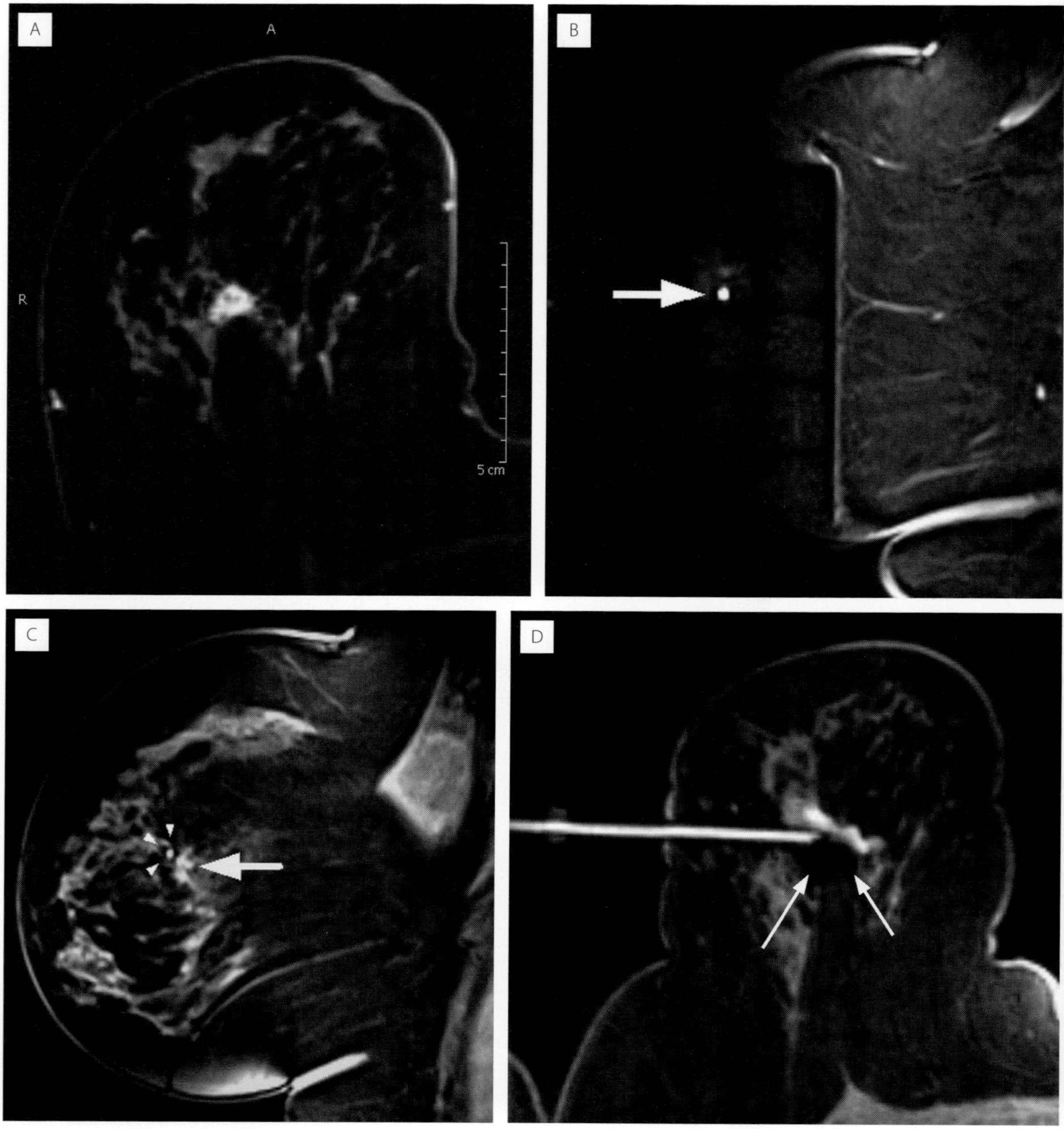

Fig. 4.2 MRI-guided biopsy: (A) Post-contrast axial fat-suppressed T1-weighted image showing a 12 mm spiculated mass. Lesion was located on sagittal scans, distance to skin surface determined, and entry point for the trochar and sheath chosen using the biopsy worksheet. After replacing the trochar with the obturator, post-contrast sagittal fat-suppressed T1-weighted image (B) at skin surface shows indentation by grid with SenoRx Visiloc obturator (arrow) in position. Obturator was tracked on sequential sagittal images to the tip (corresponding to center of biopsy chamber), with image (C) confirming good position of tip (small arrowheads) relative to target (arrow) and allowing selection of optimal biopsy arc, in this case towards the chest wall. After taking 12 × 10-gauge samples, axial image (D) shows signal void due to air in biopsy cavity (arrows), but bright signal from acute hematoma is difficult to distinguish from residual enhancing mass. Lesion was considered to be adequately sampled with histology of cores confirming IDC.

(iii) At the target lesion, which can itself become displaced by hematoma – this is avoided by use of suction in the cavity, and checking for a hematoma collection prior to further sampling.

Tissue shift in dense parenchyma

This problem arises because of the large gauge needles used for VAB, particularly when in combination with resistant dense breast tissue. This tendency for bunching and tissue shift distal to the trochar tip during insertion pushes the target beyond the original position. This displacement becomes clear on axial scans when the obturator position is first checked, and necessitates an adjustment to the calculated depth. To prevent tissue shift occurring, the probe assembly should always be advanced with a gentle back-and-forth rotational movement. If the target location permits, in a dense breast it is often easier to position the tip slightly beyond the lesion (add 5–10 mm to the initial depth calculation) and then pull back if needed. Gently tapping the end of the trochar assembly can also help to penetrate through dense tissue. For devices which offer the option, using a spring-loaded mechanism to "fire" the biopsy needle into the target lesion may be an advantage in dense tissue.

Obturator visualization

The plastic obturator devices used in VAB appear as signal voids and can sometimes be difficult to see against the background of dark fat on fat-suppressed T1-weighted images, particularly in the sagittal plane. The SenoRx Visiloc obturator overcomes this problem by showing as bright signal on fat-suppressed T1-weighted images (the device is essentially a plastic tube filled with contrast agent).

Posterior lesions

For posterior lesions, particularly those in the axillary tail, the patient is rolled to bring the lesion more anteriorly, a technique routinely used for stereotactic biopsy [11]. Where a posterior target still lies just outside the grid, the VAB probe is positioned as close to the lesion as possible. With the collection chamber then directed posteriorly during sampling, the suction effect may be enough for the target to be retrieved [10]. In some instances, a second or third biopsy arc may need to be performed.

Where available, the pillar-and-post method may be preferred because the device can be extended beyond the range of the grid, closer to the chest wall and can be angled as required [18]. As a last resort, if a small posterior lesion cannot be accessed, a marker clip can be deployed just anteriorly. This can then be used as a target for x-ray stereotactic hookwire localization so that further material can be obtained by surgical excision between the marker clip and pectoral fascia.

Retroareolar lesions

The difficulty with anterior and retroareolar lesions is that the breast may not be adequately stabilized by compression plates or padding. The breast is also thinner anteriorly and good local anesthesia can be more difficult to achieve, while in dense breasts there is the additional problem of tissue shift. Therefore, while the pillar-and-post method may be preferred for VAB, hookwire localization is sometimes the better option.

Small "thin" breasts

Small breasts can become very thin after applying even just the moderate side-to-side compression required to immobilize the breast for MRI-guided VAB. In a thin compressed breast, no matter how the approach is adjusted, the target lesion remains close to one or other skin surface. Probes which allow a "half-sample" to be taken (a short core of ~10 mm compared with ~20 mm for a full core) by only partly opening the side aperture are invaluable in these circumstances. As a guide, a practical lower limit of ~3 cm thickness of the compressed breast has been suggested for VAB to be technically feasible [7]. However, this may be reduced to as little as ~2 cm with a half-sample option.

Superficial lesions

Target lesions which are close to the skin surface pose particular problems for VAB, particularly in small breasts as described above. For a superficial lesion on the side of skin entry, the collection chamber of the VAB probe must be covered to maintain the vacuum. Injecting copious local anesthetic helps to increase the depth of subcutaneous tissue, and a slightly tight skin incision will maintain an airtight seal with the introducer sheath.

Conversely, with a superficial lesion close to the opposite surface of the breast, there is a risk of causing an exit wound during insertion of the sharp trochar or with the VAB probe during sampling. In x-ray stereotactic biopsy, applying pressure on the opposite side of the breast with a reverse-compression paddle is used to overcome this problem. Such a device has a central space in the paddle, allowing tissue and skin displaced by the VAB needle to bulge into it without piercing the skin. For MRI-guided VAB, having both medial and lateral grids in place enables the one on the far side to take over this function, with tissue bulging into the opposite grid space [12]. Where available, the option of a blunt-tipped VAB probe prevents an exit wound arising in the overlying skin during tissue sampling.

Assessment of sampling adequacy

Whether sampling was judged to be successful, based on post-biopsy imaging, should be recorded for purposes of subsequent histologic–pathologic correlation. An immediate post-biopsy MR sequence is required with a further injection of gadolinium if necessary [14]. However, while the location of the biopsy cavity is usually apparent from the presence of blood clot and/or air, even a small hematoma can obscure the lesion, making it difficult to determine if sampling was adequate or not [24]. Hematoma formation can also displace the lesion from its original location. Therefore, thorough vacuuming of the cavity is recommended prior to the post-biopsy series. Comparison is then made between pre- and post-biopsy images, using anatomic landmarks to decide whether the target has been included in the biopsy.

Sampling can be classified as (i) complete (blood/air at the biopsy site but no residual enhancing lesion), (ii) sampled (lesion still visible but clearly smaller) or (iii) possibly missed (lesion is apparently unchanged without a reduction in size) [25]. Lee *et al.* reported complete removal of the enhancing target in 30% of all MRI-guided VABs showing cancer, rising to ~50% for target lesions of up to 10 mm in diameter [26]. However, complete removal of the target lesion by VAB did not imply total histologic excision, with residual invasive cancer or DCIS found on final surgical pathology in about two-thirds of cases [26].

Clip placement and migration

An assessment should also be made as to whether the marker clip is present at the target location. This is important because if histopathology dictates that excision is required, the marker clip may be suitable as a target for x-ray stereotactic hookwire localization. To determine this, when VAB sampling is complete and the clip deployed, a last sequence may be performed to show the relationship of the clip to the biopsy cavity/residual lesion. In practice, identifying the clip among blood and air artifact can be challenging. A post-procedure XRM can help by confirming that the clip location coincides with air in the biopsy cavity. If the marker clip is clearly remote from the biopsy site, this has to be taken into account.

Migration of biopsy site marker clips is not uncommon in x-ray stereotactic VAB, attributed to the *concertina effect*, which can magnify any placement error when breast compression is released after the procedure. This might be expected to be less problematic after MRI-guided biopsy where only mild compression is applied to the breast. However, displacement of the marker clip of >1 cm away from the target lesion appears to be common, even after successful MRI-guided VAB sampling [24].

Clip artifact

While the marker clip inserted after VAB must be identifiable on MRI, it should not cause so much artifact that a significant lesion could be completely obscured ("clipped out"). In a study using clips placed in gelatin phantoms, the signal void artifact created by commercially available clips on a 3D gradient-echo T1-weighted sequence was at least double the actual clip sizes of 2–3 mm [27]. Applying fat-suppression adds banding artifacts which may be clinically significant for some clips. Care should then be taken in choosing a marker clip for routine use and in selecting suitable sequences to display it. Titanium clips produce minimal artifact and can be difficult to locate, so that stainless steel markers tend to be more practical.

Choosing a vacuum-assisted biopsy system

All VAB probes have in common a basic needle design with a side collection chamber and a central rotating or oscillating cutter which advances to take the specimen. The collection chamber can be turned to face in any direction to allow "around the clock" sampling. It is important that the vacuum effect which can be applied is efficient in pulling tissue in to the chamber. In most cases this function is achieved by the use of a free-standing vacuum console which remains outside the MRI suite and is connected to the biopsy probe by plastic tubing. The vacuum console also provides the ability to apply suction to the cavity to remove any accumulating hematoma.

Several MRI-compatible VAB systems are now commercially available, and the various features of each have recently been reviewed by O'Flynn *et al.* [28]. Some key design features to consider when choosing a VAB system are now briefly discussed.

Table 4.10 outlines a shortlist of factors which may help as a starting point when considering which system may be most suitable.

The Mammotome system was the first to be developed for stereotactic core biopsy and was then adapted by adding an MRI-compatible attachment. This probe is essentially a double-lumen rather than a truly co-axial device, which means that the probe caliber is considerably larger than the size of the cores obtained. For example, the outer diameter of the Mammotome probe used to obtain 11-g cores is about equivalent to 7 g size. After each core has been taken, the needle has to be backed out to allow each individual sample to be retrieved manually. Therefore, as the Mammotome is not a closed system, there is the potential risk of blood contamination of personnel and equipment.

The Hologic Suros ATEC Breast Biopsy System offered significant advantages over the Mammotome device, notably the ability to sample continuously without backing out the needle to retrieve cores. With this fully closed design, all core samples accumulate in a collection chamber for easy transfer to a specimen pot after completion of the procedure. The Suros design also features a small, light, pneumatically driven handheld driver assembly which is completely disposable, and offers continuous saline lavage of the cavity. Full and half-sampling are available on different probe needles, while an atraumatic rounded tip option prevents an exit wound in a small thin breast. The newer Hologic Eviva model has an offset rather than a central position of the needle, a helpful feature when accessing lesions close to the chest wall [28].

The SenoRx EnCor (SenoRx, Aliso Viejo, CA, USA) system has similar design characteristics to the Hologic system, although with a heavier electric driver in the probe head, into which a disposable needle is fitted. Instead of the usual rotating cutter, the mechanism of the EnCor device has an oscillating scissor action [29]. The sharp Tri-Concave tip design used in the trochar and probe needle appears particularly effective in penetrating dense parenchyma with minimal tissue shift (some users even report that they no longer use a scalpel to nick the skin). For VAB using the grid method, the SenoRx EnCor has locking devices at both grid/needle block and needle block/depth-stop unions to prevent any backing out of the sheath during the procedure. Full and half-sample options are available in the same needle, and a slower speed of rotation can be selected for cutting dense tissue [29]. The SenoRx EnCor allows pre-programmed sampling which can, for example, take six cores around the clock in under 60 seconds at one press of a button.

Table 4.10 Some factors to consider in MRI-guided VAB systems

Ease of use – particularly important if only used occasionally
Performance – good tissue penetration and cutting ability paramount
Functionality – amount of tissue obtained per needle insertion is key
Portability – important if biopsies are to be performed at multiple sites
Safety – contamination risk (advantage of fully closed VAB systems)
Economics – consider purchase cost and ongoing cost of consumables

The Bard Vacora System (Bard Biopsy Systems, Tempe, AZ, USA) offers an alternative concept to the three previous console-based vacuum systems. Instead, the Bard Vacora is a handheld device with vacuum provided by an integrated 20 ml syringe powered by a rechargeable lithium-ion battery [30]. The advantage is that, with no attached cable or tubing, the device is very compact, light and easy to handle. Furthermore, without the need for a console vacuum system, the Bard Vacora is extremely portable and much less costly. Half-sampling is permitted for superficial lesions or small breasts, and a "pierce" option can be used to fire the probe through dense tissue. Downsides are having to completely remove the probe from the introducer sheath to retrieve each core, [28] the absence of a channel to allow additional deep local anesthetic to be administered [28] and the inability to vacuum the cavity to control bleeding, which may result in shift of the target lesion due to hematoma [31].

In a study by Schrading *et al.*, average procedure time was only ~40 minutes using the Suros ATEC console system compared with ~70 minutes using the Bard Vacora device [18]. The authors considered that the major reason for the longer procedure time with the handheld device was weaker suction. The stronger vacuum effect of the console system made targeting less critical and helped maintain a good tissue yield throughout the procedure by preventing hematoma from accumulating at the biopsy site [18]. The reported incidence of significant pain experienced during the biopsy procedure is also higher for the Bard Vacora device when compared with console systems [18, 32]. Finally, interrupted function of the

Bard Vacora device due to magnetic field effects has been reported at 1.5T, restored by retreating to a distance of 1.5 meters from the magnet [31].

Furthermore, Schrading *et al.* found that the advantages of the console-based system meant that radiologists were more confident to biopsy small masses (average diameter ~10 mm compared with ~19 mm for the handheld device) [18]. As a consequence, when only the Bard Vacora device was available, 29% of MRI-only lesions were sampled by VAB and 71% by hookwire localization. In contrast, when the console-based Suros ATEC system was available, 88% of MRI-only lesions were sampled using VAB [18].

Despite these disadvantages, the Bard Vacora could be an acceptable and economic option for low throughput sites performing relatively few MRI-guided interventions. The concept of a fully integrated handheld VAB device remains very attractive and it is interesting to note that Bard Biopsy Systems recently acquired the SenoRx company. Some of the key features of the four different systems discussed above are summarized in **Table 4.11**.

Radiologic–pathologic correlation

When correlating a pathology result with imaging, the first step is to ensure that the lesion in question was adequately sampled. A major drawback with all MRI-guided biopsy procedures is the inability to unequivocally confirm successful lesion retrieval, because MRI enhancement cannot be reproduced in an ex vivo specimen. Conventional imaging is not usually helpful, as the very reason for using MRI guidance is for targets that are MRI-only lesions. Not surprisingly then, specimen radiography reveals the lesion in only a small minority of cases. Furthermore, ~85% of malignant lesions shown by MRI have no gross pathologic correlate [33]. Consequently, after MRI-guided VAB, the entire specimen should be processed for microscopic examination, [33] and radiologic–histologic correlation becomes all the more important in deciding if the tissue sample is representative of the lesion as a whole.

For imaging correlation purposes, histopathologic results can be classified as (i) malignant, (ii) high-risk or borderline histopathology or (iii) benign. Both the malignant and high-risk categories will lead to surgical excision, either for definitive treatment or because of the possibility of a pathologic upgrade.

Radiologic–pathologic discordance is present when the histologic findings do not satisfactorily account for the imaging appearances. In particular, benign results have to be carefully reviewed with all available imaging, conventional and MRI, to decide if they are concordant or discordant. In most instances, a benign but discordant correlation will lead to either a repeat MRI-guided VAB or a diagnostic open surgical biopsy.

Malignant histopathology

A malignant histopathologic result, either DCIS or invasive cancer, is usually accepted as concordant. A discordant result can arise where invasive cancer was expected but only DCIS was found, suggesting

Table 4.11 Key features of MRI-guided VAB systems

	Bard Vacora	Mammotome	Hologic	SenoRx
Design	Handheld	Console-based	Console-based	Console-based
Motor type	Rechargeable battery	Mains electric	Pneumatic	Mains electric
Cutting action	Rotating	Rotating	Rotating	Oscillating scissor
Core gauge	10	11 or 8	12 or 9	10 or 7
Core retrieval	Single cores, removing probe for each sample	Single cores, but probe remains in position	Closed system, multiple cores from single probe insertion	Closed system, multiple cores from single probe insertion
Cut cycle time	N/A, probe is removed	~5 seconds per core, but manual remove for each	~5 seconds per core, each manually initiated	~10 seconds per core, either manual or pre-programmed
Half-sample	Yes, in same needle	No	Yes, in different needle plus atraumatic round tip option	Yes, in same needle plus atraumatic round tip option
Offset needle	Yes	Yes	Yes, on Eviva model but not on original Suros ATEC	Yes
Cavity vacuum	No	Yes	Yes, with full saline lavage	Yes, with option of sample chamber lavage
Anesthetic	No delivery channel	Allows deep local delivery	Allows deep local delivery	Allows deep local delivery

that the lesion may have been only partially sampled. Nevertheless the patient can generally proceed to definitive surgery. In such cases, the possibility of undersampling should be noted, and a satisfactory relationship between the marker clip and target lesion confirmed prior to x-ray stereotactic localization. The consequence of missing an invasive component is that the patient may require an additional surgical procedure (SLNB), after DCIS excision.

Of course, with any biopsy yielding DCIS, there is the possibility of invasion being found in the surgically excised specimen. In their study of 34 lesions yielding DCIS after MRI-guided 9-gauge VAB, Lee *et al.* reported an upgrade rate to invasive cancer of ~20% [34]. As expected, larger areas of non-mass enhancement were more likely to be associated with an upgrade to invasion (60% for lesions over 60 mm) [34]. In another series of 538 MRI-guided 11-gauge VAB procedures, Perlet *et al.* found a lower rate of 3/64 (5%) for DCIS upgrades to invasion [7].

High-risk or borderline histopathology

For a small group of pathologic lesions, it is well known that an upgrade can occur on surgical excision, and a result in this category will lead to surgical open biopsy (Table 4.12). Experience with stereotactic biopsy has shown that VAB has a much lower rate of undersampling of high-risk lesions than does CNB, which is directly attributable to the larger volume of tissue obtained.

The most common high-risk lesion is ADH, found as the only histopathologic abnormality in ~5% of MRI-guided VAB procedures [7, 35]. About two-thirds of cases appear as non-mass enhancement, and most of the remainder as mass lesions. Upgrades to DCIS on surgical excision were reported by Perlet *et al.* in 5/17 (29%) of 11-gauge MRI-guided VABs yielding ADH, [7] while Liberman *et al.* found upgrades to DCIS in 5/13 (38%) of 9-gauge MRI-guided VABs [35]. Strigel *et al.* reported on 62 high-risk lesions detected by MRI and biopsied by various methods, observing upgrades in 11/34 (32%) of ADH on surgical excision, of which 5 had an invasive component [36]. Therefore, an upgrade on excision can be expected in about one-third of ADH lesions found at MRI-guided VAB.

Papillary lesions are relatively frequently encountered in MRI-guided VAB, presenting as intensely enhancing, small intraductal or intracystic masses. While surgical excision is still widely recommended [37], some argue that if multiple cores from a radiologically benign lesion confirm a simple papilloma, the risk of malignancy may be low enough to avoid surgery [38]. This is more likely true for smaller lesions and larger core samples, and complete lesion removal by VAB could be the optimal management in selected cases [39].

Currently though, if there are atypical radiologic or pathologic features in relation to a papillary lesion, surgery is indicated. Although solitary small intraductal papillomas close to the nipple are frequently benign, given the subtlety of atypical findings on histopathology of core samples, some experts recommend direct excision for all intraductal masses [40].

There are only very limited MRI-specific data regarding less common high-risk lesions (ALH, LCIS and radial scar), but significant upgrade rates on excision have been documented from experience with stereotactic biopsy. As there are no specific features to predict upgrade of high-risk lesions, [36] surgical excision is usually recommended when such pathologic findings present in biopsies of MRI-detected lesions.

Table 4.12 Pathologic lesions recommended for excision after MRI-guided VAB

Lesion type	Key radiologic and pathologic features
ADH	Non-mass enhancement, mass or focus, ~30% upgrade rate usually to DCIS
Lobular neoplasia	Non-mass enhancement, ~20% upgrade rate from stereotactic VAB data
Radial scar	Stellate mass, ~20% upgrade rate to either DCIS or invasive cancer
Papillary lesion	Intraductal or intracystic mass, 14–38% upgrade rate usually to ADH or DCIS

Discordant benign histopathology

Radiologic–pathologic correlation is paramount in this group, where it must be decided whether or not a benign result satisfactorily accounts for all the imaging findings. Across several series, discordant results arise in 5–7% of MRI-guided VAB procedures [12, 13, 25, 29]. In the study by Lee *et al.*, surgical excision in 20 discordant lesions yielded malignancy in 6 (30%), of which 4 were invasive cancer with DCIS and 2 were DCIS only [25].

When there is discordance between imaging and histology after MRI-guided VAB, the first step is to review the adequacy of sampling. Lee *et al.* found a significantly higher discordance rate if sampling of the target was classified as "possibly missed" (discordant in 43%) rather than "sampled" (discordant in 7%). Where the target was considered to have been completely removed at MRI-guided biopsy, only 1/92 (1%) was discordant [25].

If the lesion was "possibly missed," the options lie between a repeat attempt at VAB or hookwire localization for open surgical biopsy. In doubtful cases, a repeat MRI scan at a short interval after biopsy may help to determine if the lesion was adequately sampled, using the marker clip and the morphology of any residual enhancement as a guide. However, even at only 24 hours post-VAB, reactive enhancement in surrounding tissue may be present, with the potential to interfere with lesion identification [31]. It may then be preferable to defer a follow-up contrast study to assess sampling for about 1 month [25].

If MRI at 1 month confirms absence of any enhancement (complete removal) or a significant reduction in lesion size (suggesting representative sampling), the case may, after multidisciplinary discussion, be considered suitable for further MRI follow-up at 6 months. If, on the other hand, there is persisting doubt as to the adequacy of VAB sampling, and depending on the individual patient preference, excision biopsy may be preferred. Again, the location of the marker clip to the residual lesion should be checked to ensure that it can be used for x-ray stereotactic targeting.

Concordant benign histopathology

In instances where benign pathology is accepted as concordant, a follow-up MRI at 6 months is mandatory to ensure lesion stability. In a study by Li *et al.*, 17/177 (10%) of benign concordant lesions were rebiopsied with VAB, of which 4 (24%) were malignant (2 IDC with DCIS, 2 DCIS only) [24]. Of note, one of the invasive cancers, a 7 mm enhancing mass, was stable on MRI at 11 months after initial VAB while concerning XRM and US findings prompted further biopsy. This case underscores the value of correlating all available imaging and suggests the need for MRI follow-up to at least 2 years before assuming benignity.

The authors observed that 6 months was appropriate for the first follow-up study, as enlargement of malignant lesions could not be detected at shorter intervals [24]. It was also noted that VAB marker clips had often deployed > 1 cm away from the target

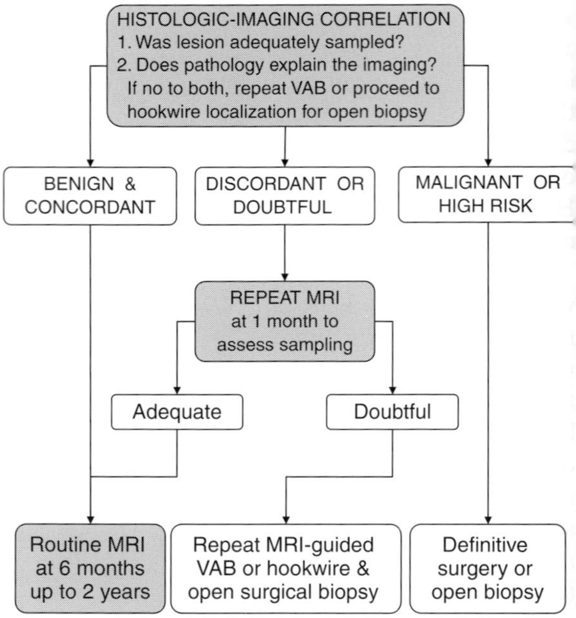

Fig. 4.3 Flow chart for correlation of imaging and histopathology after MRI-guided VAB.

lesion even when sampling was ultimately shown to be representative. A flow chart guide to management for histologic-imaging correlation after MRI-guided VAB is given in Fig. 4.3.

Histopathologic lesions which mimic malignancy on MRI

The second step in histologic-imaging correlation is to confirm that the tissue diagnosis does indeed fit the imaging findings. Apart from the initial difficulty in proving that an MRI-only lesion has been retrieved (because ex vivo imaging of the specimen is impossible), a further problem in correlating MRI-guided VAB results is that a wide range of benign pathology can cause enhancement on MRI. Occasionally even normal breast tissue could account for some non-specific findings, e.g., hormonally related focus, focal area or region of non-mass enhancement. Among false-positive lesions in one series of MRI-guided hookwire localizations, Langer *et al.* found variants of normal breast tissue accounted for two-thirds (20/29) [41].

Fundamentally then, the size and type of the MRI lesion must be taken into account in deciding if there is satisfactory histopathologic correlation and a concordant result. For example, a 3 mm papilloma seen on histopathology is likely to be incidental and should not be taken as concordant in the presence of a 10 mm stellate mass with washout. In fact, for mass lesions of 10 mm or greater, histopathologic correlation is usually rather straightforward with the major differential for invasive cancer being fibroadenoma or a complex sclerosing lesion (radial scar > 1 cm). However, a wider range of possibilities exists for small masses or foci.

Knowledge of the spectrum of benign lesions which simulate malignancy on MRI and lead to false-positive benign biopsies is then essential for radiologic–pathologic correlation. Equally, it is important to know when a benign result may not be acceptable. In this regard, caution is advised when a histologic diagnosis of non-specific fibrosis is obtained. In the study by Lee *et al.*, in 4/6 malignant discordant lesions at MRI-guided VAB, initial histopathology had shown non-specific fibrosis [25]. Stromal fibrosis was also the initial histologic result in one of the invasive cancers reviewed by Li *et al.* after having initially been accepted as a concordant benign result [24]. Therefore, due consideration should be given to further sampling where only fibrosis is obtained on MRI-guided VAB. In particular, the presence of significant architectural distortion as an imaging feature usually warrants surgical excision (Wendie Berg, personal communication, 2011).

Table 4.13 Benign causes for suspicious enhancing lesions

Focus or small mass
Focal adenosis – range of fibrocystic glandular proliferations especially sclerosing adenosis
Fibroadenomatoid hyperplasia
Fibroadenoma – internal septations usually not visible in small lesions
Papilloma – often rapid initial enhancement, may have associated ectatic duct
Normal intramammary lymph node – fatty hilus, characteristic morphology and location
Radial scar
PASH (pseudoangiomatous stromal hyperplasia)
Post-surgical scarring or focal fat necrosis
Other non-specific focal mastitis or inflammatory lesion
Non-mass enhancement
Usual ductal hyperplasia, CAPSS (columnar cell change), ADH
Non-specific proliferative fibrocystic changes
Lobular neoplasia – ALH and LCIS (lobular intraepithelial neoplasia)
PASH (pseudoangiomatous stromal hyperplasia)
Post-surgical reparative changes and fat necrosis
Other non-specific focal area of mastitis or inflammatory lesion

Focus or small mass on MRI

Enhancing foci and small masses < 5 mm in diameter have a generally low risk of malignancy and can often be safely followed up, [41, 42] particularly if kinetics are also benign (see Chapter 3) [43]. Benign proliferative fibrocystic change, or more accurately *focal adenosis*, is the most frequent offender in causing more "suspicious" foci leading to MRI-guided intervention. Several specific benign lesions, including fibroadenomas, papillomas and normal intramammary lymph nodes are often responsible for small masses. Some benign lesions which would be concordant with the MRI finding of a focus or small mass are given in Table 4.13.

Non-mass enhancement on MRI

The differential diagnosis of non-mass enhancement, discussed in Chapter 3, includes DCIS and ILC, while benign possibilities include the whole spectrum of proliferative fibrocystic changes from usual epithelial hyperplasia through to CAPSS lesions and ADH, together with lobular neoplasia. However, in the presence of a typical segmental or linear-ductal distribution of non-mass enhancement with clumped internal architecture, the PPV for DCIS is such that a purely benign histopathologic result may not be acceptable as concordant. A list of some benign pathologies which would be concordant with less specific MRI findings (focal area or region of stippled enhancement) is given in Table 4.13.

MULTIPLE CHOICE QUESTIONS

4.1 Answer true or false to the following statements

A. An advantage of MRI-guided VAB over 14-gauge CNB is the larger amount of tissue per core.
B. For patients on full anticoagulation, MRI-guided hookwire localization is often preferred to VAB.
C. Firm compression of the breast is essential before targeting small lesions at MRI-guided VAB.
D. The high technical failure rate of MRI-guided hookwire localization led to replacement by VAB.
E. MRI-guided VAB is the biopsy method of choice for a lesion adjacent to a silicone implant.

4.2 Answer true or false to the following statements
A. A marker clip at 10 mm from the biopsy site after MRI-guided VAB implies a missed target.
B. The "vanishing target phenomenon" refers to complete removal of a lesion at MRI-guided VAB.
C. For discordant benign pathology at MRI-guided VAB, 6-month follow-up MRI is recommended.
D. Histology showing a 5 mm papilloma would be considered concordant for an enhancing focus.
E. Histology showing stromal fibrosis satisfactorily accounts for a 5 mm enhancing stellate mass.

See page 189 for answers.

References

1. Daniel BL, Birdwell RL, Ikeda DM, *et al.* Breast lesion localization: a freehand, interactive MR imaging-guided technique. *Radiology* 1998; **207**: 455–63.
2. Orel SG, Schnall MD, Newman RW, *et al.* MR imaging-guided localization and biopsy of breast lesions: initial experience. *Radiology* 1994; **193**: 97–102.
3. Slanetz PJ, Jain R, Kline JL, *et al.* CT-guided preoperative needle localization of MR imaging-detected mammographically occult lesions. *AJR Am J Roentgenol* 1999; **172**: 160–2.
4. Kuhl CK, Morakkabati N, Leutner CC, *et al.* MR imaging–guided large-core (14-gauge) needle biopsy of small lesions visible at breast MR imaging alone. *Radiology* 2001; **220**: 31–9.
5. van den Bosch MAAJ, Daniel BL. MR-guided interventions of the breast. *Magn Reson Imaging Clin N Am* 2005; **13**: 505–17.
6. Perlet C, Heinig A, Prat X, *et al.* Multicenter study for the evaluation of a dedicated biopsy device for MR-guided vacuum biopsy of the breast. *Eur Radiol* 2002; **12**: 1463–70.
7. Perlet C, Heywang-Köbrunner SH, Heinig A, *et al.* Magnetic resonance-guided, vacuum-assisted breast biopsy. Results from a European multicenter study of 538 lesions. *Cancer* 2006; **106**: 982–90.
8. Lehman CD, Eby PR, Chen X, *et al.* MR imaging-guided breast biopsy using a coaxial technique with a 14-gauge stainless steel core biopsy needle and a titanium sheath. *AJR Am J Roentgenol* 2003; **181**: 183–5.
9. Chen X, Lehman CD, Dee KE. MRI-guided breast biopsy: clinical experience with 14-gauge stainless steel core biopsy needle. *AJR Am J Roentgenol* 2004; **182**: 1075–80.
10. Liberman L, Morris E, Dershaw DD, *et al.* Fast MRI-guided vacuum-assisted breast biopsy: initial experience. *AJR Am J Roentgenol* 2003; **181**: 1283–93.
11. Lehman CD, DePeri ER, Peacock S, *et al.* Clinical experience with MRI-guided vacuum-assisted breast biopsy. *AJR Am J Roentgenol* 2005; **184**: 1782–7.
12. Liberman L, Bracero N, Morris E, *et al.* MRI-guided 9-gauge vacuum-assisted breast biopsy: initial clinical experience. *AJR Am J Roentgenol* 2005; **185**: 183–93.
13. Orel SG, Rosen M, Mies C, *et al.* MR imaging-guided 9-gauge vacuum-assisted core-needle breast biopsy: initial experience. *Radiology* 2006; **238**: 54–61.
14. Heywang-Köbrunner SH, Sinnatamby R, Lebeau A, *et al.* Interdisciplinary consensus on the uses and technique of MR-guided vacuum-assisted breast biopsy (VAB): results of a European consensus meeting. *Eur J Radiol* 2009; **72**: 289–94.
15. Han B, Schnall MD, Orel SG, *et al.* Outcome of MRI-guided breast biopsy. *AJR Am J Roentgenol* 2008; **191**: 1798–804.
16. Morris EA, Liberman L, Dershaw DD, *et al.* Preoperative MR imaging-guided needle localization of breast lesions. *AJR Am J Roentgenol* 2002; **178**: 1211–20.
17. Hefler L, Casselman J, Amaya B, *et al.* Follow-up of breast lesions detected by MRI not biopsied due to absent enhancement of contrast medium. *Eur Radiol* 2003; **13**: 344–6.
18. Schrading S, Simon B, Braun M, *et al.* MRI-guided breast biopsy: influence of choice of vacuum biopsy system on the mode of biopsy of MRI-only suspicious breast lesions. *AJR Am J Roentgenol* 2010; **194**: 1650–7.
19. Meeuwis C, Peters NH, Mali WP, *et al.* Targeting difficult accessible breast lesions: MRI-guided needle localization using a freehand technique in a 3.0 T closed bore magnet. *Eur J Radiol* 2007; **62**: 283–8.
20. Morris EA, Liberman L, editors. *Breast MRI Diagnosis and Intervention*. New York, Springer, 2005.
21. Landheer ML, Veltman J, van Eekeren R, *et al.* MRI-guided preoperative wire localization of nonpalpable breast lesions. *Clin Imaging* 2006; **30**: 229–33.
22. Bedrosian I, Schlencker J, Spitz FR, *et al.* Magnetic resonance imaging-guided biopsy of mammographically and clinically occult breast lesions. *Ann Surg Oncol* 2002; **9**: 457–61.

23. Noroozian M, Gombos EC, Chikarmane S, *et al.* Factors that impact the duration of MRI-guided core needle biopsy. *AJR Am J Roentgenol* 2010; **194**: W150–7.

24. Li J, Dershaw DD, Lee CH, *et al.* MRI follow-up after concordant, histologically benign diagnosis of breast lesions sampled by MRI-guided biopsy. *AJR Am J Roentgenol* 2009; **193**: 850–5.

25. Lee J, Kaplan JB, Murray MP, *et al.* Imaging-histologic discordance at MRI-guided 9-gauge vacuum-assisted breast biopsy. *AJR Am J Roentgenol* 2007; **189**: 852–9.

26. Lee J, Kaplan JB, Murray MP, *et al.* Complete excision of the MRI target lesion at MRI-guided vacuum-assisted biopsy of breast cancer. *AJR Am J Roentgenol* 2008; **191**: 1198–202.

27. Genson CG, Blane CE, Helvie MA, *et al.* Effects on breast MRI of artifacts caused by metallic tissue marker clips. *AJR Am J Roentgenol* 2007; **188**: 372–6.

28. O'Flynn EAM, Wilson ARM, Michell MJ. Image-guided breast biopsy: state-of-the-art. *Clin Radiol* 2010; **65**: 259–70.

29. Mahoney MC. Initial clinical experience with a new MRI vacuum-assisted breast biopsy device. *J Magn Reson Imaging* 2008; **28**: 900–5.

30. Ghate SV, Rosen EL, Soo MSC, *et al.* MRI-guided vacuum-assisted breast biopsy with a handheld portable biopsy system. *AJR Am J Roentgenol* 2006; **186**: 1733–6.

31. Hauth EA, Jaeger HJ, Lubnau J, *et al.* MR-guided vacuum-assisted breast biopsy with a handheld biopsy system: clinical experience and results in postinterventional MR mammography after 24 h. *Eur Radiol* 2008; **18**: 168–76.

32. Salem C, Sakr R, Chopier J, *et al.* Pain and complications of directional vacuum-assisted stereotactic biopsy: comparison of the Mammotome and Vacora techniques. *Eur J Radiol* 2009; **72**: 295–9.

33. Carlson JW, Birdwell RL, Gombos EC, *et al.* MRI-directed, wire-localized breast excisions: incidence of malignancy and recommendations for pathologic evaluation. *Hum Pathol* 2007; **32**: 1754–9.

34. Lee J, Kaplan JB, Murray MP, *et al.* Underestimation of DCIS at MRI-guided vacuum-assisted breast biopsy. *AJR Am J Roentgenol* 2007; **189**: 468–74.

35. Liberman L, Holland AE, Marjan D, *et al.* Underestimation of atypical ductal hyperplasia at MRI-guided 9-gauge vacuum-assisted breast biopsy. *AJR Am J Roentgenol* 2007; **188**: 684–90.

36. Strigel RM, Eby PR, DeMartini WB, *et al.* Frequency, upgrade rates, and characteristics of high-risk lesions initially identified with breast MRI. *AJR Am J Roentgenol* 2010; **195**: 792–8.

37. Bernik SF, Troob S, Ying BL, *et al.* Papillary lesions of the breast diagnosed by core needle biopsy: 71 cases with surgical follow-up. *Am J Surg* 2009; **197**: 473–8.

38. Philpotts LE, Shaheen NA, Jain KS, *et al.* Uncommon high-risk lesions of the breast diagnosed at stereotactic core-needle biopsy: clinical importance. *Radiology* 2000; **216**: 831–7.

39. Maxwell AJ. Ultrasound-guided vacuum-assisted excision of breast papillomas: review of 6-years experience. *Clin Radiol* 2009; **64**: 801–6.

40. Berg WA. Image-guided breast biopsy and management of high-risk lesions. *Radiol Clin North Am* 2004; **42**: 935–46.

41. Langer SA, Horst KC, Ikeda DM, *et al.* Pathologic correlates of false positive breast magnetic resonance imaging findings: which lesions warrant biopsy? *Am J Surg* 2005; **190**: 633–40.

42. Liberman L, Mason G, Morris EA, *et al.* Does size matter? Positive predictive value of MRI-detected breast lesions as a function of lesion size. *AJR Am J Roentgenol* 2006; **186**: 426–30.

43. Eby PR, DeMartini WB, Gutierrez RL, *et al.* Characteristics of probably benign breast MRI lesions. *AJR Am J Roentgenol* 2009; **193**: 861–7.

Chapter 5

High-risk screening using breast MRI

Chapter outline

- Introduction
- Defining risk categories and identifying risk factors
- Women in the high-risk category
- Women in other risk subgroups
- Principles and limitations of XRM screening
- Performance of breast MRI in high-risk screening
- Principles and limitations of high-risk screening using breast MRI
- How long to screen for and at what internal

Introduction

The practical and the interpretative skills required to conduct a breast MRI program have been addressed in earlier chapters. In many centers, screening of women at high risk of breast cancer is now the commonest indication for performing breast MRI. This chapter will review breast screening concepts in general, and consider which women should be targeted for MRI screening. As gatekeepers of a precious resource, radiologists engaged in breast MRI screening, in close consultation with genetics experts and surgical colleagues, need to develop clear local guidelines on when MRI is considered appropriate. Other management options and issues relating to women at high risk of breast cancer are also addressed.

Defining risk categories and identifying risk factors

The likelihood of developing breast cancer is commonly expressed as *lifetime risk*, which for an average woman with no known risk factors is ~10%. Risk estimates vary between different populations, and the exact figure also depends on whether a lifetime is taken as up to age 70, 75, 80 or even 85 years. A risk estimate given for a specified time period is termed an *absolute risk*. When "lifetime risk" is determined at a particular age, this is the *absolute risk for the remainder of the defined life expectancy, and is more correctly termed cumulative residual lifetime risk*. Breast cancer is rare in the first three decades, so at age 30 years lifetime risk and cumulative residual lifetime risk are virtually identical. In later decades (despite the fact that incidence increases with age), residual lifetime risk actually decreases as more time elapses without breast cancer developing.

Definitions of what constitutes "high risk" are variable. In guidelines published in 2007, the ACS defined three categories, based on lifetime risk, for the purposes of decision-making in regard to which women should have screening breast MRI.

Risk categories defined by the ACS using lifetime risk:

High risk = lifetime risk 20–25% or greater

Moderate risk = lifetime risk 15–20%

Average or "normal" risk = lifetime risk not more than 10–15%

The ACS recommended annual breast MRI in addition to XRM screening for those at 20–25% or greater lifetime risk as estimated using any one of several mathematical models (Gail, Claus, Tyrer–Cuzick, BRCAPRO, BOADICEA) [1]. This advice included women with a high probability of carrying either a BRCA1 or BRCA2 gene mutation. Based on expert consensus opinion, women with other rare gene mutations strongly associated with breast cancer and a small group of women who had previously received RT to the chest for Hodgkin's disease or other malignancy were also recommended to have annual supplementary screening MRI.

Recognizing that there was insufficient evidence to make a recommendation either for or against MRI in women with 15–20% lifetime risk, the ACS suggested screening decisions should be made on a case-by-case basis. The ACS recommended against

MRI screening for those women considered to be at only average risk.

For clinical purposes it is helpful to give women an absolute risk estimate for a foreseeable period, e.g., the next 10 years, as this is more easily understood than a residual lifetime risk estimate. The 10-year absolute risk for breast cancer is age-dependent, increasing from <0.05% at age 20 years to ~2.5% at age 60 years for an average-risk woman (Table 5.1). Another advantage of a 10-year absolute risk estimate is that it will remain reasonably accurate when subdivided, e.g., if the 10-year absolute risk is 10%, the 5-year risk will be ~5% and the *annual risk* over that decade will be ~1%. Such risk estimates derived from mathematical models can also be used to define risk categories, e.g., a 5-year risk by the Gail model of >2% is often considered as "high risk" by clinicians.

Table 5.1 Defining breast cancer risk categories

Average risk = lifetime risk < 15% or relative risk less than 2 × average
Age 20 10-year absolute risk < 0.05%
Age 30 10-year absolute risk < 0.5%
Age 40 10-year absolute risk ~1.5%
Age 50 10-year absolute risk ~2.0%
Age 60+ 10-year absolute risk ~2 5%
Moderate risk = lifetime risk 15–20% or relative risk of 2–3 × average
Single first degree relative diagnosed with breast cancer < 50 years
Personal history of postmenopausal breast cancer (or > 50 years)
BI-RADS 3 density in isolation (heterogeneously dense or 50–75%)
Risk 15–20% by Claus, BRCAPRO, Tyrer–Cuzick models
Absolute risk of 3–5% over next 10 years by Tyrer–Cuzick model
High risk = lifetime risk > 20% or relative risk of at least 3–4 × average
Known mutation carrier (BRCA1/2, Li-Fraumeni, Cowden, Peutz-Jegher's)
Untested first degree relative of known carrier (50% risk of mutation)
From 8 years after RT to chest or mediastinum at age 10–30 years
LCIS (based on estimated absolute risk of 10–20% after 15–20 years)
ADH, particularly with a first degree family history (RR ~9×) or with breast density
Personal history of premenopausal breast cancer (or < 50 years)
BI-RADS 4 density (extremely dense or > 75%, RR 4–6×)
Combination of BI-RADS 3 density with family history or other risk factor
Risk > 20% by Claus, BRCAPRO, Tyrer–Cuzick models
Absolute risk of > 5% over next 10 years by Tyrer–Cuzick model

Risk factors are often quantified by *relative risk*, the ratio of the likelihood of developing cancer with the particular risk factor to the risk without it, e.g., the estimates of relative risk associated with a spectrum of pathologic diagnoses on breast biopsy given in Chapter 2. One alternative definition of "high risk" is any individual factor or combination of factors conferring an increase in relative risk of 3-fold or greater [2]. However, there is no agreed standard, and in Australia the NBOCC classifies a relative risk of 2- to 4-fold as "moderate" and greater than 4-fold as "strong" [3]. Comparing relative risks with the ACS categories, taking average lifetime risk as ~10%, a doubling of relative risk (to around ~20%) equates to at least the moderate-risk category.

In reality, of course, there is a continuous spectrum of risk across the population and the division into average-, moderate- and high-risk groups based on any particular known risk factor becomes inevitably rather arbitrary. As will be seen, several factors will influence the global risk for a given individual (Table 5.2). Neither lifetime risk, relative risk nor the assignment to a broad risk category readily captures the real implications of these factors for an individual woman at a given point in her life. It can then be appreciated why when communicating risks to women, absolute risk estimates for a 5- or 10-year period are the most meaningful [4].

Risk categories defined by relative risk:

High risk = relative risk of 3- to 4-fold or greater
Moderate risk = relative risk of 2- to 3-fold
Average risk = relative risk not more than 2-fold

Table 5.2 Risk factors for breast cancer

Age
BRCA1, BRCA2 or other breast cancer gene mutation
Breast density
History of chest, mediastinal, or axillary RT before age 30 years
Prior biopsy showing LCIS, ALH, ADH, proliferative fibrocystic changes
Strong family history (risk estimates by accepted mathematical models)
Personal history of breast cancer
Reproductive history (menarche, parity, breast-feeding, menopause)

Women in the high-risk category

Women in the following groups are considered to be high risk:

- known BRCA mutation or other gene strongly associated with breast cancer
- previous chest RT
- lifetime risk of 20–25% or greater by accepted mathematical models.

Cancer risks associated with BRCA mutations

The breast cancer risks for BRCA carriers are substantial, even for very young women. For a BRCA1 carrier at age 20 years the 10-year absolute risk for breast cancer is ~2%, already equivalent to that for an average-risk woman at age 50 years. By age 30 years the 10-year absolute breast cancer risk for a BRCA1 carrier has risen to ~10% and by age 40 years it is ~20% (Table 5.3).

Overall lifetime risk estimates to age 70 years for breast cancer have been placed at 57–65% for BRCA1 and 40–45% for BRCA2 in meta-analyses [5, 6]. Women who are known BRCA mutation carriers also face a higher incidence of ovarian cancer, an effect which is much greater for BRCA1 (lifetime risk to age 70 years 40–50%) than BRCA2 (lifetime risk 10–20%) [5, 6]. Male breast cancer is much more frequent in BRCA2 gene mutation carriers, with a lifetime risk to age 70–80 years of 6–9% (roughly equal to an average-risk woman) [7]. Mutations in BRCA2 are also associated with increased risk of a variety of other malignant tumors in both men and women, notably prostate and pancreatic cancer (Table 5.4) [8, 9]. The risks for developing cancers other than breast and ovary in BRCA1 mutation carriers are more modest, although women may be at increased risk of endometrial (RR ~ 2.7) and cervical cancer (RR ~3.7) [10].

Table 5.3 Indicative 10-year absolute risks for BRCA-related breast and ovarian cancer

	BRCA1 breast	BRCA2 breast	BRCA1 ovary	BRCA2 ovary
Age 20	2%	1%	1%	0.2%
Age 30	10%	7%	2%	0.5%
Age 40	20%	15%	7%	2%
Age 50	20%	15–20%	15%	5%
Age 60	20%	15–20%	22%	10%

Chen *et al* [6].

Table 5.4 Other reported BRCA2-associated cancers

Prostate cancer (before age 65 years, RR ~7)
Male breast cancer (RR ~100)
Pancreatic (RR ~3.5)
Gastric (RR ~2.5)
Gallbladder and bile duct (RR ~5)
Melanoma (RR ~2.5)

Breast Cancer Linkage Consortium [8], van Asperen *et al.* [9]

After an initial breast cancer diagnosis, BRCA women also have a greatly increased risk of developing contralateral breast cancer. A recent study showed that BRCA1 carriers have a ~4.5-fold and BRCA2 carriers a ~3.5-fold increased risk compared to non-carriers [11]. For a BRCA carrier with a first diagnosis of breast cancer before age 35 years the 10-year absolute risk for developing cancer in the opposite breast is ~30% or about 3% per year.

It should then be apparent why *primary prevention* strategies to reduce risk (RRSO, BPM and chemoprevention, see Appendix 7) are strongly recommended to these women once childbearing is complete. However, increased surveillance using breast MRI screening offers the best possible *secondary prevention* until such time as women are prepared to consider the more drastic primary preventive options. The untested first degree relatives of a proven BRCA mutation carrier each have a 50% chance of carrying the mutation and should also be recommended for high-risk surveillance with MRI pending the results of genetic testing.

In most other cases, the possibility of a BRCA gene is suggested by a strong family history or by a mathematical risk model, as discussed below. Occasionally, genetic testing may be considered based on a personal history of breast cancer diagnosed at a young age but without an extensive family history. In such cases, histopathologic data can be helpful for predicting a BRCA1 mutation. The probability that a woman diagnosed with breast cancer at age 30–35 years harbors a BRCA1 mutation is ~5%. However, if the histology showed this was a grade 3, ER-negative breast cancer, the chance of finding a BRCA1 mutation is increased to 25–30% [12, 13], and may be higher in the presence of a typical triple-negative phenotype [14]. Other rare genes associated with high breast cancer risk as part of known clinical syndromes are listed in Appendix 8.

Risk after previous radiation therapy to the chest

Women who have received mantle RT to the chest for Hodgkin's disease are a very high-risk subgroup, comparable to BRCA mutation carriers and recommended for MRI screening by the ACS [1]. However, the individual risk varies widely according to several factors including age at diagnosis, number of years since diagnosis and exact type of therapy used, with chemotherapy and pelvic radiation having a protective effect relating to ovarian suppression [1, 15–17].

For a woman treated for Hodgkin's lymphoma at age 25 years, with a chest radiation dose of 40 Gy, the absolute risk of breast cancer is ~1.5% after 10 years, ~10% after 20 years and ~30% after 30 years [17]. Accordingly, as with BRCA mutation carriers, patients should be counseled regarding primary preventive strategies such as prophylactic mastectomy or chemoprevention. Similar levels of increased risk may apply to chest RT given for other tumors in childhood or adolescence [18]. Annual screening MRI is recommended to commence from age 25 years for childhood exposure, or from 8 years after completion of RT for adults [1, 19].

After chest RT there is a high incidence of bilateral tumors, with synchronous or metachronous cancers seen in 20–30% of patients [20]. The cancers are more often located in the medial quadrants than is typical (40–50% versus 20% in a sporadic distribution) [20]. Cancers in this group of women are reported to be visible on XRM in ~90% of cases, with this unusually high sensitivity reflecting the presence of microcalcification in 62–72% of abnormal mammograms [19]. Screening XRM is therefore recommended despite young age and frequent breast density, as the potential benefit for a 30-year-old woman having an annual XRM to age 50 years is estimated to exceed the risk of cancer induction by a factor of 100-fold [19].

Women assessed as high risk using mathematical models

A further category recommended for MRI screening by the ACS is women with a lifetime risk of 20–25% or greater by accepted mathematical models. Such algorithms are widely used by clinicians to help quantify risk and advise women on appropriate management options, but they are also potentially valuable to radiologists in selecting women for MRI screening. All are based on family history, which to a large extent is used as a surrogate indicator for the possible presence of a BRCA mutation. Some models allow inclusion of other risk factors and so can provide a more global breast cancer risk estimate. There is though, considerable variation in design and accuracy of the various models, and not all are suited to the task of selecting women for MRI screening in a radiology practice setting.

Among the available models, the original and clinically still widely used 1989 Gail model is not suitable because it includes only affected first degree maternal-side relatives and does not take into account age at diagnosis. When evaluating familial breast cancer, because BRCA mutations show autosomal dominant inheritance, the maternal- and paternal-side history are equally important (but also independent, i.e., the number of affected relatives on each side cannot be added together). Cases of breast or ovarian cancer should be sought in first degree (mother, sister, daughter, father, brother, son) and second degree relatives (grandparents, aunts and uncles, nieces and nephews). Furthermore, both the Gail and the Claus models are known to significantly underestimate future breast cancer risk, [21] and neither can be used to predict the risk of a BRCA mutation.

The 2004 Tyrer–Cuzick model (IBIS Risk Evaluator) addressed the deficiencies of earlier algorithms by including an extensive family history, reproductive/hormonal factors and previous high-risk biopsy (atypical hyperplasia and LCIS) in a single software package [21–23]. This includes most of the information radiologists need to (i) estimate global risk (for MRI screening) and (ii) estimate BRCA mutation risk (for referral for genetic counseling). The BRCAPRO and BOADICEA models were developed specifically to predict the likelihood of a BRCA mutation being present, and are more suited to use by genetic counselors.

The easy-to-use format of the Tyrer–Cuzick software is well suited to use in a radiology practice, allowing rapid data input and automatically generating a family pedigree chart. Results are given as both a residual lifetime risk and a 10-year absolute risk, together with probability estimates for BRCA1 and BRCA2 mutations. The Tyrer–Cuzick model has been shown to be consistently more accurate in predicting breast cancer risk than the Gail, Claus or Ford (BRCAPRO) models, [21] and it shows close correlation with observed incidences in BRCA1 and BRCA2 families [24]. The ability of the Tyrer–Cuzick model to predict BRCA mutations has also been validated against other models used by genetic counselors [25].

Women in other risk subgroups

For the great majority of women, i.e., the > 95% who are not clearly at high risk because of a known breast cancer gene or previous chest RT, the challenge is to categorize their global risk. To do this, a range of risk factors need to be considered, which fall into four main groups [22]:

- family history
- reproductive history
- history of previous "high-risk" biopsy
- breast density.

Family history

The BRCA1/2 mutations and other known breast cancer genes together explain only about half of all familial breast cancer cases, with the remainder probably attributable to a range of more common but less powerful polygenes acting in combination, including some which act by influencing breast density. Therefore, family history is a common and important risk factor in its own right, and not just a surrogate for a possible BRCA or other high-risk gene.

From meta-analysis, we know that lifetime risk estimates to age 80 years for women with zero, one or two first degree relatives affected by breast cancer are about 8%, 13% and 21% respectively [26]. Based on this, women with two or more affected first degree relatives (~1% of the population) can be placed in the high-risk category. However, a complicating factor to consider is that exact risk for a given individual with a family history is significantly age-dependent, as will become apparent.

The relative risk for a woman aged 50 years with a single first degree affected relative is ~2-fold, with two affected first degree relatives is ~3-fold and for three or more ~4-fold [26]. For a woman aged < 35 years, the relative risk with a single affected first degree relative is at least 3-fold, but by age 60 years has fallen to ~1.5-fold. With two affected first degree relatives, the relative risk for a woman aged < 45 years is > 5-fold but is just over 2-fold for a woman aged > 65 years [26]. The age at which affected family members developed breast cancer further influences risk, so that a woman aged 40–45 years with a single first degree relative diagnosed before age 40 years has a 3-fold relative risk (Fig. 5.1) [26].

As can be seen, risk evaluation of family history is complex, and probability algorithms like the Tyrer–Cuzick model are invaluable to make the task easier. Lifetime risk or 10-year absolute risk estimates can be used to guide screening strategies in line with individual women's requirements and local circumstances. Genetic testing may be considered if the probability of finding a BRCA mutation is at least 10–15% (Appendix 8), and radiologists should be aware of other specific clinical features which might prompt referral for genetic counseling (Table 5.5).

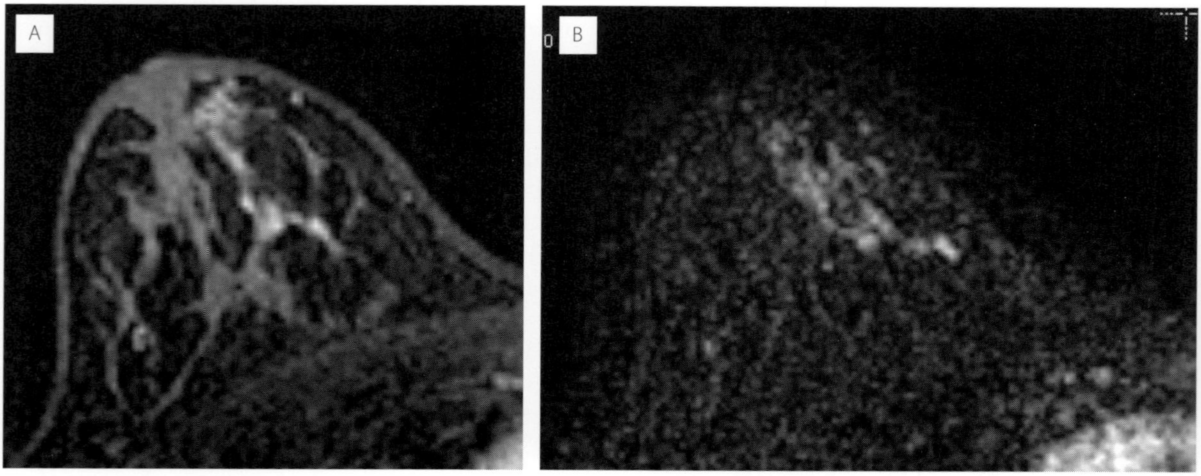

Fig. 5.1 Screen-detected pure DCIS: Second round screening MRI in a 39-year-old woman with family history of breast cancer: mother in 50s and sister at age 38 years. By Tyrer–Cuzick model lifetime risk was 22%, 10-year absolute risk was 4% and BRCA1/2 risk < 5%. Axial fat-suppressed T1-weighted image (A) and subtracted image (B) show segmental distribution of clumped non-mass enhancement with reticular architectural pattern. XRM and TUS were normal, with MRI-guided hookwire excision revealing high-grade DCIS. Patient opted for bilateral mastectomy with final histopathology showing 50 mm of high-grade DCIS without invasion.

Table 5.5 Some factors prompting referral to a genetic counselor for possible testing

Untested first degree relative of known BRCA mutation carrier (50% risk of carrying gene)
At least two first or second degree relatives with premenopausal breast cancer or ovarian cancer
Close relative with bilateral breast cancer or history of breast and ovarian cancer in same woman
Close relative with male breast cancer (suggests BRCA2)
Ashkenazi Jewish descent (or similar group with known founder mutation)
BRCA mutation risk of > 10–15% by Tyrer–Cuzick model
Personal history of breast cancer < 50 years plus relative with premenopausal breast or ovarian cancer
Personal history of grade 2 or 3 ER –ve breast cancer diagnosed < 40 years, especially if triple-negative

Reproductive history and hormonal factors

In essence, it is the sustained effects of estrogen which increase risk (menstruation and HRT), while factors which suppress ovulation (multiple pregnancies and prolonged breast-feeding) are protective. For most women the effects on risk are modest compared to the influence of family history [3, 22, 26]. Nevertheless, they are significant risk modifiers in some women and their inclusion in global risk assessment models is important.

The following hormonal factors may confer an up to 2-fold increase in risk:

(i) increased duration of menstruation (menarche age < 12 years, menopause age > 55 years)
(ii) oral contraceptive pill (controversial) – risk normal by 10 years after cessation
(iii) HRT (especially estrogen/progestogen) – risk normal by 1 year after cessation
(iv) high postmenopausal endogenous estrogen levels (may relate to obesity).

The following features in the reproductive history contribute to slightly reduced risk:

(i) having one child reduces risk by ~20% versus nulliparous
(ii) having four children versus one child reduces risk by a further ~20%
(iii) first child at age < 20 years reduces risk by ~30–40% versus first child at age > 30 years
(iv) breast-feeding reduces risk by 4–5% for each cumulative year.

History of previous high-risk biopsy

Relative risks associated with a range of possible benign findings on breast biopsy have been discussed in Chapter 2 (Table 2.7). Non-proliferative breast disease (fibrosis, cysts, duct ectasia, fat necrosis, mastitis) have no increased risk, while proliferative fibrocystic changes and benign lesions without atypia are associated with ~2.0-fold increased risk (usual duct hyperplasia, solitary papilloma, simple fibroadenoma, radial scar). The risk may be as high as 3- to 4-fold for some lesions (sclerosing adenosis, multiple peripheral papillomas, complex fibroadenoma), but all can be included in the "hyperplasia without atypia" field using the Tyrer–Cuzick model, and global risk estimated in the context of age and family history. The presence of "atypia" (ADH or ALH) is considered to confer a 4–5-fold relative risk, while for ADH combined with a first degree family history, risk multiplies to ~9-fold [27].

Meanwhile, LCIS is estimated to confer up to 10-fold increased cancer risk [22]. A single study in the literature addresses the role of MRI in lobular neoplasia. From MRI screening over 6 years, Port *et al.* detected cancer occult to XRM in 5/135 (4%) of women with LCIS. All cancers were TNM stage 0 or I in women aged 39–55 years, of which one also had a first degree family history [28]. For lobular neoplasia in young women particularly then, MRI may be appropriate even with no other risk factors (Fig. 5.2). Favoring use of MRI is that lobular neoplasia usually progresses to ILC, a subtype often occult to XRM, particularly in dense breasts.

Breast density

A major risk factor not routinely included in mathematical models to date is breast density. Density is a strong independent risk factor with a predominantly hereditary mechanism, which is not simply due to masking effect and is not just confined to young women [29–34]. Breast density of at least moderate degree is so widely prevalent that, after age and BRCA mutation, it is probably the most important breast cancer risk factor on a population basis.

Incidence studies suggest that women with the most dense breasts (BI-RADS class 4) have an increased breast cancer risk of 4- to 6-fold compared to women in the least dense quintile (< 10%) [29, 30, 35, 36]. Despite inherent limitations in deriving % density estimates from 2D mammographic area measurements, [36] the use of Cumulus software is currently the best-validated

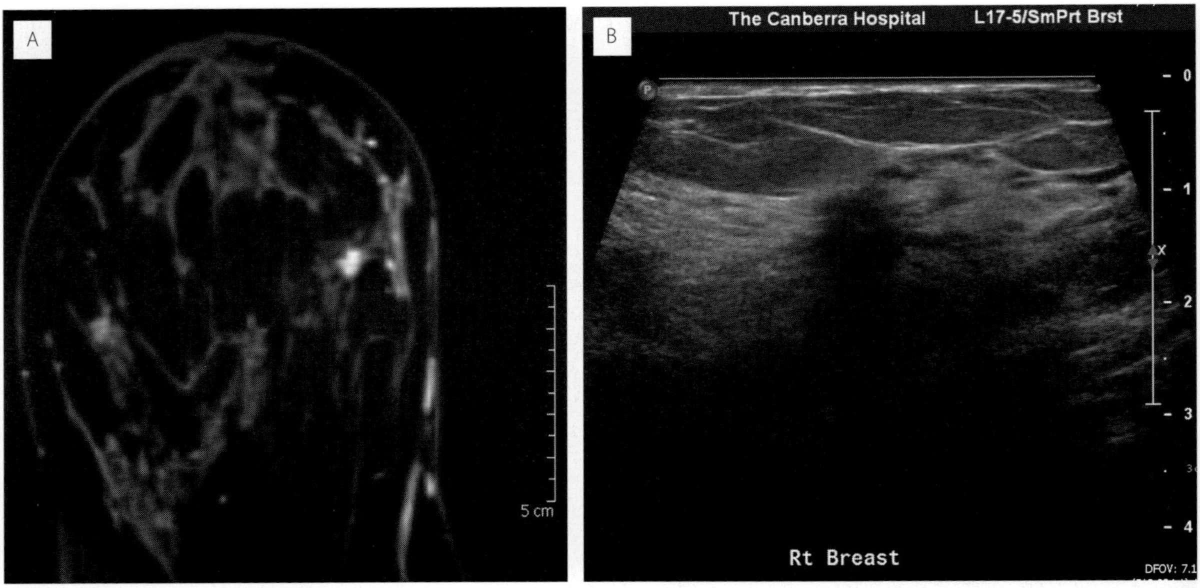

Fig. 5.2 Screen-detected invasive cancer: First round screening MRI in a 44-year-old woman with history of previous biopsy revealing ALH in left breast (normal XRM). (A) Early post-contrast axial fat-suppressed T1-weighted image shows solitary 5 mm focus/small mass medially in right breast which displayed a type 3 curve (washout kinetics). (B) Image from TUS showing a corresponding 7 mm hypoechoic stellate mass, found to be grade 2 invasive cancer on 14-gauge CNB.

technique for predicting breast cancer risk [29, 35, 37]. Even crude visual estimates of the proportion of dense tissue appear useful, particularly when both mammographic views are assessed [37]. This is important given that the visual BI-RADS classification is so widely used in clinical practice.

Recently, sophisticated software algorithms such as R2 Quantra (Hologic, Bedford, MA, USA) have become available for automatically calculating % volume estimates from digitally acquired mammograms, and have been integrated into commercially available CAD systems.

While most estimates have used % density, it is very possible that the absolute amount of dense tissue present may be the most accurate predictor of risk. This would fit well with an observed decrease in lifetime risk of ~40% after breast reduction surgery [38]. There is also epidemiologic evidence of a higher incidence of premenopausal breast cancer in young women with low BMI and large bra cup size (i.e., high absolute amount of dense tissue), but not in overweight or obese women with large breasts [39].

Work to validate methods for evaluating breast density is ongoing, and it is anticipated that density will be incorporated into risk assessment algorithms. Meanwhile, an acceptable workaround for the Tyrer–Cuzick model at least is to use the "hyperplasia without atypia" and "atypical hyperplasia" fields to respectively approximate risks for BI-RADS 3 and 4 density (Jack Cuzick, personal communication, 2011). This assumes that for BI-RADS class 3 risk is about 2- to 3-fold, and for density, BI-RADS class 4 density about 4- to 5-fold. The combination of dense breasts with an additional risk factor such as a first degree family history would then frequently constitute high risk (Fig. 5.3). Intuitively, BI-RADS 4 density alone could be considered to confer high risk, particularly when the masking effect is taken into account, but data from prospective studies using MRI in this subgroup are needed to better guide management.

Previous breast cancer diagnosis

A further group of women, steadily increasing in number as breast cancer treatment has improved, are the survivors from a previous breast cancer diagnosis. This is a factor not considered in most mathematical models which are designed only to predict a first breast cancer episode.

Women with a personal history of breast cancer have at least a 2- to 3-fold relative risk of developing a second primary in the contralateral breast (compared to the risk of unaffected women developing a first breast cancer), with 10-year absolute risk at 6–7% [40, 41]. If the first cancer was diagnosed before

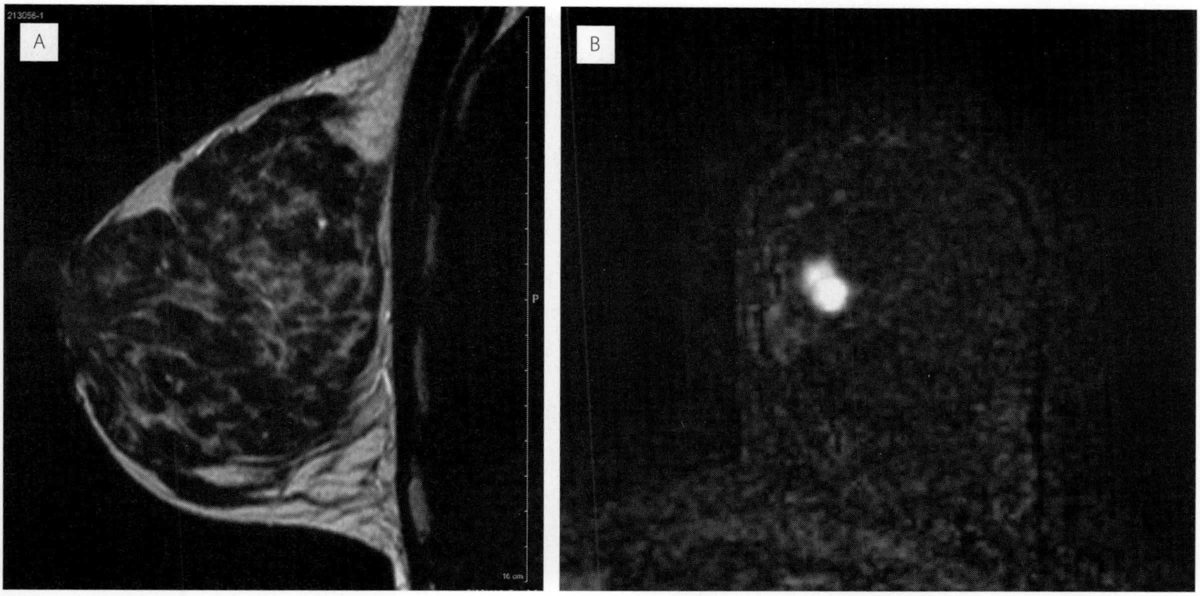

Fig. 5.3 **Screen-detected invasive cancer:** First round screening MRI in a 48-year-old woman with history of maternal breast cancer at age 53 years and BI-RADS 4 density evident on (A) sagittal T2-weighted image. By Tyrer–Cuzick model, 10-year absolute risk was < 5%, rising to > 15% after checking the "atypical hyperplasia" field to approximate risk associated with extreme density. (B) Early post-contrast axial subtracted image shows irregular mass with rapid wash-in. Both XRM and TUS were normal, with MRI-guided VAB showing IDC, treated with wide local excision. Final histopathology confirmed a 15 mm grade 2 IDC with negative SLNB.

age 40 years, this rises to >4-fold relative risk (Fig. 5.4) and increases further with a positive family history [40]. The use of chemotherapy for the index cancer lessens risk, while the addition of endocrine therapy (tamoxifen) reduces the risk of ER-positive contralateral cancer by about 50%. For a BRCA mutation carrier diagnosed before age 40 years there is 16-fold relative risk of contralateral cancer (Fig. 5.5).

Although data are limited, studies which have included women with a personal history of breast cancer in MRI screening have shown significant yields in this subgroup [42, 43]. In a recent study, among a cohort of 144 women (mean age 49 years) undergoing routine MRI surveillance solely on the basis of a personal history of breast cancer (i.e., with no family history), cancer was identified in 12% after a mean 2.7 years follow-up (range 1–9 years). Almost 60% were minimal cancers (DCIS or node-negative invasive cancer < 1 cm) and the PPV of biopsy was ~40% [44].

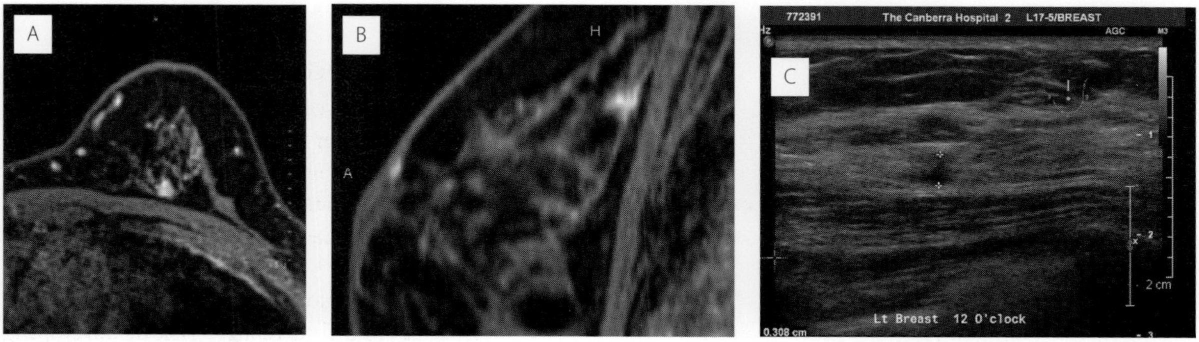

Fig. 5.4 **Screen-detected invasive cancer**: Fourth round screening MRI in a 41-year-old woman with previous left breast cancer diagnosed at age 35 years, treated with wide local excision and RT. Genetic testing had shown no BRCA mutation. (A) Axial and (B) sagittal fat-suppressed T1-weighted images of left breast show solitary 6 mm enhancing deep zone lesion (normal XRM). (C) TUS shows corresponding small deep zone hypoechoic lesion shown to be IDC on 14-gauge CNB. Patient opted for bilateral mastectomy with final pathology showing 5 mm grade 2 IDC, ER/PR +ve, HER2 –ve with background extensive low-grade DCIS (occult to XRM and MRI).

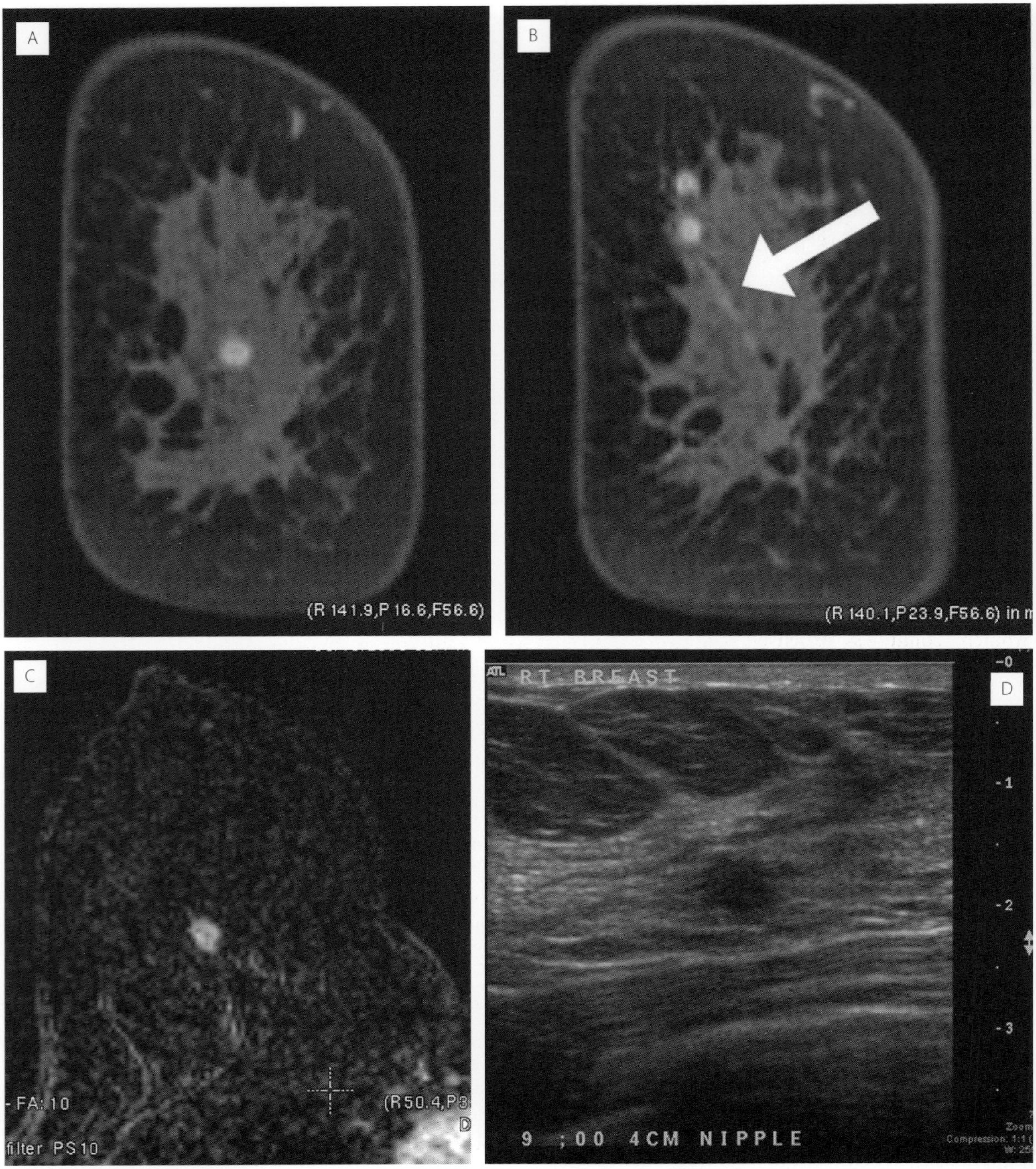

Fig. 5.5 Screen-detected multicentric cancer: Screening MRI in a 38-year-old woman with history of multifocal left breast cancer diagnosed 3 years earlier, treated with left mastectomy, ALND, anthracycline-based chemotherapy, ovarian ablation with goserelin and continuing tamoxifen. Patient refused XRM screening, previous screening MRI of right breast was normal. Post-contrast coronal T1-weighted images (A and B) show three new enhancing masses, the largest centrally showing fine linear enhancement consistent with lymphatic tumor bridging (arrow) to two further small lesions in UOQ. (C) Axial post-contrast subtracted image of central mass shows rim enhancement and spiculated margins. (D) On TUS, a relatively non-specific hypoechoic lesion corresponded to the central mass, with 14-gauge CNB showing IDC. Final pathology showed multicentric grade 3 IDC, 4–7 mm diameter, ER/PR +ve, HER2 –ve. Patient had further right mastectomy with 0/4 nodes involved on SLNB. Genetic testing, based on young patient age with contralateral breast cancer (despite absence of a family history), revealed a BRCA2 mutation.

Screening with MRI can then be recommended, for women with a premenopausal breast cancer history, and in women diagnosed over age 50 years if there are other risk factors, e.g., family history or breast density. A history of previous ILC or of IDC/DCIS which was occult to XRM may be particularly appropriate candidates for MRI screening.

Principles and limitations of XRM screening

Having reviewed the key factors which influence breast cancer risk, it should be clear that for only a small percentage of women does a single strong factor (BRCA mutation or other genetic syndrome, prior chest RT) place them in the high-risk category. In many more women, combinations of more common but less powerful risk factors may confer a similar level of risk, and mathematical modeling can help to quantify the individual effect. Before exploring the potential role of MRI, it is worth reviewing the basic principles of XRM screening and then considering the question that if XRM is not adequate for some women, could less expensive adjunctive measures such as US be successfully employed?

Screening means applying a diagnostic test to an apparently normal, healthy population. Only those individuals who are actually found to have the target disease stand to benefit. To be considered for population screening, the target disease must be common enough and serious enough to warrant the use of resources, and early intervention must be able to significantly improve prognosis. The disease should then have a predictable course with the opportunity for detection both before symptoms occur and before it is too late to alter outcomes. In breast cancer screening, this means a significant number of cases detected must be EBC (TNM Stage II or less) when there is the prospect of surgical cure. Finding small invasive cancers with negative axillary nodes confers the best hope of achieving an overall population survival benefit. Data on more than 50 000 women with node-negative invasive cancers < 10 mm in diameter shows breast cancer-related deaths at just 4% after 10 years [45].

In breast cancer screening, a complicating factor is that the target disease is remarkably heterogeneous. At one end of the spectrum there is life-threatening, aggressive, high-grade invasive cancer while at the other is low-grade DCIS which might never progress to invasive cancer in any given patient's lifetime. Those patients with "cancer" that would not have become clinically apparent or shortened their lives are overtreated by screening programs, enduring significant bodily harm and psychologic stress without benefit.

Furthermore, in the case of breast cancer, not only is the target disease heterogeneous but so also is the target population, which in reality consists of many individuals with widely differing risk profiles due to genetic and environmental factors. Some women may be "over-screened" because their risk is so low, while for others at very high risk, screening mammography alone is probably inadequate for effective surveillance.

To date, XRM is the only imaging test which has been extensively applied to population screening for breast cancer. There is clear evidence of a mortality reduction in screened populations, with most estimates in the range of 25–35% for women aged 50–70 years. However, at least one-third (and possibly closer to two-thirds) of this overall benefit may be due to improved treatment, particularly adjuvant chemotherapy [46, 47]. The proportion of "lives saved" attributable to XRM screening alone is therefore uncertain.

Despite XRM being the only breast screening test associated with a proven mortality reduction, some still argue that its use is not justified. A Cochrane review, evaluating seven trials involving some half a million women, estimated the mortality reduction benefit from XRM alone to be 15–20%, and concluded that, taking into account over diagnosis and overtreatment of some patients, it was "not clear whether screening does more good than harm" [48]. Furthermore, a meta-analysis of data from several national screening programs estimated the rate of over diagnosis to be as high as 50%, so that 1 in 3 cancers might be overtreated [49]. Including all DCIS cases in the "cancer" definition is the major source of over diagnosis while some forms of invasive disease, e.g., tubular carcinoma, likely also contribute. Unfortunately, we cannot yet reliably distinguish the potentially lethal cancers from those which might be better thought of as "pathologic cancer, but not clinical disease."

So, despite a wealth of accumulated data, controversy persists as to whether screening XRM is even worthwhile. Recently significant changes have been made in evidence-based mammographic screening recommendations by the US Preventive Services Task Force which aim to maximize benefit and minimize harm. Biennial (not annual) screening is proposed from 50 to 74 years, while selective risk-based application of biennial screening is preferred to routine screening from age 40 to 50 years [50].

For the typical target population of women over age 50 years undergoing XRM screening, an overall invasive cancer detection rate of ~4 per 1000 is an appropriate benchmark (easily remembered as 5 malignant diagnoses per 1000 women including 20% DCIS). Recall rates of ~10% are considered acceptable for the first screening (prevalence) round, while ~5% is probably optimal for subsequent (incidence) rounds. The higher first round recall rate reflects not only the prevalence of cancer in hitherto unscreened women, but also the difficulty in interpretation of XRM in the absence of a prior study for comparison. Biopsy in a screening XRM program aims for a PPV of at least 25% (benign to malignant biopsy ratio of 3:1). Over half of malignancies detected should be small node-negative invasive cancers or DCIS (TNM Stage 0 or I) in order to achieve the expected long-term survival benefit.

Limitations of screening XRM in young women and dense breasts

High sensitivity for the target disease is a fundamental requirement for a screening test. In breast cancer screening, the "detection" definition of sensitivity is applied whereby a screen-detected cancer is a true-positive result, and any cancer detected in the interval between screens is a false-negative.

One meta-analysis estimated the overall sensitivity of XRM to be in the range of 83–95% (median 90%) for annual screening [51]. However, sensitivity fell to only ~70% where 2-yearly screening was performed, reflecting the longer interval which allows more "missed" cancers to appear. That study also noted that the sensitivity of screening XRM in women below age 50 years was, on average, 10 percentage points lower than for women aged 50 to 59 years. Therefore for women in the 40–50 years age group, sensitivity is expected to reduce to ~60% with a 2-yearly screening interval. About 25% of women presenting with breast cancer are below age 50 years.

The primary cause of reduced mammographic sensitivity in young women is increased breast density. More than half of women aged < 50 years and at least a third of women aged > 50 years have BI-RADS 3 or 4 breast density (Table 1.8), with studies confirming that XRM sensitivity falls to as low as only 30–56% in the densest breasts [52–54].

Furthermore, XRM screening has a general bias towards the detection of slower-growing invasive cancers. Faster-growing cancers are more likely to escape XRM detection and present as interval cancers, with potentially poorer outcomes. Unfortunately, high-grade invasive cancers with rapid tumor growth occur more frequently in younger women, compounding the problem of the reduced sensitivity of XRM in this group [55, 56]. It is then not surprising that the benefit from screening XRM in women aged 40–50 years is more marginal, with best estimates of 15–25% mortality reduction in this age-group [57, 58]. It has also been estimated that a decade of annual two-view screening XRM commencing before the age of 40 years could result in a net increase in breast cancer deaths [59].

High specificity is also important for a screening test in order to minimize potential harm caused by false-positive results. Specificity in breast screening programs is determined by the percentage of screened subjects recalled for further assessment but subsequently shown not to have cancer. Due to the cumulative effect, over 10 rounds of screening XRM about half of all women receive a false-positive recall, while almost 20% will have had a negative biopsy [60]. False-positive recalls are more frequent in younger women, those with dense breasts or on HRT, and those with a family history [61, 62]. In one study, false-positive recalls after nine screening rounds varied from only 5% for women at low risk up to 100% for women with multiple risk factors [62]. These findings add support for a tailored approach to screening, with a pressing need to improve the sensitivity for cancer detection in young dense breasts.

Possible measures to improve screening in young, dense breasts

Breast self-examination and clinical breast examination

A Cochrane review from 2003, which assessed data from two large trials, suggested no benefit from screening by BSE. Rather, a potential for harm was identified due to an increased number of benign biopsies [63]. In a study comparing performance of CBE, US and XRM in almost 28 000 screening episodes, Kolb and coworkers found that CBE independently detected "extremely few cancers" [52]. Therefore, neither BSE or CBE appear to be effective for screening of the general population.

In women at high risk, interval cancers first palpated by the patient are more frequently encountered, but cancers detected only by routine CBE remain relatively few. Despite this, 6-monthly CBE is included in many high-risk surveillance programs. Since the incidence of self-detected cancers is much higher than in the general population, some high-risk programs also strongly encourage frequent and regular BSE [64].

Digital mammography

In the ACRIN DMIST, almost 50 000 women from over 33 centers underwent both conventional film-screen and digital XRM [65, 66]. Although overall diagnostic accuracy of digital and film XRM was similar, there was a statistically significant detection benefit of digital XRM in women under the age of 50 years and in those with dense breasts. Taking a BI-RADS score of 4 or 5 as a positive result (and with 12-month follow-up to allow for interval cancers) the sensitivity of digital XRM in women below age 50 years was 78% compared with 51% for film XRM. For all women with BI-RADS class 3–4 density, digital XRM sensitivity was 70% compared with 55% for film XRM. It is then possible that digital technology may overcome some of the limitations of XRM screening in young women with dense breasts, while new techniques like contrast-enhanced digital XRM and tomosynthesis may also have a significant impact.

Screening ultrasound

Used as a screening test adjunctive to XRM, US has the capability to significantly increase detection rates for invasive cancer in women with dense breasts, with incremental yields of 39–57% across several large studies [52, 53, 67–69]. The majority of additional cancers shown by US are small early-stage invasive cancers, with around 70% < 10 mm in size and ~90% being axillary node negative [52, 67]. The major limitation of US as a screening test is the very substantial number of false-positive biopsies generated, with reported PPVs of 10% at best (9:1 benign to malignant biopsy ratio) [52, 67, 68].

The ACRIN 6666 trial recruited asymptomatic women over age 25 years with BI-RADS class 3–4 breast density by XRM, plus at least one additional significant risk factor [67]. Among 2637 women, the addition of screening US to XRM increased the cancer yield by over 50%, but again the PPV for an US biopsy recommendation was low at only ~9%. Nevertheless, the sensitivity of XRM alone in this study was only 50%, increasing to 78% for the combination of XRM and US.

Given the limited availability of MRI, screening US additional to digital XRM offers an option for women with breast density in the moderate-risk category. Current problems are logistical factors in service delivery and the low reported PPV for US-generated biopsies. The advent of automated whole breast US is likely to make the task technically easier and may improve accuracy.

Performance of breast MRI in high-risk screening

Women who are known or suspected to carry a BRCA1 or BRCA2 gene mutation have been the obvious target group for assessment of the efficacy of screening breast MRI. Meta-analysis suggests the risk of developing breast cancer by age 70 years is ~65% for women with BRCA1 mutations and ~45% for BRCA2 mutations, although the risk may be substantially higher in some families [5]. Given that up to half of all BRCA women develop breast cancer before menopause, a reliable means of cancer detection in dense breasts is vital. In young women generally, and in BRCA mutation carriers particularly, invasive cancers are often high grade, show a rapid growth pattern and present as circumscribed or ill-defined non-spiculated masses [55, 70]. Furthermore, XRM sensitivity for DCIS is low among BRCA women, even with fatty breasts, because microcalcification is often absent (Fig. 5.6) [71]. Therefore, a number of tumor characteristics and frequent breast density contribute to poor performance of XRM, while the aggressive nature of tumors in BRCA carriers suggests that prognosis could be adversely affected by delayed diagnosis. For mutation carriers screened only by annual XRM, almost half present as interval cancers and up to 50% of those are axillary lymph node positive [72–74].

Women placed in the high-risk category are usually recommended to begin annual XRM screening at age 25–30 years, or at least 5 years earlier than the age of the youngest affected relative. For BRCA1 carriers, screening from as early as age 20–25 years has been considered reasonable [75]. At such young age, however, the risk of radiation-induced breast cancer is considerably increased, and this is a particular concern in women with BRCA mutations, who by definition have faulty DNA-repair genes and may be particularly susceptible to the effects of ionizing radiation. One epidemiologic study found ~50% increase in breast cancer risk for BRCA mutation carriers after any exposure to chest x-rays, [76] while a recent meta-analysis of six studies suggests a 2.5-fold increased risk from either XRM or chest x-rays performed

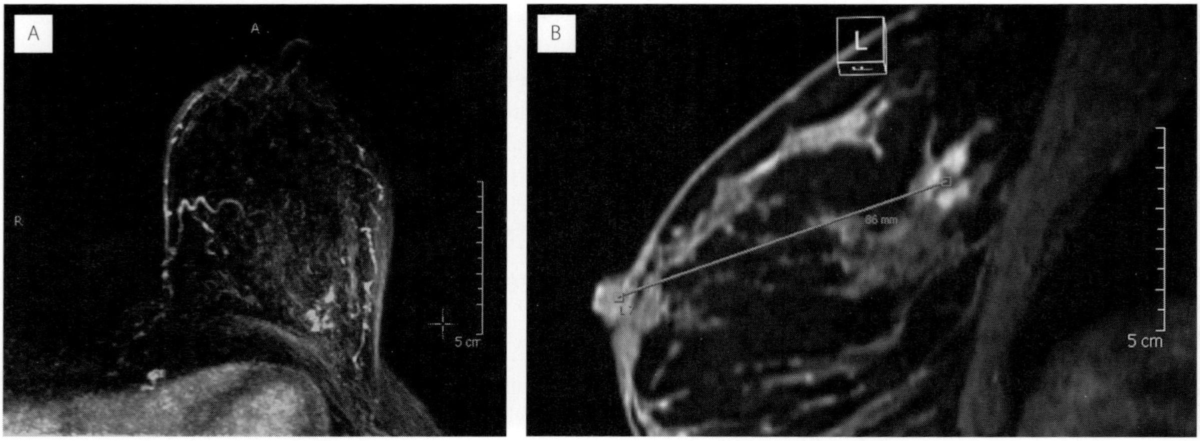

Fig. 5.6 Screen-detected pure DCIS: Third round screening MRI in a 47-year-old BRCA1 carrier. (A) Axial MIP and (B) sagittal oblique reformatted fat-suppressed T1-weighted image show 20 mm focal area of clumped enhancement which had no XRM or TUS correlate. MRI-guided VAB revealed high-grade DCIS and the patient opted for bilateral mastectomy. Histopathologic extent of high-grade DCIS without invasion exactly correlated with size estimated by MRI.

before age 20 years. It does then seem particularly likely that for young BRCA mutation carriers (below age 35 years), annual XRM screening may cause significant harm [77].

Not surprisingly then, when breast MRI became established as a sensitive method for the detection of invasive breast cancer, its potential for use in BRCA mutation carriers was soon considered, leading to a number of trials being launched in the mid to late 1990s. Several such studies are now available from which we can assess the performance of breast MRI in asymptomatic women at high risk of familial breast cancer.

First published was a study from Germany, by Kuhl *et al.* in 2000, comprising 192 known or suspected gene mutation carriers [78]. Screening MRI identified cancer in nine women, while US and XRM combined detected only four of the nine cases. All nine cancers were node negative, Stage 0 or I, with the invasive cancers having a mean diameter of 10.5 mm. In 2005, the same group reported additional data on 529 women amongst whom 19 cancers were detected only by MRI, comprising 5 high-grade DCIS and 14 node-negative invasive cancers with a mean size of 7.5 mm [79]. Sensitivity of MRI was 91% compared with 49% for both XRM and US combined.

Another single-center study from Canada examined a cohort of 236 women, all of whom were proven BRCA mutation carriers, and found 22 cancers [80]. The sensitivity of MRI was 77%, more than double that of XRM, which detected only 36% of cancers. Screening US was also included and had a sensitivity of 33%, while combined sensitivity of XRM and US was 67%. Of all invasive cancers detected, 90% were node negative.

The largest published series, by Kriege *et al.*, was the Dutch (MRISC) multicenter study which screened 1909 women with estimated lifetime risk of at least 15%, including 358 mutation carriers [81]. This study also compared findings with two age-matched control groups, the first drawn from sporadic cancers in the general population, and the second derived from unscreened patients with a lifetime risk of > 15% based on family history. Importantly, the incidence of node-positive invasive cancers observed in the screened population was 21% versus 52% and 56% in the sporadic and high-risk control groups respectively. In the screened group, 43% of invasive cancers were less than 10 mm in diameter, which was > 3-fold the number of subcentimeter cancers found in each of the two control groups.

A further multicenter study of 649 women from the UK (MARIBS) selected only women aged < 50 years who were either known gene mutation carriers, a first degree relative of a carrier or had at least a 1% annual risk of breast cancer [82]. This design then combined both high familial risk and an age demographic with the highest expected prevalence of breast density. Mean size of invasive cancers was 15 mm, with 38% less than 10 mm in diameter, while ~80% were node negative.

These four large trials (German, Canadian, Dutch and UK) were all prospective, each detected in excess of 20 cancers, and all had the follow-up data required to allow an accurate estimation of the sensitivity and specificity of MRI as summarized in Table 5.6. Together, the sensitivity of MRI was in the range of 71–91%, with specificity of 81–97%. Over all the studies, 151 cancers were detected, of which 67 were found only by MRI, giving ~80% incremental sensitivity, with very few interval cancers reported. A good yield of small node-negative invasive cancers was seen across all studies. In all but the UK study, the PPV for a biopsy generated by an MRI finding averaged 50% (a 1:1 benign to malignant biopsy ratio).

Another important feature to underscore is the high NPV of MRI in the screening setting. In the German and Canadian single-center studies, NPV was documented at 97% and 99% respectively. Therefore, in the absence of any suspicious enhancing lesion, the risk of a missed invasive cancer is extremely low, so a normal result is very reassuring for the patient. The same cannot be said for XRM, even in the general population, where the reality is that a large number of women are falsely reassured about the absence of cancer.

Furthermore, it should be noted that despite much higher sensitivity of MRI in these trials, overall the specificity of MRI was only slightly lower than for XRM. The lowest specificity, and lowest PPV for MRI-generated biopsy at 25% (benign to malignant biopsy ratio of 3:1), was in the UK MARIBS trial. However, that study involved 22 different centers, so that the MRI experience of individual radiologists was probably less than in the other studies.

Detection of DCIS by MRI screening

It has long been known that MRI could sometimes demonstrate DCIS, and that in some instances this was non-calcified disease, occult to XRM. However, early reports of MRI sensitivity for DCIS were very variable, with a range of 40–100% quoted in the literature.

Across the four high-risk screening trials, spanning 1996–2004, rates of DCIS detection by MRI varied significantly. Although the number of pure DCIS cases was small, the German and Canadian single-center trials found MRI to be more sensitive than XRM. Kuhl *et al.* reported that 3/9 (33%) of cases with pure DCIS were shown by XRM versus 8/9 (89%) with MRI [79]. In the Canadian study, meanwhile, XRM showed 3/6 pure DCIS cases (50%) while MRI showed 4/6 (67%) [80]. In the Dutch and UK studies though, 5/6 pure DCIS cases in each were shown by XRM, with MRI showing only 1/6 and 2/6 respectively. So why this discrepancy? Warner and Causer commented that a higher sensitivity of XRM for DCIS was also the initial Canadian experience, but added that "since becoming more adept at diagnosing the subtle signs of DCIS on MRI, we have found MRI to be much more sensitive than mammography, with a differential similar to what we see with invasive cancer" [83]. To improve DCIS detection by MRI, the importance of high spatial resolution and interpretation based on enhancement patterns became increasingly recognized, while kinetic curves were found to be of limited value.

Table 5.6 Summary of study data on high-risk screening using MRI

	Germany [80]	Canada [81]	Netherlands [82]	UK MARIBS [83]
Number of centers	1	1	6	22
Study period	Feb 1996–Feb 2002	Nov 1997–Mar 2003	Nov 1999–Oct 2003	Aug 1997–May 2004
Number of women	529 (8% BRCA)	236 (100% BRCA)	1909 (19% BRCA)	649 (18% BRCA)
Age range	27–59 (mean 42)	25–65 (mean 47)	25–70 (mean 40)	35–49 (median 40)
Total of all cancers	43	22	51	35
DCIS only (% of total)	9 (21%)	6 (27%)	6 (12%)	6 (18%)
Cancers found only by MRI	19 (44%)	7 (32%)	22 (43%)	19 (54%)
XRM sens & spec	33% & 97%	36% & 99%	40% & 95%	40% & 93%
US sensitivity	40%	33%	Not applicable	Not applicable
MRI sensitivity	91%	77%	71%	77%
MRI specificity	97%	95%	90%	81%
PPV of Bx due to MRI	50%	46%	57%	25%

In 2007, Kuhl *et al.* published results of a prospective study showing overall 92% sensitivity for MRI versus 56% for XRM in 193 women with pure DCIS [84]. For high-grade DCIS, MRI performed particularly strongly with double the sensitivity of XRM. However, some low-grade DCIS cases are only detected as mammographic microcalcification. Therefore the highest overall yield of DCIS in a screening context is likely to be achieved by using both MRI and XRM in combination, which has been the general recommendation for high-risk surveillance. In a review of all cancers missed by MRI in the Dutch study, over one-third were non-enhancing DCIS cases shown only by XRM [85].

Principles and limitations of high-risk screening using breast MRI

From these initial trials then, it became apparent that MRI outperformed a combination of even XRM and screening US, with the prospect of a widening differential as detection of DCIS by MRI was significantly improving. So exactly how then, should this powerful tool be best applied and what are its limitations?

Cancer yields from high-risk screening using breast MRI

The yield from high-risk screening programs will depend on the exact inclusion criteria and rates will also be higher in the incident round compared to subsequent follow-up rounds. From 1015 screening episodes in a cohort of purely proven BRCA mutation carriers, Causer *et al.* reported a total yield of 41 cancers (4%) from multimodality screening [86]. An evidence-based review by Granader *et al.* found cancer detection rates in BRCA-positive women were 2.7% by MRI, 1.0% by XRM and 3.1% for a combination of both. Among women at increased risk but without a BRCA gene, detection rates were substantially lower at 1.1% by MRI, 0.5% by XRM, and 1.2% for both combined [87]. Additional cancers revealed by MRI are of the greatest importance, which would have gone undetected by conventional surveillance. The best quality studies of MRI screening in typical mixed high-risk populations report yields of "MRI-only" cancers between 1.5% and 2.0% [43, 79, 80, 88, 89].

It is worth noting that while the cost of breast MRI may be higher than for XRM, the cancer yield from high-risk screening with MRI is 2- to 8-fold that of XRM screening in the general population, making the *cost per cancer diagnosed* comparable for the two scenarios.

Cancers missed by MRI screening

As already mentioned, MRI fails to detect a proportion of DCIS cases which may manifest as microcalcification and therefore be amenable to XRM detection. Any slow-enhancing cancer, whether it appears as a mass (usually invasive) or as a non-mass enhancement (usually DCIS), can be obscured by marked background enhancement. A small proportion (up to 5%) of invasive cancers, usually low-grade histologic types, may fail to show any significant enhancement.

Obdeijn *et al.* recently reported on 21 cancers missed by MRI in the Dutch study [85]. In 12 of the 21 there was no MRI-enhancing lesion even on review, of which 8 were DCIS cases detected only by XRM as microcalcification (2 low grade, 2 intermediate grade and 4 high grade). Some missed IDCs were attributed to small lesions being rendered inconspicuous due to intense background enhancement, while in one case the MRI study was deemed to be technically inadequate.

For 6/21 missed lesions in the MRISC study, interpretative errors were considered to be responsible. In all but one of these, a BI-RADS 4 or 5 score was given on review of the MRI, suggesting that these misses reflected the learning curve in this multicenter study. These included five masses of 9–15 mm diameter (three showing rim enhancement and a type 3 curve) while another was a 50 mm DCIS showing a segmental distribution.

Another potential limitation of MRI screening in the target population of young high-risk women is in detecting rapidly growing high-grade cancers. Among BRCA mutation carriers, cancers may have doubling-times as short as 28 days [55]. Tumor growth is particularly rapid in BRCA1 carriers, and in the MRISC study 5 of 7 palpable interval cancers arose in that subgroup, although only one (a 12 mm grade 3 IDC presenting 10 months after screening) had an entirely normal MRI scan on review. Achieving optimum sensitivity from MRI screening requires that interpreting radiologists have the requisite level of training and experience. A high index of suspicion is essential to detect early high-grade cancers which may appear only as non-specific foci or small rounded masses. There is, however, no doubt that a proportion of cancers in high-risk populations (typically in BRCA1 carriers) attain a large size within a 12-month screening interval [55] (Fig. 5.7).

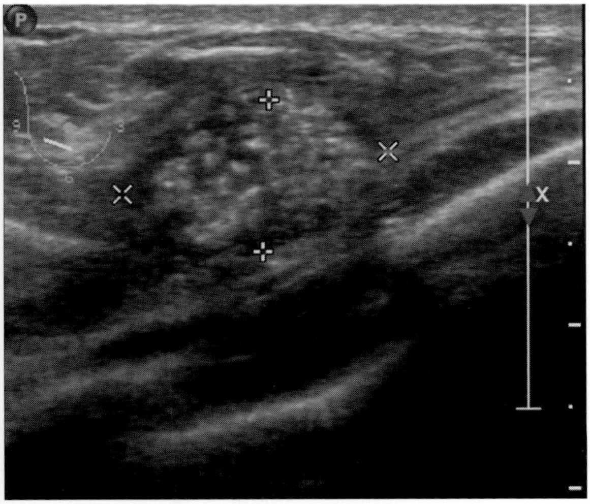

Fig. 5.7 Interval cancer: An untested 42-year-old woman with two sisters proven to have a BRCA1 mutation presented with a 2–3 week history of a lump in the inferior right breast. US image shows circumscribed ovoid 20 mm diameter predominantly echogenic mass with punctate foci consistent with calcification. A 14-gauge CNB showed high-grade DCIS and invasive cancer. Screening MRI from 6 months earlier was normal, even on retrospective review. Surgical pathology showed triple-negative grade 3 IDC and high-grade DCIS with luminal necrosis and calcification, SLNB 0/4 nodes positive.

False-positive recalls and biopsies

The downside of maintaining a high index of suspicion to maximize the sensitivity of MRI in a high-risk MRI population is, of course, a tendency to lower specificity due to recalls for relatively non-specific or subtle findings. In addition to foci or small masses (~5 mm), other causes of false-positive MRI recalls in the high-risk setting include myxoid fibroadenomas and non-mass enhancement due to either cyclical hormonal effects or benign proliferative fibrocystic changes.

As with XRM screening, having a prior examination for comparison improves specificity. Recall rates for additional imaging may be in the range of 8–17% for the initial screening MRI round, but typically fall below 10% in subsequent rounds [1]. Similarly, in one recent study recommendations for short interval follow-up reduced from 10% after the first round to less than 3% in the following rounds [90]. Granader *et al.* reported that false-positive recall rates were the same for both BRCA and non-BRCA high-risk groups at 10% for MRI and 5% for XRM [88]. This seems very acceptable for the additional cancer yield from MRI, with pooled results of several studies confirming a PPV for biopsy of at least 50% [91].

An important part of managing a breast MRI screening program is audit of in-house results on an ongoing basis. This includes monitoring of recall rates, cancer detection rates and benign to malignant biopsy ratios. Complete pathologic data should also be recorded on abnormal findings, and protocols devised for periodically obtaining information on interval cancers where possible.

Will breast MRI screening reduce mortality in high-risk women?

Direct evidence of a reduction in breast cancer mortality due to MRI screening could only be obtained from large-scale, long-term prospective RCTs allocating high-risk women into groups with and without the use of MRI surveillance, using mortality as the endpoint. Such trials are expensive to administer, require participation of very large numbers of women to achieve sufficient statistical power and may not deliver an answer for many years.

Given the evidence already to hand, it is very unlikely that such an RCT to assess the impact of MRI screening on mortality in high-risk women would now be considered ethical. As such, surrogate endpoints are needed, with probably the best indicators of benefit from surveillance including MRI being the proportion of (i) small invasive cancers and (ii) node-negative cancers (Stage 0 or I) detected.

In this regard, the Dutch trial, in which more than 3-fold as many subcentimeter invasive cancers were found versus the two control groups, was encouraging. Another prospective study comparing cancer detection in 413 women in a multimodality high-risk screening program (using XRM, US and MRI) with similar risk women outside the program, found that 85% were pre-invasive or less than 2 cm in diameter (compared with 44% outside the program) while 83% were node negative (48% outside the program) [88].

In a pooled review of the German, Canadian, Dutch and UK trials together with their own prospective data from the HIBCRIT trial (a total of 3571 women screened), Sardanelli and Podo reported that < 20% of MRI-detected invasive cancers were node positive, whereas in results for high-risk screening without MRI, 30–45% of cancers were node positive [91]. So, although evidence remains limited, there are data which suggest that a stage shift to the left does occur where MRI screening is used, and a benchmark of 80% appears to be reasonable for the overall proportion of node-negative cancers detected. A further strong indicator of likely benefit is the significant reduction in interval cancer rates compared to XRM screening, providing evidence that breast MRI detects clinically significant disease.

Computer modeling could also be useful in extrapolating long-term results from available pathologic data. Lee *et al.* used a mathematical model to compare projected clinical outcomes of different screening strategies in women with the BRCA1 gene mutation [92]. Using annual XRM, median invasive tumor diameter was 19 mm, but with the addition of MRI this reduced to 11 mm. The projected reduction in breast cancer mortality improved from around 17% for XRM alone to 22% for both techniques combined.

While it should not automatically be assumed that mortality reduction will be achieved by MRI screening of high-risk women, intuitively it seems probable that this will be the case. However, there is evidence that cancers behave more aggressively in young women and in BRCA mutation carriers, calling into question whether MRI will impact on mortality to the extent anticipated, despite earlier diagnosis [55, 93]. This is particularly a concern in regard to the basal-like molecular subtype characteristic of women with BRCA1 mutations which show a propensity for early vascular invasion (see Chapter 3).

How long to screen for and at what interval

In known or suspected mutation carriers, XRM screening is widely recommended to begin 10 years before the age of the youngest affected relative or from as early as age 20–25 years [75]. Given the greater sensitivity of MRI screening with no radiation risks, similar guidelines can be reasonably applied, keeping in mind that the 10-year absolute breast cancer risk for a 20-year-old BRCA1 carrier is about 2%, equivalent to average-risk women of age 50 years (Tables 5.1 and 5.3). A 12-month interval has been almost universally adopted for MRI screening and appears to be effective in the high-risk group. However, given the concerns in relation to rapid tumor progression in BRCA1 carriers, the possibility of using a 6-month MRI screening interval in this subgroup has been raised.

Since the increased benefit from MRI is still apparent in postmenopausal women at high risk, MRI screening could reasonably continue to age 70, although 2-yearly screening is probably adequate in the seventh decade (Ellen Warner, personal communication, 2010).

Is high-risk screening using only breast MRI feasible?

Other multicenter studies from Norway, Italy (HIBCRIT study) and most recently Germany (EVA trial) have added further data on high-risk MRI screening [43, 89, 94]. A recent pooled analysis of nine series comprising 4485 high-risk women showed that XRM alone detected only 36% of cancers while the addition of MRI increased sensitivity more than 2.5-fold to 93% [75]. The superior sensitivity of MRI over US has also been confirmed, with Berg *et al.* suggesting that screening US has no additional role where MRI is appropriately used for high-risk screening [67]. In accordance with this view, screening ultrasound was removed from the multimodality protocol adopted for surveillance of BRCA women by the Toronto group who published the original Canadian study [86].

Furthermore, the 2008 review by Granader *et al.* found any small gain in sensitivity from using MRI and XRM combined versus MRI alone was offset by an increase in false-positive rates [87]. The authors concluded that MRI had an "essential role" in high-risk screening, and commented that the decision on the trade-offs in using XRM in addition to MRI "ultimately rests with the local provider." In short, a case was emerging for using breast MRI as a stand-alone primary screening technique for high-risk women, at least in experienced centers.

Updated results from Toronto on 355 BRCA mutation carriers (189 BRCA1 and 166 BRCA2) show 41 cancers detected after 1015 screening episodes giving a 4% cancer yield. Among these, MRI missed five lesions prospectively of which two were small DCIS lesions shown as microcalcification on XRM [86]. Therefore while MRI alone found 36/41 (88%) and XRM alone found 11/41 (27%) cancers, adding XRM to MRI contributed only two additional cancers which MRI had missed, increasing sensitivity from 88% to 95% with both methods combined.

In the EVA trial, 687 women at 20% or greater lifetime risk underwent a total 1679 annual screening rounds. The combination of XRM and US together yielded 7.7 cancers/1000 screens while the yield from MRI alone was about double at 15/1000. The yield from MRI increased only marginally to 16/1000 by adding XRM and did not change by adding US.

Kuhl *et al.* concluded that in women undergoing quality-assured annual MRI, neither XRM, 6-monthly US or CBE added to the cancer yield achieved by MRI alone [89]. The reported PPVs for a malignant diagnosis (BI-RADS 4 or 5 score) were 36% for US, 39% for XRM and 48% for MRI.

So, for high-risk screening in expert hands, only a small proportion (~5%) of cancers (almost exclusively DCIS) are missed by MRI but detected as microcalcifications on XRM (German study 1/40, Canadian study 2/41 and 2/27 in the EVA trial) [79, 86, 89]. In the young age-group particularly, where the risks of radiation are more significant, there is then a strong argument for eliminating use of screening XRM. That is not to say XRM should not be used at all, but analogous to TUS, its role might be restricted to workup views for MRI-detected lesions, particularly indeterminate non-mass enhancement. In the learning phase though, continued use of MRI and XRM screening in combination has to be recommended, although a possible compromise in women below age 40 years may be to perform only a single digital MLO view of each breast to minimize the radiation dose [91].

Is screening MRI in women at average risk appropriate?

For any screening technique, the lower the incidence of the target disease in the tested population, the less cost-effective the test becomes. This is particularly important for an expensive undertaking like breast MRI. The rate of false-positive biopsy results will also increase if the pre-test probability of breast cancer being present is reduced. Even in the most developed countries, there are insufficient resources to provide MRI screening to all women, even if this were considered to be appropriate. It is therefore essential to have a clear understanding of the factors which influence breast cancer risk, in order to advise women on the possible benefits of breast MRI in their individual case (Table 5.7).

In some clinical situations, even though women may only be at average risk, breast MRI may have a potential role because the effectiveness of XRM is known to be compromised. In such cases, it might be reasonable to perform MRI at 2-yearly intervals, with the option of adding limited digital XRM (e.g., single MLO view) to detect possible microcalcification. The following groups of women are included in this category, where MRI offers a viable alternative to XRM as a primary screening method:

Table 5.7 Suggested criteria for MRI screening

BRCA1, BRCA2 or other high-risk genetic syndrome and their untested close blood relatives
History of chest or mediastinal RT before age 30 years (commence after interval > 8 years)
Based on assessment by accepted mathematical models, e.g., lifetime risk of ~20% or more
Absolute risk of > 5% over next 10 years by accepted mathematical models
Personal history of breast cancer especially diagnosed < 50 years +/− breast density
Prior biopsy with LCIS, ADH, ALH, atypical papillary lesion +/− family history or breast density
Breast density (BI-RADS class 3 or 4), +/− family history, e.g., affected first degree relative
Average risk but compromised XRM – implants, mammographic intolerance, small breast size

(i) Breast implants: There is no evidence that implants are associated with increased breast cancer risk. In fact, women with implants appear to have a slightly reduced risk, perhaps because the absolute amount of dense breast tissue present is generally lower. Nevertheless, implants make XRM technically difficult to perform, frequently resulting in often inadequate coverage (see Chapter 8). Meanwhile, the absorbed radiation dose can be doubled [95] and diagnostic sensitivity is reduced to less than 50% [96]. For women with painful fibrous contracture, XRM becomes intolerable.

(ii) Intolerance to mammography: Although very difficult to standardize, pain is the most frequently cited reason for women declining screening mammography [97]. Some 25–35% of women undergoing XRM report at least discomfort or moderate pain relating to breast compression, and for some women the procedure is intolerable [98].

(iii) Small breast size: In women with small breasts, it may be technically impossible to achieve adequate coverage using XRM. This is a particularly frequent problem in some Asian populations and is often compounded by extreme breast density.

To what extent MRI screening will be adopted for other women at average risk remains to be seen, with some bold predictions that MRI will indeed become the method of choice [99]. Certainly, an increasing number of radiologists now have substantial expertise with breast MRI screening, with Kuhl observing that "there is no medical reason for these radiologists to withhold breast MRI from asymptomatic women at average risk who, after careful explanation of the possible advantages and disadvantages of this approach, choose for themselves to undergo the most sensitive test that is currently available for diagnosing breast cancer" [100]. Recently, Kuhl has also shown the feasibility of using a limited screening breast MRI protocol (T2-weighted sequence, static pre- and early post-constrast T1-weighted sequence), taking only a few minutes to perform and interpret (Christiane Kuhl, personal communication, 2011). Women with positive findings could then be recalled for multimodality imaging work-up including biopsy as required, similar to current mammographic assessment clinics.

MULTIPLE CHOICE QUESTIONS

5.1 Answer true or false to the following statements

A. The sensitivity of XRM in extremely dense breasts (BI-RADS 4) is at least 80%.

B. Previous chest RT confers a breast cancer risk similar to that for a BRCA mutation.

C. Low-grade DCIS represents a major cause of overtreatment in XRM screening programs.

D. Breast cancer diagnosed before age 40 confers >4-fold risk of contralateral breast cancer.

E. Breast implants significantly increase the risk of developing invasive ductal breast cancer.

5.2 Answer true or false to the following statements

A. Annual MRI screening is known to offer a clear survival benefit in BRCA mutation carriers.

B. In high-risk screening, US has the advantage of a higher PPV of biopsy compared to MRI.

C. Among MRI-detected cancers in high-risk screening, about 80% are node negative.

D. In combined high-risk screening, XRM always detects more DCIS cases than does MRI.

E. A family history of male breast cancer suggests the possibility of a BRCA2 mutation.

See page 189 for answers.

References

1. Saslow D, Boetes C, Burke W, *et al.* American Cancer Society guidelines for breast screening with MRI as an adjunct to mammography. *CA Cancer J Clin* 2007; **57**: 75–89.
2. Berg WA. Beyond standard mammographic screening: mammography at age extremes, ultrasound, and MR imaging. *Radiol Clin North Am* 2007; **45**: 895–906.
3. National Breast and Ovarian Cancer Center (NBOCC). *Breast Cancer Risk Factors: A Review of the Evidence.* Surry Hills, NSW, National Breast and Ovarian Cancer Center, 2009.
4. Elmore JG, Gigerenzer G. Benign breast disease – the risks of communicating risk. *N Engl J Med* 2005; **353**: 297–9.
5. Antoniou A, Pharoah PDP, Narod SA, *et al.* Average risks of breast and ovarian cancer associated with mutations in BRCA1 or BRCA2 detected in case series unselected for family history: a combined analysis of 22 studies. *Am J Hum Genet* 2003; **72**: 1117–30.
6. Chen S, Parmigiani G. Meta-analysis of BRCA1 and BRCA2 penetrance. *J Clin Oncol* 2007; **25**: 1329–33.
7. Evans DGR, Susnerwala I, Dawson J, *et al.* Risk of breast cancer in male BRCA2 carriers. *J Med Genet* 2010; **47**: 710–11.
8. Breast Cancer Linkage Consortium. Cancer risks in BRCA2 mutation carriers. *J Natl Cancer Inst* 1999; **91**: 1310–16.
9. van Asperen CJ, Brohet RM, Meijers-Heijboer EJ, *et al.* Cancer risks in BRCA2 families: estimates for sites other than breast and ovary. *J Med Genet* 2005; **42**: 711–19.
10. Thompson D, Easton DF, The Breast Cancer Linkage Consortium. Cancer incidence in BRCA1 mutation carriers. *J Natl Cancer Inst* 2002; **94**: 1358–65.
11. Malone KE, Begg CB, Haile RW, *et al.* Population-based study of the risk of second primary contralateral breast cancer associated with carrying a mutation in BRCA1 or BRCA2. *J Clin Oncol* 2010; **28**: 2404–10.
12. Lakhani SR, van de Vijver MJ, Jacquemier J, *et al.* The pathology of familial breast cancer: predictive value of immunohistochemical markers estrogen receptor, progesterone receptor, HER-2, and p53 in patients with mutations in BRCA1 and BRCA2. *J Clin Oncol* 2002; **20**: 2310–18.
13. Lidereau R, Eisinger F, Champeme M, *et al.* Major improvement in the efficacy of BRCA1 mutation screening using morphoclinical features of breast cancer. *Cancer Res* 2000; **60**: 1206–10.
14. Vargas AC, Da Silva L, Lakhani SR. The contribution of breast cancer pathology to statistical models to predict mutation risk

in BRCA carriers. *Familial Cancer* 2010; **9**: 545–53.

15. van Leeuwen FE, Klokman WJ, Stovall M, *et al.* Roles of radiation dose, chemotherapy, and hormonal factors in breast cancer following Hodgkin's disease. *J Natl Cancer Inst* 2003; **95**: 971–80.
16. Travis LB, Hill DA, Dores GM, *et al.* Breast cancer following RT and chemotherapy among young women with Hodgkin disease. *JAMA* 2003; **290**: 465–75.
17. Travis LB, Hill D, Dores GM, *et al.* Cumulative absolute breast cancer risk for young women treated for Hodgkin lymphoma. *J Natl Cancer Inst* 2005; **97**: 1428–37.
18. Kenney LB, Yasui Y, Inskip PD, *et al.* Breast cancer after childhood cancer: a report from the childhood cancer survivor study. *Ann Intern Med* 2004; **141**: 590–7.
19. Ralleigh G, Given-Wilson R. Breast cancer risk and possible screening strategies for young women following supradiaphragmatic irradiation for Hodgkin's disease. *Clin Radiol* 2004; **59**: 647–50.
20. Clemons M, Loijens L, Goss P. Breast cancer risk following irradiation for Hodgkin's disease. *Cancer Treat Rev* 2000; **26**: 291–302.
21. Amir E, Evans DG, Shenton A, *et al.* Evaluation of breast cancer risk assessment packages in the family history evaluation and screening programme. *J Med Genet* 2003; **40**: 807–14.
22. Cuzick J. Assessing risk for breast cancer. *Breast Cancer Res* 2008; **10** (Suppl 4): S13.
23. Tyrer J, Duffy SW, Cuzick J. A breast cancer prediction model incorporating familial and personal risk factors. *Stat Med* 2004; **23**: 111–23.
24. Mann GJ, Thorne H, Balleine RL, *et al.* Analysis of cancer risk and BRCA1 and BRCA2 mutation prevalence in the kConFab familial breast cancer resource. *Breast Cancer Res* 2006; **8**: R12.
25. Antoniou AC, Hardy R, Walker L, *et al.* Predicting the likelihood of carrying a BRCA1 or BRCA2 mutation: validation of BOADICEA, BRCAPRO, IBIS, Myriad and the Manchester scoring system using data from UK genetics clinics. *J Med Genet* 2008; **45**: 425–31.
26. Collaborative Group on Hormonal Factors in Breast Cancer. Familial breast cancer: collaborative reanalysis of individual data from 52 epidemiological studies including 58 209 women with breast cancer and 101 986 women without the disease. *Lancet* 2001; **358**: 1389–99.
27. Arpino G, Laucirica R, Elledge RM. Premalignant and in situ breast disease: biology and clinical implications. *Ann Intern Med* 2005; **143**: 446–57.
28. Port ER, Park A, Borgen PI, *et al.* Results of MRI screening for breast cancer in high-risk patients with LCIS and atypical hyperplasia. *Ann Surg Oncol* 2007; **14**: 1051–7.
29. McCormack VA, dos Santos Silva I. Breast density and parenchymal patterns as markers of breast cancer risk: a meta-analysis. *Cancer Epidemiol Biomarkers Prev* 2006; **15**: 1159–69.
30. Boyd NF, Dite GS, Stone J, *et al.* Heritability of mammographic density, a risk factor for breast cancer. *N Engl J Med* 2002; **347**: 886–94.
31. Martin LJ, Boyd NF. Mammographic density. Potential mechanisms of breast cancer risk associated with mammographic density: hypotheses based on epidemiological evidence. *Breast Cancer Res* 2008; **10**: 201.
32. Boyd NF, Martin LJ, Rommens JM, *et al.* Mammographic density: a heritable risk factor for breast cancer. *Methods Mol Biol* 2009; **472**: 343–60.
33. Martin LJ, Melnichouk O, Guo H, *et al.* Family history, mammographic density, and risk of breast cancer. *Cancer Epidemiol Biomarkers Prev* 2010; **19**: 456–63.
34. Odefrey F, Stone J, Gurrin LC, *et al.* Common genetic variants associated with breast cancer and mammographic density measures that predict disease. *Cancer Res* 2010; **70**: 1449–58.
35. Boyd NF, Guo H, Martin LJ, *et al.* Mammographic density and the risk and detection of breast cancer. *N Engl J Med* 2007; **356**: 227–36.
36. Kopans DB. Basic physics and doubts about relationship between mammographically determined tissue density and breast cancer risk. *Radiology* 2008; **246**: 348–53.
37. Duffy FJ, Nagtegaal ID, Astley SM, *et al.* Visually assessed breast density, breast cancer risk and the importance of the craniocaudal view. *Breast Cancer Res* 2008; **10**: R64.
38. Baasch M, Nielsen SF, Engholm G, *et al.* Breast cancer incidence subsequent to surgical reduction of the female breast. *Br J Cancer* 1996; **73**: 961–3.
39. Kusano AS, Trichopoulos D, Terry KL, *et al.* A prospective study of breast size and premenopausal breast cancer incidence. *Int J Cancer* 2006; **118**: 2031–4.
40. Fowble B, Hanlon A, Freedman G, *et al.* Second cancers after conservative surgery and radiation for stages I-II breast cancer: identifying a subset of women at increased risk. *Int J Radiat Oncol Biol Phys* 2001; **51**: 679–90.
41. Gao X, Fisher SG, Emami B. Risk of second primary cancer in the contralateral breast in women treated for early-stage breast cancer: a population-based study.

Int J Radiat Oncol Biol Phys 2003; **56**: 1038–45.

42. Morris EA, Liberman L, Ballon DJ, *et al.* MRI of occult breast carcinoma in a high-risk population. *AJR Am J Roentgenol* 2003; **181**: 619–26.
43. Sardanelli F, Podo F, D'Agnolo G, *et al.* Multicenter comparative multimodality surveillance of women at genetic-familial high risk for breast cancer (HIBCRIT Study): interim results. *Radiology* 2007; **242**: 698–715.
44. Brennan S, Liberman L, Dershaw DD, *et al.* Breast MRI screening of women with a personal history of breast cancer. *AJR Am J Roentgenol* 2010; **195**: 510–16.
45. Hanrahan EO, Gonzalez-Angulo AM, Giordano SH, *et al.* Overall survival and cause-specific mortality of patients with stage T1a, bN0M0 breast carcinoma. *J Clin Oncol* 2007; **25**: 4952–60.
46. Early Breast Cancer Trialists' Collaborative Group (EBCTCG). Effects of chemotherapy and hormonal therapy for early breast cancer on recurrence and 15-year survival: an overview of the randomised trials. *Lancet* 2005; **365**: 1687–717.
47. Berry DA, Cronin KA, Plevritis SK, *et al.* Effect of screening and adjuvant therapy on mortality from breast cancer. *N Engl J Med* 2005; **353**: 1784–92.
48. Gøtzsche PC, Nielsen M. Screening for breast cancer with mammography. *Cochrane Database Syst Rev* 2006; **4**: CD001877.
49. Jørgensen KJ, Gøtzsche PC. Overdiagnosis in publicly organised mammography screening programmes: systematic review of incidence trends. *BMJ* 2009; **339**: 2587–94.
50. Nelson HD, Tyne K, Naik A, *et al.* Screening for breast cancer: an update for the U.S. Preventive Services Task Force. *Ann Intern Med* 2009; **151**: 727–37.
51. Mushlin AI, Kouides RW, Shapiro DE, *et al.* Estimating the accuracy of screening mammography: a meta-analysis. *Am J Prev Med* 1998; **14**: 143–53.
52. Kolb TM, Lichy J, Newhouse JH. Comparison of the performance of screening mammography, physical examination, and breast US and evaluation of factors that influence them: an analysis of 27,825 patient evaluations. *Radiology* 2002; **225**: 165–75.
53. Leconte I, Feger C, Galant C, *et al.* Mammography and subsequent whole-breast sonography of nonpalpable breast cancers: the importance of radiologic breast density. *AJR Am J Roentgenol* 2003; **180**: 1675–9.
54. Mandelson MT, Oestreicher N, Porter PL, *et al.* Breast density as a predictor of mammographic detection: comparison of interval- and screen-detected cancers. *J Natl Cancer Inst* 2000; **92**: 1081–7.
55. Tilanus-Linthorst M, Obdeijn IM, Hop WCJ, *et al.* BRCA1 mutation and young age predict fast breast cancer growth in the Dutch, United Kingdom, and Canadian magnetic resonance imaging screening trials. *Clin Cancer Res* 2007; **13**: 7357–62.
56. Weedon-Fekjær H, Lindqvist BH, Vatten LJ, *et al.* Breast cancer tumor growth estimated through mammography screening data. *Breast Cancer Res* 2008; **10**: R41.
57. Moss SM, Cuckle H, Evans A, *et al.* Effect of mammographic screening from age 40 years on breast cancer mortality at 10 years' follow-up: a randomised controlled trial. *Lancet* 2006; **368**: 2053–60.
58. Armstrong K, Moye E, Williams S, *et al.* Screening mammography in women 40 to 49 years of age: a systematic review for the American College of Physicians. *Ann Intern Med* 2007; **146**: 516–26.
59. Berrington de Gonzalez A, Reeves G. Mammographic screening before age 50 years in the UK: comparison of the radiation risks with the mortality benefits. *Br J Cancer* 2005; **93**: 590–6.
60. Elmore JG, Barton MB, Moceri VM, *et al.* Ten-year risk of false positive screening mammograms and clinical breast examinations. *N Engl J Med* 1998; **338**: 1089–96.
61. Kavanagh AM, Davidson N, Jolley D, *et al.* Determinants of false positive recall in an Australian mammographic screening program. *The Breast* 2006; **15**: 510–18.
62. Christiansen CL, Wang F, Barton MB, *et al.* Predicting the cumulative risk of false-positive mammograms. *J Natl Cancer Inst* 2000; **92**: 1657–66.
63. Kosters JP, Gøtzsche PC. Regular self-examination or clinical examination for early detection of breast cancer. *Cochrane Database Syst Rev* 2003; **2**: CD003373.
64. DeMichele A, Weber BL. Risk management in BRCA1 and BRCA2 mutation carriers: lessons learned, challenges posed. *J Clin Oncol* 2002; **20**: 1164–6.
65. Pisano ED, Gatsonis C, Hendrick E, *et al.* Diagnostic performance of digital versus film mammography for breast-cancer screening. *N Engl J Med* 2005; **353**: 1773–83.
66. Pisano ED, Hendrick RE, Yaffe MJ, *et al.* Diagnostic accuracy of digital versus film mammography: exploratory analysis of selected population subgroups in DMIST. *Radiology* 2008; **246**: 376–83.
67. Berg WA, Blume JD, Cormack JB, *et al.* Combined screening with ultrasound and mammography vs mammography alone in women at elevated risk of breast cancer. *JAMA* 2008; **299**: 2151–63.
68. Corsetti V, Houssami N, Ferrari A, *et al.* Breast screening with ultrasound in women with

mammography-negative dense breasts: evidence on incremental cancer detection and false positives, and associated cost. *Eur J Cancer* 2008; **44**: 539–44.

69. Buchberger W, Niehoff A, Obrist P, *et al.* Clinically and mammographically occult breast lesions: detection and classification with high resolution sonography. *Semin Ultrasound CT MR* 2000; **21**: 325–6.

70. Tilanus-Linthorst M, Verhoog L, Obdeijn I, *et al.* A BRCA1/2 mutation, high breast density and prominent pushing margins of a tumour independently contribute to a frequent false-negative mammography. *Int J Cancer* 2002; **102**: 91–5.

71. Bigenwald RZ, Warner E, Gunasekara A, *et al.* Is mammography adequate for screening women with inherited BRCA mutations and low breast density? *Cancer Epidemiol Biomarkers Prev* 2008; **17**: 706–11.

72. Komeneka IK, Ditkoff B, Joseph K, *et al.* The development of interval breast malignancies in patients with BRCA mutations. *Cancer* 2004; **100**: 2079–83.

73. Brekelmans CTM, Seynaeve C, Bartels CCM, *et al.* Effectiveness of breast cancer surveillance in BRCA1/2 gene mutation carriers and women with high familial risk. *J Clin Oncol* 2001; **19**: 924–30.

74. Scheuer L, Kauff N, Robson M, *et al.* Outcome of preventive surgery and screening for breast and ovarian cancer in BRCA mutation carriers. *J Clin Oncol* 2002; **20**: 1260–8.

75. Berg WA. Tailored supplemental screening for breast cancer: what now and what next? *AJR Am J Roentgenol* 2009; **192**: 390–9.

76. Andrieu N, Easton DF, Chang-Claude J, *et al.* Effect of chest x-rays on the risk of breast cancer among BRCA1/2 mutation carriers in the International BRCA1/2 Carrier Cohort Study. *J Clin Oncol* 2006; **24**: 3361–6.

77. Berrington de Gonzalez A, Berg CD, Visvanathan K, *et al.* Estimated risk of radiation-induced breast cancer from mammographic screening for young BRCA mutation carriers. *J Natl Cancer Inst* 2009; **101**: 205–9.

78. Kuhl CK, Schmutzler RK, Leutner CC, *et al.* Breast MR imaging screening in 192 women proved or suspected to be carriers of a breast cancer susceptibility gene: preliminary results. *Radiology* 2000; **215**: 267–79.

79. Kuhl CK, Schrading S, Leutner CC, *et al.* Mammography, breast ultrasound, and magnetic resonance imaging for surveillance of women at high familial risk for breast cancer. *J Clin Oncol* 2005; **23**: 8469–76.

80. Warner E, Plewes DB, Hill KA, *et al.* Surveillance of BRCA1 and BRCA2 mutation carriers with magnetic resonance imaging, ultrasound, mammography and clinical breast examination. *JAMA* 2004; **292**: 1317–25.

81. Kriege M, Brekelmans CTM, Boetes C, *et al.* Efficacy of MRI and mammography for breast-cancer screening in women with a familial or genetic predisposition. *N Engl J Med* 2004; **351**: 427–37.

82. Leach MO, Boggis AK, Dixon AK, *et al.* Screening with magnetic resonance imaging and mammography of a UK population at high familial risk of breast cancer: a prospective multicenter cohort study (MARIBS). *Lancet* 2005; **365**: 1769–78.

83. Warner E, Causer PA. MRI surveillance for hereditary breast-cancer risk. *Lancet* 2005; **365**: 1747–9.

84. Kuhl CK, Schrading S, Bieling HB, *et al.* MRI for diagnosis of pure ductal carcinoma in situ: a prospective observational study. *Lancet* 2007; **370**: 485–92.

85. Obdeijn IM, Loo CE, Rijnsburger AJ, *et al.* Assessment of false-negative cases of breast MR imaging in women with a familial or genetic predisposition. *Breast Cancer Res Treat* 2010; **119**: 399–407.

86. Causer PA, Jong RA, Warner E, *et al.* Breast cancers detected with imaging screening in the BRCA population: emphasis on MR imaging with histopathologic correlation. *RadioGraphics* 2007; **27**: S165–82.

87. Granader EJ, Dwamena B, Carlos RC. MRI and mammography surveillance of women at increased risk for breast cancer: recommendations using an evidence-based approach. *Acad Radiol* 2008; **15**: 1590–5.

88. Schmutzler RK, Rhiem K, Breuer P, *et al.* Outcome of a structured surveillance programme in women with a familial predisposition for breast cancer. *Eur J Cancer Prev* 2006; **15**: 483–9.

89. Kuhl C, Weigel S, Schrading S, *et al.* Prospective multicenter cohort study to refine management recommendations for women at elevated familial risk of breast cancer: the EVA trial. *J Clin Oncol* 2010; **28**: 1450–7.

90. Abramovici G, Mainiero MB. Screening breast MR imaging: comparison of interpretation of baseline and annual follow-up studies. *Radiology* 2011; **259**: 85–91.

91. Sardanelli F, Podo F. Breast MR imaging in women at high-risk of breast cancer. Is something changing in early breast cancer detection? *Eur Radiol* 2007; **17**: 873–87.

92. Lee JM, Kopans DB, McMahon PM, *et al.* Breast cancer screening in BRCA1 mutation carriers: effectiveness of MR imaging – Markov Monte Carlo Decision Analysis. *Radiology* 2008; **246**: 763–71.

93. Hamilton LJ, Evans AJ, Cornford EJ, *et al.* Will MRI screening deliver the expected survival advantage in BRCA1 carriers? *Clin Radiol* 2009; **64**: 1045–7.

94. Hagen AI, Kvistad KA, Maehle L, *et al.* Sensitivity of MRI versus conventional screening in the diagnosis of BRCA-associated breast cancer in a national prospective series. *The Breast* 2007; **16**: 367–74.

95. Smathers SL, Boone JM, Lee LJ, *et al.* Radiation dose reduction for augmentation mammography. *AJR Am J Roentgenol* 2007; **188**: 1414–21.

96. Miglioretti DL, Rutter CM, Geller BM, *et al.* Effect of breast augmentation on the accuracy of mammography and cancer characteristics. *JAMA* 2004; **291**: 442–50.

97. Elwood M, McNoe B, Smith T, *et al.* Once is enough – why some women do not continue to participate in a breast cancer screening programme. *N Z Med J* 1998; **111**: 180–3.

98. Miller D, Livingstone V, Herbison GP. Interventions for relieving the pain and discomfort of screening mammography. *Cochrane Database Syst Rev* 2008; **1**: CD002942.

99. Hall FM. The rise and impending decline of screening mammography. *Radiology* 2008; **247**: 597–601.

100. Kuhl CK. Current status of breast MR imaging. Part 2. Clinical applications. *Radiology* 2007; **244**: 672–91.

Chapter 6

Preoperative staging with breast MRI

Chapter outline

- Introduction
- Overview of early-stage breast cancer management
- Mapping local disease extent with MRI
- Staging the lymph nodes with MRI
- Identifying distant metastases
- The controversy over routine preoperative MRI

Introduction

The issue as to whether MRI should be used routinely for preoperative staging of newly diagnosed breast cancer has become one of the most controversial in current practice. To place the potential role of breast MRI as a staging tool in context, this chapter begins with an overview of the principles of breast cancer management. Evidence that MRI is the imaging method of choice for determining disease extent is then reviewed and important features in reading staging breast MRI examinations are highlighted. Finally arguments are considered in the controversy over whether it is appropriate to recommend MRI for staging routinely, selectively or not at all.

Overview of early-stage breast cancer management

What is early-stage disease?

Most definitions of *early-stage breast cancer* (EBC) include invasive cancers up to 5 cm in diameter and those with involved but mobile axillary lymph nodes, corresponding to clinical TNM Stages I–IIA (**Appendix 3**). In the era of mass screening mammography, most new breast cancer cases (up to about 80%) present with early-stage disease. Of those, about 20% will have only DCIS (Stage 0), while a majority of invasive cancers are small or even *minimal cancers* (pathologic size < 10 mm), of which only a minority will have spread to the axillary nodes. Implicit in the designation as EBC is that the disease is operable, i.e., amenable to surgical cure.

In some definitions, cancers > 5 cm (T3), even with fixed or matted nodes (N2), i.e., up to TNM Stage IIIA, may be included as "early-stage" because with neoadjuvant (preoperative) systemic therapy it may be possible to down-stage some of these locally extensive tumors into the operable category.

Regardless of any size criteria, invasive cancers with chest wall or skin involvement (T4) constitute Stage IIIB *locally advanced breast cancer*. Level III (infraclavicular) node involvement (N3) defines Stage IIIC, while distant metastases (M1) indicate Stage IV. Prognosis is significantly poorer in these groups, with treatment aimed at control of disease to prolong survival with good quality of life.

The three major factors that determine the prognosis of invasive breast cancer are tumor size, extent of spread at presentation (regional nodes or distant metastases) and histologic grade. Additional biologic markers such as ER and HER2 expression are also routinely used to further assess prognosis and to guide the use of adjuvant systemic therapy (Appendix 6). Even for Stage I–II breast cancer, prognosis varies considerably. Key clinico-pathologic features of invasive cancers associated with potentially poorer prognosis are summarized in Table 6.1.

Probably the most significant advance in breast cancer management in recent decades has been establishing that breast-conserving surgery should be the treatment aim for the majority of EBC cases. Evidence for this comes from six large prospective RCTs comparing mastectomy and BCT with whole breast RT for Stage I and II breast cancer, which have shown no significant difference in overall mortality [1]. Local RT to the whole breast is standard treatment after BCT, and is intended to deal with any residual microscopic

Table 6.1 Adverse prognostic factors for invasive breast cancer

Young patient age
High number of positive lymph nodes
High tumor grade
Large tumor size
Unfavorable histologic type
Presence of LVI
Extensive DCIS (EIC) with "dirty" margins
ER/PR-negative status
HER2-positivity
Markers of basal-like tumors
High Ki-67 index
Known BRCA1 mutation

disease in order to minimize the risk of future local recurrence.

The 20-year follow-up results of the NSABP B-06 trial (published in 2002) showed no difference in overall survival between women with Stage I–II disease randomly assigned to either mastectomy, lumpectomy with breast irradiation or lumpectomy alone [2]. However, the incidence of ipsilateral breast recurrence was 14% in women who received BCT with irradiation compared with 39% in those who only had lumpectomy [2]. A prerequisite for NSABP B-06 was that tumor margins were negative after BCT, and in current practice patients with positive margins on histopathology are returned to the operating room for further tissue to be shaved from the appropriate wall of the cavity. It is generally accepted that the addition of RT in BCT should never be used as an excuse to accept pathologically involved ("dirty") margins.

Many women with invasive cancer (but not pure DCIS) receive adjuvant chemotherapy to address possible systemic disease, depending on their overall risk of disease recurrence. Even patients with positive axillary nodes appear to gain no survival benefit from having mastectomy compared with BCT, provided chemotherapy is given in addition to RT (NSABP B-06 and Milan I trials) [1]. Adding systemic therapy also reduces the likelihood of local recurrence after BCT for invasive cancer. With current selection criteria and new adjuvant therapies, local recurrence rates after BCT are generally low, typically 5–10% at 10 years [3]. In later NSABP trials (conducted after B-06), the ipsilateral breast recurrence rate in node-negative women receiving systemic therapy in addition to RT was ~6% after 10 years of follow-up [2].

Table 6.2 Factors favoring selection of mastectomy over BCT

Large tumor size relative to breast size preventing satisfactory cosmesis
Tumors with nipple or significant skin involvement or chest wall fixation
Multicentric disease or multiple invasive foci with separation >2–3 cm
Invasive cancer associated with extensive DCIS component
Medical contraindications, e.g., scleroderma preventing RT
BRCA mutation carrier or similar risk level (bilateral prophylactic)
Individual preference for low recurrence risk over cosmetic/psychologic factors

Accordingly, BCT is the treatment goal for EBC. Around two-thirds of all women with newly diagnosed breast cancer (70% of mammographically detected and 50% of clinically detected cancers) receive BCT. In the remaining one-third of women, mastectomy may be recommended because local disease extent precludes conservation. Large tumor size is only a relative contraindication to BCT, with the practical upper limit (where adequate resection is likely to result in a poor cosmesis) usually set at around 5 cm. However, this depends on the individual breast size, and even a relatively large tumor in a small breast may be amenable to BCT following neoadjuvant chemotherapy. Women who have multicentric disease or extensive DCIS (particularly involving the nipple) are among those who are generally not candidates for BCT (Table 6.2).

Management of DCIS

A striking change since the advent of widespread mammographic screening in developed countries has been the increasing incidence of DCIS, from once an uncommon condition to now at least 20% of newly diagnosed breast cancers. For women with only DCIS, surgical treatment aims to prevent future local recurrence (although distant metastases may arise in a few percent of patients due to occult invasive disease). Even untreated, 10-year survival exceeds 95% and the current dilemma is deciding on appropriate management when it is not yet possible to reliably predict which cases are likely to progress to invasion. Women with DCIS are overtreated if invasive cancer would not have occurred during their lifetime. On the other hand, finding cancer at the pre-invasive stage offers a unique window of opportunity for surgical cure in those women who would otherwise have subsequently presented with invasive cancer. The development of markers which will more clearly predict the biologic aggressiveness of DCIS is a high research priority.

While DCIS was traditionally treated with mastectomy, with increasingly frequent early detection by mammographic screening, the need for such radical surgery was called into question. Following the significant proven benefit from including RT in BCT for invasive cancer, three prospective trials of local excision with or without RT for DCIS were launched in the 1980s (NSABP B-17, EORTC 10853 and a third between the UK, Australia and New Zealand), all of which showed a substantial reduction in local recurrence rates from adding RT [4]. At 10-year follow-up, results of the EORTC 10853 trial found that 15% of women who received RT had experienced a recurrence compared with 26% in the group without RT, representing an ~50% risk reduction for those patients receiving RT in addition to lumpectomy [5].

Currently, there is still no clearly defined subset of DCIS patients where excision alone constitutes satisfactory management [6–8]. After BCT with whole breast RT for DCIS, the risk of local recurrence is ~10% at 10 years, [9] which manifests as invasive disease in ~50% of cases [5]. Patients who have large areas of high-grade DCIS are at the highest risk for developing recurrent DCIS or invasive cancer after incomplete excision. However, a report on 30-year follow-up of 28 women who had histologically low-grade DCIS treated by excisional biopsy alone showed that 11 (39%) developed invasive cancer (all in the same breast and quadrant as the initial biopsy). Furthermore, 5 of the 11 women died from distant metastatic disease within 1–7 years of the invasive cancer diagnosis [10]. Therefore, even histologically low-grade disease is a significant health issue if left untreated, despite its generally more indolent course.

The risk of recurrence after local excision of DCIS is strongly related to the surgical margin status. What constitutes an acceptable clear margin is rather controversial, but 2–3 mm is often accepted as adequate if RT is going to be used, with a minimum of 10 mm if no RT is planned. In one cohort of 272 women with DCIS treated by excision alone (margins at least 10 mm but with no RT), the local recurrence rate was 14% at 12 years [11]. On the other hand, another recent prospective trial of local excision without RT (margins again at least 10 mm) showed that even for small (< 25 mm) non-high grade DCIS there was a high recurrence rate of 12% after 5 years. Therefore it appears that RT offers potential benefit in reducing the incidence of recurrence in all DCIS cases. So, extent of DCIS, nuclear grade, margin status and use of RT are all factors influencing the risk of local recurrence (Table 6.3). Patient age at diagnosis is a further particularly important prognostic factor for DCIS, with a recent study showing the incidence of breast cancer events at 5 years to be 43% for women aged < 36 years compared with only 8% for women aged > 65 years [12].

Table 6.3 Risk factors for recurrence after BCT for DCIS

Young patient especially age < 40 years
DCIS extent > 30–40 mm, particularly if multifocal
High nuclear grade and/or presence of comedonecrosis
Positive or close margins
Treatment by excision without RT
ER-negative status
HER2-positive status
High Ki-67 proliferation index

In practice, RT is often omitted for older women with small (<10 mm) low-grade DCIS excised with clear margins, as the absolute benefit in reducing risk of recurrence is small. Meanwhile, at the other end of the spectrum, with high-grade DCIS of > 30–40 mm extent, many surgeons will perform SLNB because of the risk that occult invasion may already be present.

At least for ER-positive DCIS, tamoxifen appears to further reduce the risk of local recurrence [13], and trials of local excision and RT combined with newer agents such as aromatase inhibitors are now in progress. Positive HER2 status is associated with a higher risk of progression to invasion and recurrence, and the possible role of the anti-HER2 monoclonal antibody trastuzumab is also being explored.

Management of locoregional recurrence

So, while systemic therapy is required to address possible metastatic disease and improve survival after a breast cancer diagnosis, excision with clear margins and RT are vital in minimizing the risk of local disease recurrence in the breast, chest wall or axilla. While there has been no discernible difference in long-term survival, in four of the six trials of mastectomy versus BCT with whole breast RT for invasive cancer, there was a significant reduction in the risk of locoregional recurrence after mastectomy, an effect which persisted in pooled analysis [14].

The majority of local recurrences (~70%) arise within 5 years, with most successfully managed by performing completion mastectomy. Although controversial, there is evidence that these early recurrences signify a higher risk of metastatic disease and reduced survival, so that restaging may be appropriate in these women. Local recurrences continue to occur even up to 15 years after BCT.

Even DCIS treated by initial mastectomy carries a small risk of chest wall recurrence of ~1–2% at 10 years [9, 15, 16]. Most of these (~75%) arise as palpable invasive disease in close relation to the mastectomy scar. In such instances, excision is performed if possible and RT is given (this would not have been used initially after DCIS treated by mastectomy). Endocrine therapy, chemotherapy or trastuzumab may also be used as appropriate.

Assessing the regional lymph nodes

Another advance in modern breast cancer management relates to the assessment of the regional lymph nodes, reflecting that the raw number of involved axillary nodes is the single most powerful prognostic indicator for breast cancer survival. A key revision in the 2006 sixth edition of the *AJCC Staging Manual* was to redefine the major classification of lymph node status such that pathologic nodal staging essentially became pN1 = 1–3, pN2 = 4–9 and pN3 = 10 or more level I or II axillary nodes involved. Any metastases in level III axillary (infraclavicular) nodes led to an automatic pN3 classification, in recognition of the associated significantly poorer prognosis [17].

Lymph node status is also correlated to tumor size with larger tumors being more likely to have axillary nodal metastases. Indeed, it is this principle that most breast cancers enlarge to a certain point and then spread to the axilla and beyond in a predictable fashion which makes early detection worthwhile. In the past, with larger clinically detected tumors where lymph nodes were frequently positive, routine dissection and clearance of the axilla was a reasonable approach, but the shift towards EBC in the era of mass screening means that positive nodes are now less often present. Only ~30% of EBC cases have involved nodes, so most women would be overtreated by routine ALND and unnecessarily put at risk of the main complications of lymphedema and neuropathy. Nevertheless, even among minimal cancers (<1 cm or T1ab), up to ~10% may be node positive at presentation [18]. Therefore, it is important to ascertain the number of involved axillary nodes in all cases in order to estimate prognosis and the need for adjuvant chemotherapy.

With the advent of SLNB (Appendix 4), it became possible to stage the axilla with greatly reduced arm morbidity [19]. A number of clinical trials have confirmed SLNB to be a highly accurate technique, with a false-negative rate of < 10% achievable when up to three sentinel nodes are routinely sought. Accordingly, current clinical best practice for staging the axilla is to perform SLNB unless positive axillary nodes have been detected clinically or by imaging, and confirmed by biopsy. If SLNB does show positive nodes, only then is level I and II ALND performed, with retrieval of at least 10 nodes usually preferred to more limited axillary sampling. The benefit of the added yield from more nodes has to be weighed against the morbidity of more extensive dissection.

Mapping local disease extent with MRI

Assessing the extent of a known invasive cancer was among the first major applications of breast MRI, utilizing its high sensitivity to demonstrate multifocal or multicentric disease and contralateral tumors. A point to note is that TNM staging does not specifically take into account multifocality, multicentricity or extent of DCIS, while a contralateral tumor is staged separately. Consequently, purists may prefer the term "disease mapping" when considering the role of MRI in surgical planning.

Where MRI findings do change TNM stage, this is usually either because an invasive cancer is shown to be larger than expected or because abnormal lymph nodes are detected, although these findings often do not alter the surgical plan [20]. Compared to conventional breast imaging, MRI has consistently shown much better correlation with histopathologic disease extent [21, 22], confirming its potential as a pre-surgical planning tool. Overestimation of tumor size and false-positive results remain problematic, and techniques to improve lesion specificity are being developed, among which DWI shows considerable potential.

Additional disease shown by MRI in the ipsilateral breast

In two recent reviews, concordance of MRI and pathologic size was within 5 mm for 50–65% of all invasive cancers [23, 24]. As would be expected, correlation was best for cancers < 2 cm in diameter, with both these studies and others showing a tendency for overestimation by MRI as lesion size increases. In some

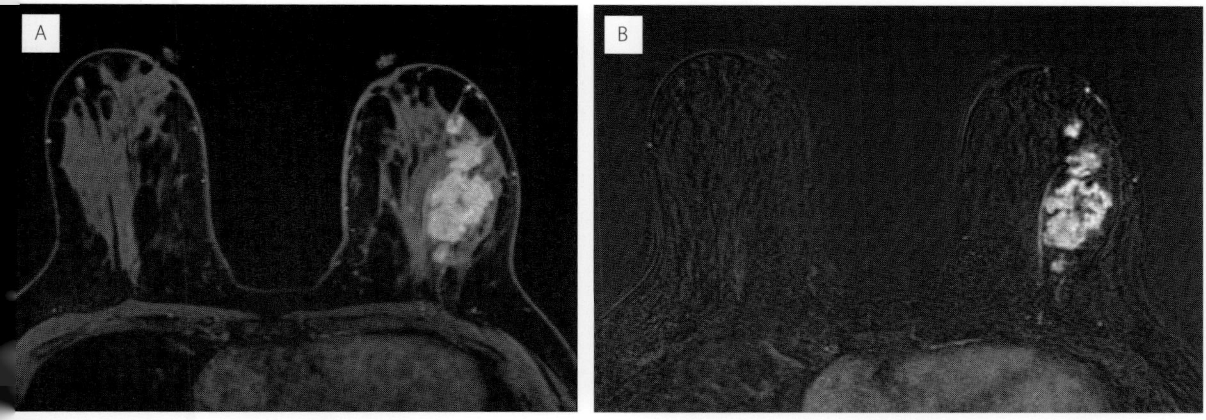

Fig. 6.1 **Defining index cancer size and multifocality:** MRI in a 46-year-old woman with dense breasts and left breast mass difficult to assess clinically and by conventional imaging (XRM and US estimated tumor size at 3–4 cm). (A) Contrast-enhanced fat-suppressed T1-weighted image and (B) subtracted image delineate a dominant 40 mm tumor mass with at least three satellite lesions giving an overall anteroposterior extent of 85 mm and transverse diameter of 35 mm. The patient was treated by subcutaneous mastectomy and ALND (grade 2 IDC with 1/12 nodes positive).

cases, overestimation can reflect significant other findings such as adjacent DCIS or satellite lesions [23, 25]. Shrinkage which occurs in fixed pathology specimens could also be a contributing factor to apparent overestimation by MRI [24].

Ipsilateral tumor foci additional to the index cancer found only by MRI are reported in up to 35% of preoperative staging studies (Fig. 6.1), with a recent meta-analysis giving an estimated mean of 16% across 19 studies totalling 2610 women (range 6–34%) [26]. In the majority of cases, additional disease is multifocal (within 2–3 cm of the index cancer or in the same quadrant), with multicentric lesions (at least 2–3 cm away from the index cancer or in another quadrant) reported in 2–15% in different series [3]. This variation is not unexpected due to differences in selection criteria, technical factors and definitions of multicentricity.

In a large single-center study, Hollingsworth *et al.* reported on 603 consecutive surgical cases with newly diagnosed breast cancer (388 IDC, 149 DCIS, 65 ILC and 1 malignant phyllodes tumor) [27]. Multicentric disease (defined as further disease at least 5 cm away from the index cancer or non-contiguously involving another quadrant) was identified in 43 patients (7%) on conventional imaging, while a further 43 cases (7%) were revealed only by MRI. This is comparable to the IBMC 6883 multicenter trial in which additional foci >2 cm from the index cancer were defined as multicentric disease, and were found only by MRI in ~10% of patients (41/423) [28].

In a meta-analysis by Houssami *et al.*, the overall PPV for malignancy of an additional MRI finding was a very creditable 66% (benign to malignant ratio of 1:2) [26]. Nevertheless, this represents a significant false-positive rate in confirming additional cancer lesions with about one-third of women undergoing benign biopsies. Despite this, it is essential that biopsy proof of possible multicentric disease is obtained whenever this could potentially alter management from BCT to mastectomy. In the meta-analysis, MRI was responsible for conversion from BCT to mastectomy in ~8% of women, while false-positive MRI findings resulted in inappropriate conversion to mastectomy in only 1% [26].

In addition to delineating tumor size and multicentricity, advanced local disease with chest wall invasion (defined as involvement of ribs, serratus anterior or intercostal muscles as distinct from only pectoral muscle infiltration) is reliably shown by MRI, and nodular skin infiltration can also be identified in some cases (Fig. 6.2).

Additional disease in the contralateral breast

A recent meta-analysis of 3250 women across 22 studies has established that contralateral cancer is shown only by MRI in 4% of cases with a PPV of ~50% (1:1 benign to malignant ratio) [29]. Where reported, additional contralateral cancers were invasive in 65% (mean size 9 mm) and DCIS in 35% (mean size 7 mm).

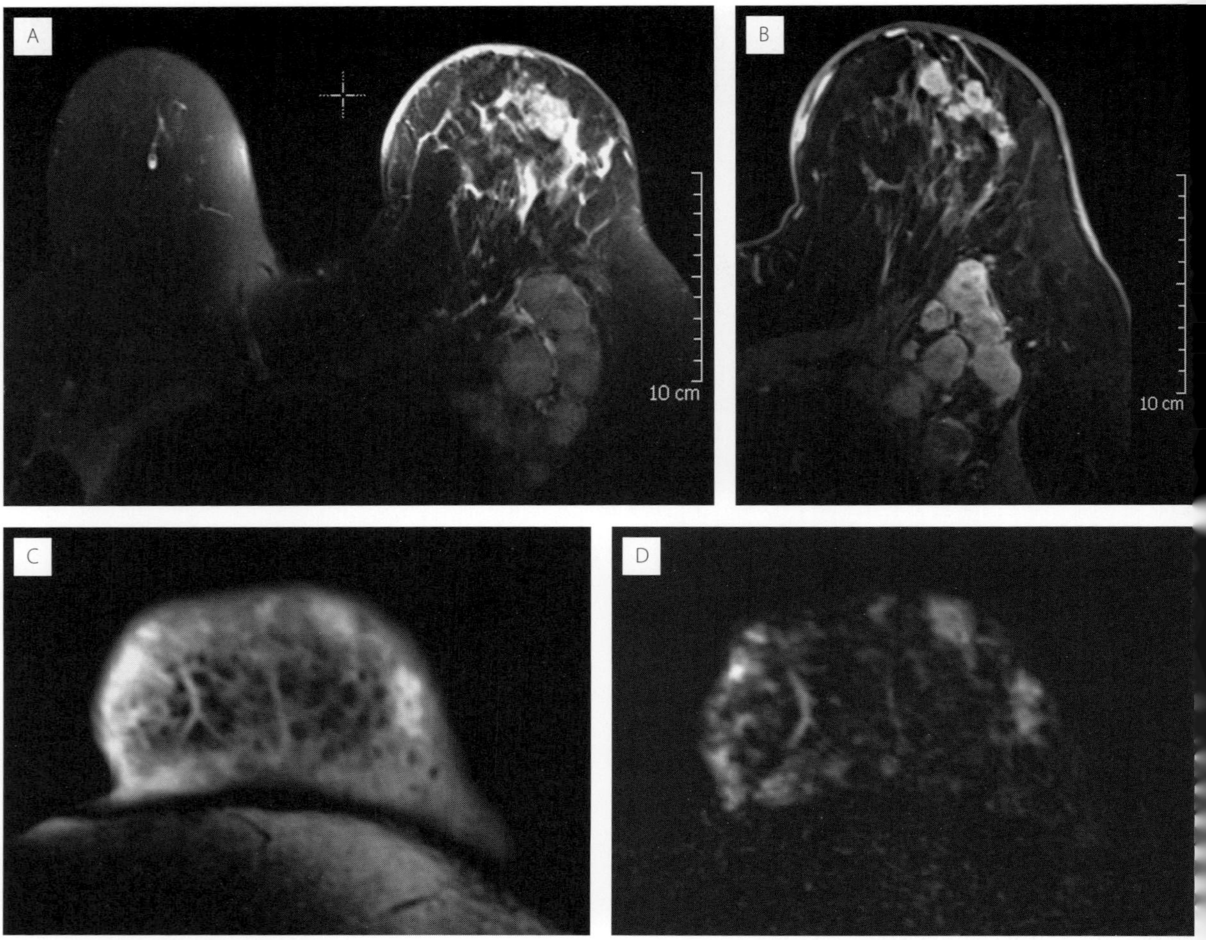

Fig. 6.2 **Inflammatory breast cancer with dermal infiltration:** (A) Non-contrast SPAIR image (fat-suppressed T2-weighted) shows skin-thickening and diffuse edema in the left breast with massive axillary lymphadenopathy. (B) Post-contrast fat-suppressed T1-weighted image shows multiple enhancing masses consistent with invasive tumor foci and coalescent axillary nodes. (C) Axial post-contrast T1-weighted and (D) subtracted images at inferior border of breast show patchy nodular dermal enhancement with tumor plugging of dermal lymphatics confirmed on punch biopsy. Tumor was accordingly T4d (inflammatory carcinoma), N2a (matted axillary nodes) and Stage IIIB. Patient was treated with neoadjuvant chemotherapy prior to mastectomy and ALND.

Where pathologic staging of the contralateral cancers was available, the great majority were either pTis or pT1 and node negative.

In the largest study to date, the multicenter ACRIN trial 6667 involving 969 women over 25 sites, MRI detected clinically and mammographically occult breast cancer in the contralateral breast in 30 women (3.1%). The sensitivity of MRI for contralateral cancer was 91%, specificity was 88% and the NPV was 99% [30]. In the single-center series reported by Hollingsworth *et al.*, contralateral cancers were evident in six cases on conventional imaging with an additional 22 cases shown only by MRI [27]. Overall 3.7% of patients had a contralateral cancer found only by MRI, with the authors observing that half of these were of equal or higher stage than the index lesion.

Invasive lobular cancer

Invasive lobular cancer is widely recognized as a distinct clinico-pathologic entity which may often present with large multifocal or multicentric tumors (Fig. 6.3) [31]. The insidious growth pattern of ILC, with only minimal fibrosis, makes this tumor notoriously difficult to diagnose on XRM, which is a contributing factor to often late diagnosis and potentially poorer outcomes.

Although ILC can be a challenging diagnosis even on MRI, the reported 93% overall sensitivity

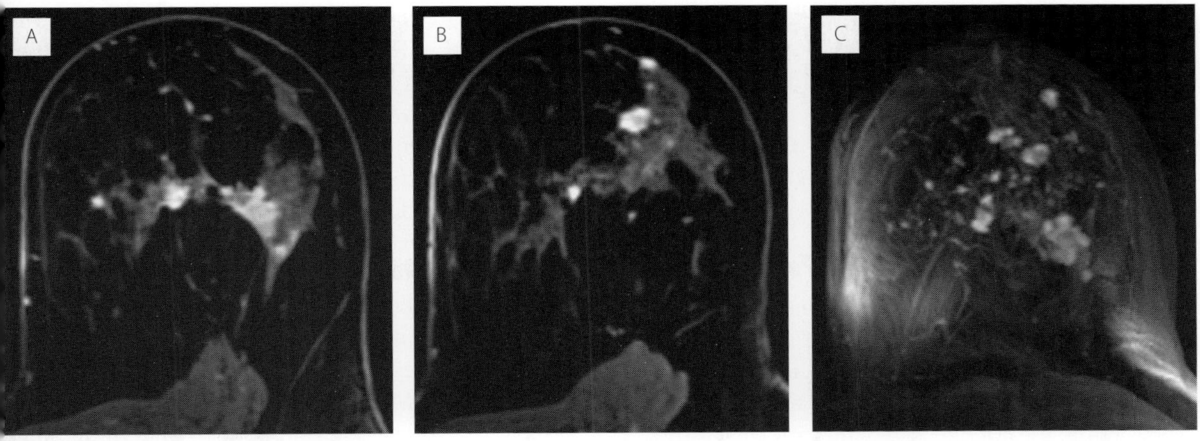

Fig. 6.3 **Multicentric invasive lobular cancer:** MRI in a 58-year-old woman after screening XRM showed non-specific asymmetric density and architectural distortion in left breast, with acoustic shadowing on US, considered to be equivocal (images not shown). Subsequent x-ray stereotactic biopsy revealed ILC but extent was unclear. (A) Post-contrast axial fat-suppressed T1-weighted image shows non-mass enhancement laterally, 10 mm central mass and enhancing focus medially with more cephalad image (B) showing further masses and foci. Composite MIP image (C) shows widely distributed lesions which involved three quadrants. Further biopsies at 12:00 and 4:00, more than 5 cm apart showed ILC at both locations. The patient underwent mastectomy with pathology confirming multicentric classical ILC, closely correlating with MRI extent.

indicates substantially better performance than conventional imaging methods, particularly XRM [32]. Nevertheless, a thorough understanding of the various patterns of presentation of ILC is vital for accurate MRI interpretation (Chapter 3), together with a recognition that ILC is more frequently subtle or even undetectable on MRI than is IDC.

Significantly higher rates of both multifocal and multicentric disease detection by MRI have been confirmed, with Liberman *et al.* finding additional mammographically occult ispilateral foci in 55% of ILC cases versus 22% for other tumor types [21]. Meanwhile, in the series by Hollingsworth *et al.*, among 65 patients with ILC, multicentricity was found in 18%, with more than two-thirds of these cases demonstrated only by MRI [27].

Correlation of MRI with pathologic size of ILC

A literature review by Mann *et al.* confirmed the superiority of MRI over conventional imaging in delineating tumor extent, with MRI showing excellent histopathologic correlation (coefficients of 0.81–0.97) and rarely overestimating lesion size [32]. Over all studies reviewed, additional ipsilateral lesions were detected only by MRI in over 30% of patients. Contralateral cancer is more frequently encountered with ILC, with tumors occult to conventional imaging and seen only by MRI in 7–8% of patients, compared with ~4% for all invasive cancer types. Overall, the MRI findings after preoperative assessment for ILC result in altered surgical management in about 28% of patients [32].

One study which specifically evaluated the accuracy of tumor size predictions for 69 surgically treated ILCs found MRI was correct within 10 mm of pathologic size in 74% and underestimated 16% [33]. Overestimation by MRI of > 10 mm occurred in 7/69 (10%), due to extensive DCIS (2 cases), LCIS (4 cases) or inflammatory reaction (1 case) [34]. Another series of 70 patients reported that MRI was correct within 5 mm of pathologic size in 56%, underestimated in 14% and overestimated by > 5 mm in 31%, comparable to the previous study after allowing for the smaller degree of tolerance [35].

Influence of MRI on surgical outcomes

Multidisciplinary guidelines for BCT indicate that patients with ILC "are candidates for conservative surgery and radiation, provided the tumor is not diffuse in the breast and that complete excision with negative margins can be achieved" [1]. In practice, difficulty in determining tumor extent has resulted in higher reported failure rates for BCT in ILC patients, frequently resulting in conversion to mastectomy. A recent large review of data from multiple trials showed an overall 72% mastectomy rate for ILC compared with 56% for IDC [31].

Mann *et al.* reported data on 267 consecutive patients with ILC of which 99 had preoperative MRI while 168 did not, and found a significantly lower re-excision rate of 9% in the MRI group compared with 27% in the non-MRI group [36]. There was no increase in the mastectomy rate which was 48% in the MRI group compared with 59% in the non-MRI group. Accordingly, MRI appears ideally suited as a preoperative planning tool whenever a histologic diagnosis of ILC is obtained.

Assessing DCIS extent

The extent of DCIS is not actually considered in TNM staging, whether in pure form or associated with invasive cancer. The traditional concept of an EIC as an adverse prognostic indicator has also been superseded by the knowledge that achieving clear surgical margins is the key to minimizing the risk of local recurrence. Nevertheless, accurately estimating DCIS extent is vital in determining whether the primary aim of BCT is achievable or if the disease is so extensive (large bidimensional measurement, multicentric or involving the NAC) that only mastectomy will be effective.

In recent years, the role of MRI in DCIS detection has become clearer, as improved resolution and greater experience have allowed the MRI signs of DCIS to be much better appreciated. It has also emerged that DCIS is frequently entirely non-calcified and mammographically occult, such that MRI consistently outperforms XRM in DCIS detection. In a key prospective study of 167 women with pure DCIS, Kuhl *et al.* showed the respective sensitivities of XRM and MRI to be 56% and 92% [37].

High-grade DCIS typically shows classical features of linear-ductal or segmental distribution with clumped architecture or clustered ring enhancement (Chapter 3) and MRI has high sensitivity in these circumstances. Kuhl *et al.* reported 98% sensitivity for high-grade pure DCIS while >80% of false-negative findings were in non-high-grade lesions [37]. The reduced sensitivity of MRI for low-grade DCIS relates to its weaker enhancement and relatively non-specific MRI features which are difficult to differentiate from associated background benign proliferative changes. This not only makes the diagnosis of low-grade DCIS challenging, but also makes estimation of disease extent problematic, with the risk of substantial overestimation by MRI [38, 39].

Correlation of MRI with pathologic size of DCIS

A recent literature review confirmed that MRI is superior to XRM for the estimation of DCIS extent either in pure form or as an EIC in association with invasive cancer (Fig. 6.4) [39]. This analysis, including all studies from 1995 to 2008, showed a wide range for rates of both underestimation and overestimation of disease extent, which is unsurprising given the variation in technical factors and study design. The authors concluded that while histopathologic extent of DCIS is more accurately demonstrated with MRI, overestimation due to benign proliferative lesions was problematic in up to 50% of cases and occurred most frequently with non-high-grade disease [39].

Many studies which have attempted to correlate DCIS size by MRI with histopathology have been based on patients presenting with mammographic calcifications, which may tend to be biased against MRI, whose key strength is in demonstrating non-calcified DCIS. Furthermore, there are inherent difficulties in obtaining an accurate histopathologic size for DCIS shown by MRI, calling into question whether this pathology is always a valid reference standard. While most IDCs are macroscopically apparent and can often be palpated at surgery, an area of non-calcified DCIS may not be visible to the naked eye and cannot be confirmed by specimen radiography. Not only is it then difficult for the surgeon to know how much to resect, but the histopathologist who later cuts the specimen for blocking may be hard-pressed to accurately document DCIS extent, particularly in a large piece of excised breast tissue.

In retrospective studies, accurate MRI estimation compared to pathologic size is reported in 57–72% of cases versus only 43–48% for XRM [33, 40, 41]. Among 66 patients (54 pure DCIS and 12 DCIS with IDC <10 mm), Schouten van der Velden and colleagues found MRI sensitivity was 94% but observed overestimation of DCIS size by more than 5 mm in 38% of cases [40].

In a prospective study of 33 patients with pure DCIS (2 low grade, 15 intermediate grade, 16 high grade) using a unilateral breast MRI examination technique, Marcotte-Bloch *et al.* found an overall 97% sensitivity for MRI [33]. Size of DCIS was correctly estimated by MRI within 5 mm of histologic size in 60% with ~20% overestimated and ~20% underestimated. The correlation coefficient for MRI in that study was 0.83 compared with only 0.67 for XRM, which was accurate within 5 mm of histologic size in only 38% of patients. In practice, combined interpretation of XRM and MRI is likely to afford the most accurate estimation of DCIS extent [41, 42]. It should be kept in mind

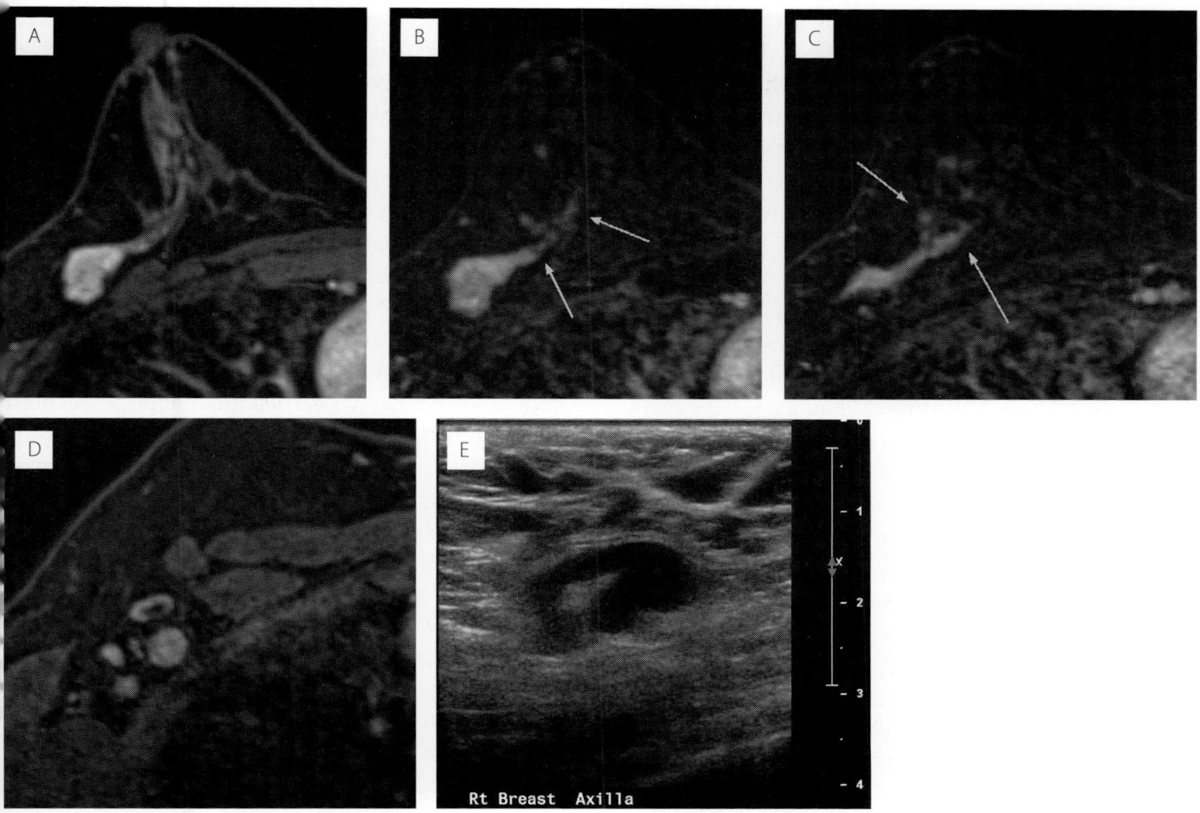

Fig. 6.4 Extent of DCIS and regional nodes: First screening MRI in a 58-year-old woman recently diagnosed as a BRCA2 mutation carrier. Screening XRM 4 months earlier was normal. (A) Early post-contrast fat-suppressed T1-weighted image shows a 22 mm mass laterally in right breast with subtracted images (B and C) showing branching linear-ductal pattern typical of DCIS extending medially (arrows) giving overall estimated size of 50 mm. (D) MRI identified six axillary lymph nodes as unequivocally involved (note only most anterior node in this group shows a normal thin cortex and preserved fatty hilum). (E) TUS confirmed MRI findings with positive FNA of multilobulated enlarged node. The patient underwent right mastectomy with ALND and prophylactic left mastectomy. MRI findings closely correlated with pathologic invasive cancer size and DCIS extent (23 mm grade 3 IDC, 25 mm high-grade DCIS, ER/PR +ve, HER2 –ve, 15/16 nodes positive, T2, pN3a, Stage IIIC disease).

that both underestimation and false-negative MRI studies do occur, even with high-grade DCIS.

Influence of MRI on surgical outcomes

Positive margins after initial surgical resection are found in 20–70% of women undergoing BCT [43], usually due to a DCIS component. Standard practice is to undertake further surgery to shave additional tissue from the appropriate location in the cavity wall. The final recourse is to mastectomy if margins remain persistently positive. In such circumstances, MRI can be used after the initial surgery in a problem-solving role, to determine if residual disease is amenable to further resection or whether mastectomy is inevitable (Chapter 7).

Other centers have adopted a prospective approach and use MRI preoperatively to predict DCIS extent. Harms reported low re-excision rates of less than 10% and improved cosmesis with BCT because better delineation by MRI allowed the appropriate surgery to be performed the first time [44]. Similarly, in a retrospective review, Schouten van der Velden *et al.* noted that among women with DCIS who had preoperative MRI, 50% had tumor-involved surgical margins after first excision compared with 80% of women who did not have MRI [40]. Harms observed that because of the ductal distribution of DCIS, "cigar-shaped excisions" after MRI-guided hookwire localization made BCT a viable option in some women who might otherwise have been candidates for mastectomy [44]. In such cases, bracketing non-mass lesions with two MRI-guided hookwires may be very helpful.

Another potential role for bilateral MRI after a biopsy diagnosis of DCIS is in detecting additional disease in the ipsilateral or contralateral breast, not apparent on conventional imaging. However, while larger invasive foci can often be detected, MRI cannot identify microinvasive foci present in background DCIS. Nonetheless, using the high NPV of MRI to exclude occult disease may allow more limited lumpectomies to be performed in women with small focal areas of DCIS [44].

Staging the lymph nodes with MRI

Although MRI cannot compete with the sensitivity of SLNB (which accurately detects metastases of 2 mm or less), it is often possible to identify morphologically abnormal axillary lymph nodes on MRI, allowing subsequent US-guided biopsy. In instances where a positive result is obtained, the need for SLNB is obviated and ALND is performed. Furthermore, MRI may have a complementary role by showing abnormal nodes which SLNB fails to detect. Some false-negative SLNB results are due to nodes being completely replaced by tumor so that they are bypassed by the lymphatic flow. Such nodes are often significantly enlarged and amenable to demonstration by MRI. The sensitivity of SLNB is also lower for involved IMC nodes, which have a deeper drainage pathway and yet may be the site of first metastasis for cancers located in the medial quadrants. As surgical sampling of IMC nodes is not routine, their detection by MRI makes a useful contribution to accurate staging.

To date, relatively little importance has been attached to the evaluation of axillary lymph nodes on MRI. Early commercially available breast coils often did not provide good axillary coverage and suffered from cardiac pulsation artifact [45]. Kvistad *et al.* emphasized the importance of coil design and Luciani *et al.* used additional surface coils to better demonstrate the axillary regions [45, 46]. Recent multichannel coils incorporate elements specifically placed to provide artifact-free axillary coverage and allow high-resolution imaging, capable of resolving the internal architecture of lymph nodes. With the technical limitations of imaging the axilla now largely overcome, radiologists can now look beyond diagnosing only grossly enlarged nodes, or those with overt extracapsular spread.

So, given that grossly abnormal morphology is seen in only a small proportion of lymph nodes which are found to be histologically malignant, are there other features which can be used to predict more subtle metastatic disease? Kvistad *et al.* suggested that the intense enhancement often seen in malignant nodes could be more reliable than morphology in discriminating between benign and malignant nodes [45]. In the context of ipsilateral invasive cancer this may be of some help, but it is common clinical experience that even benign nodes often enhance intensely and may show a type 3 kinetic curve (washout). Therefore, as is the case in characterizing other lesions on breast MRI, morphologic features need to be evaluated.

Long-axis size is not a good benign versus malignant discriminator because long thin nodes are often seen as normal. However, rounded nodes with short-axis dimensions over 5 mm become increasingly suspicious for expansion by tumor [45]. Eccentric nodular cortical thickening is another strong malignant sign (previously validated by US) reflecting that afferent lymphatic channels enter the nodal cortex peripherally. Nodular cortical expansion by metastatic deposits then leads to compression and eventual obliteration of the hilar fat (Fig. 6.4).

Signal characteristics are also important to consider. Whereas most benign nodes show bright signal on FSE T2-weighted and pre-contrast non-fat-suppressed T1-weighted images, malignant nodes exhibit low signal on these sequences. Luciani *et al.* observed that fatty hila in normal nodes were dark on fat-suppressed T2-weighted IR images, while in malignant nodes the hilar fat often showed bright signal, above that of adjacent pectoral muscle [46]. Recently, signs of involved axillary nodes have been further validated in an ex vivo study, and are summarized in Table 6.4 [47]. When used in combination, these signs offer the best overall prediction of involved axillary nodes by MRI, and this information can then be used to locate and biopsy by US. A useful practical tip is that in ~80% of cases the sentinel node is the lowest

Table 6.4 MRI features of malignant axillary nodes

Irregular outer cortical contours, spiculation, overt extracapsular spread
Low signal on FSE T2-weighted and pre-contrast T1-weighted images
Short-axis diameter > 5 mm (less sensitive but more specific if increase threshold to 10 mm)
High signal intensity of hilum > muscle on fat-suppressed T2-weighted, replacing normal dark fat signal
Abnormal cortex (thickened > 3 mm, irregular or eccentric more suspicious than uniform)
Intense enhancement (but in isolation this is a soft malignant sign even with washout)

Colour Plates

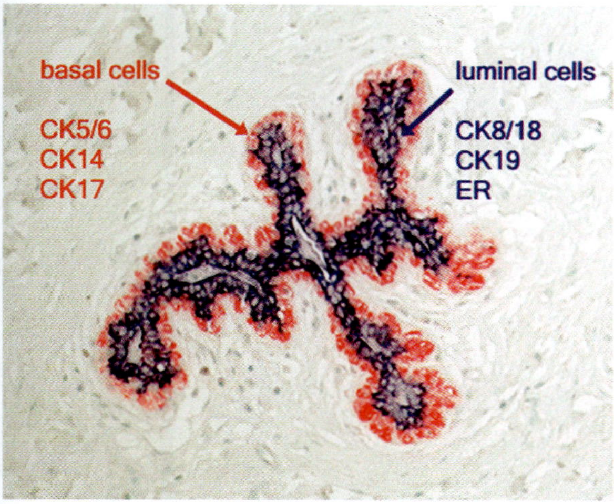

Plate 1 **Breast anatomy:** TDLU stained to show outer basal cell layer (red) with inner luminal cell layer (blue) and typical basal and luminal cytokeratins. Luminal cells also stain positive for ER. (Photomicrograph by kind permission of Professor Sunil Lakhani, University of Queensland, Brisbane). See chapter 2.

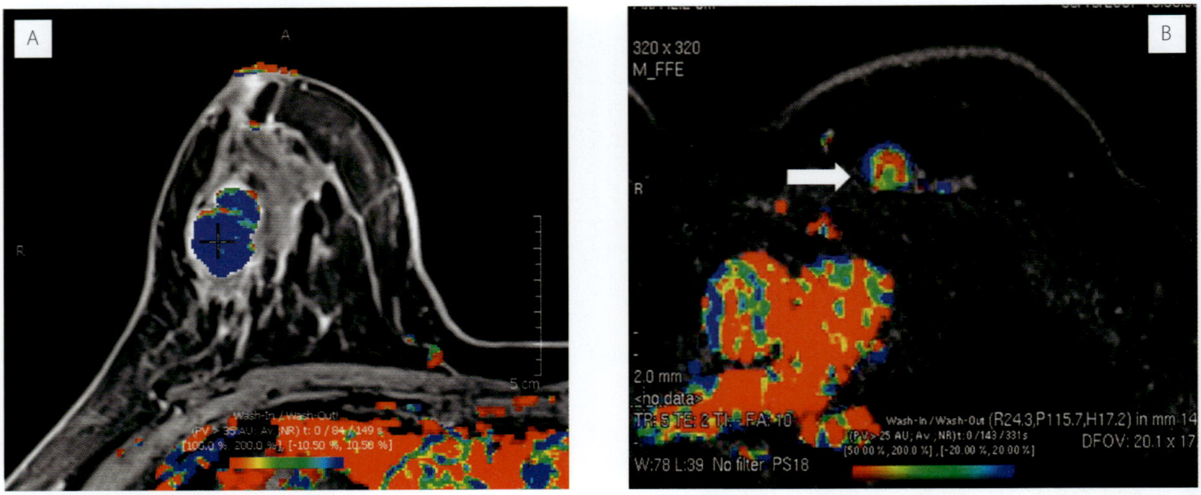

Plate 2 **Use of color-mapping in mass analysis:** (A) Color-mapping overlay on large ovoid circumscribed mass with internal septations which showed rapid initial-phase enhancement to ~200% at 90 seconds. The mass is coded blue to indicate the late-phase behavior of persistent kinetics (type 1 curve) consistent with fibroadenoma (see also Fig. 3.13). (B) In a different patient, another ovoid circumscribed mass (arrow) also showed rapid initial-phase enhancement to ~200% at 90 seconds. Color-mapping overlay shows heterogeneous late-phase pattern with areas of wash-out kinetics coded red. Biopsy showed triple-negative grade 3 IDC (see also Fig. 3.15). See chapter 3.

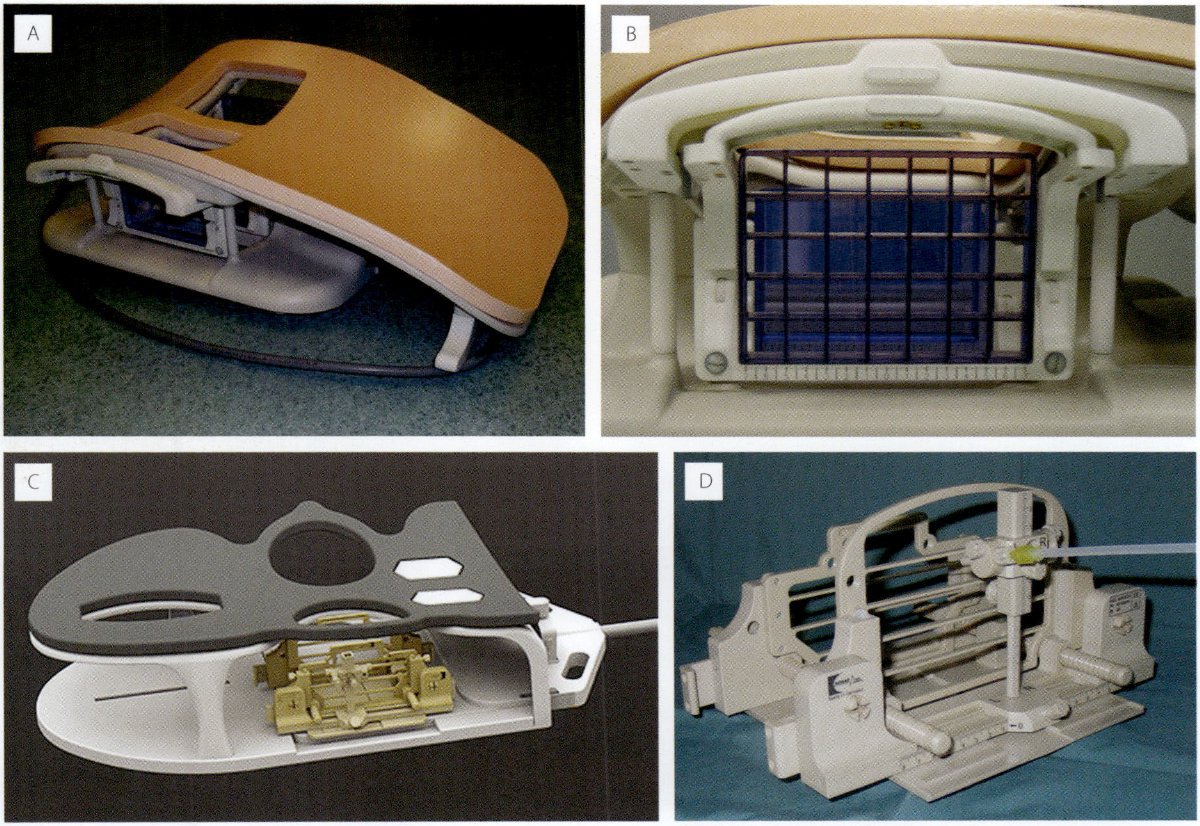

Plate 3 Interventional breast coils: (A) InVivo 7-channel coil design incorporating biopsy access with (B) detail of grid system underneath. (C) Noras 4-channel coil with biopsy device attached and detail view (D) showing set-up for hookwire procedure using pillar-and-post method. See chapter 4.

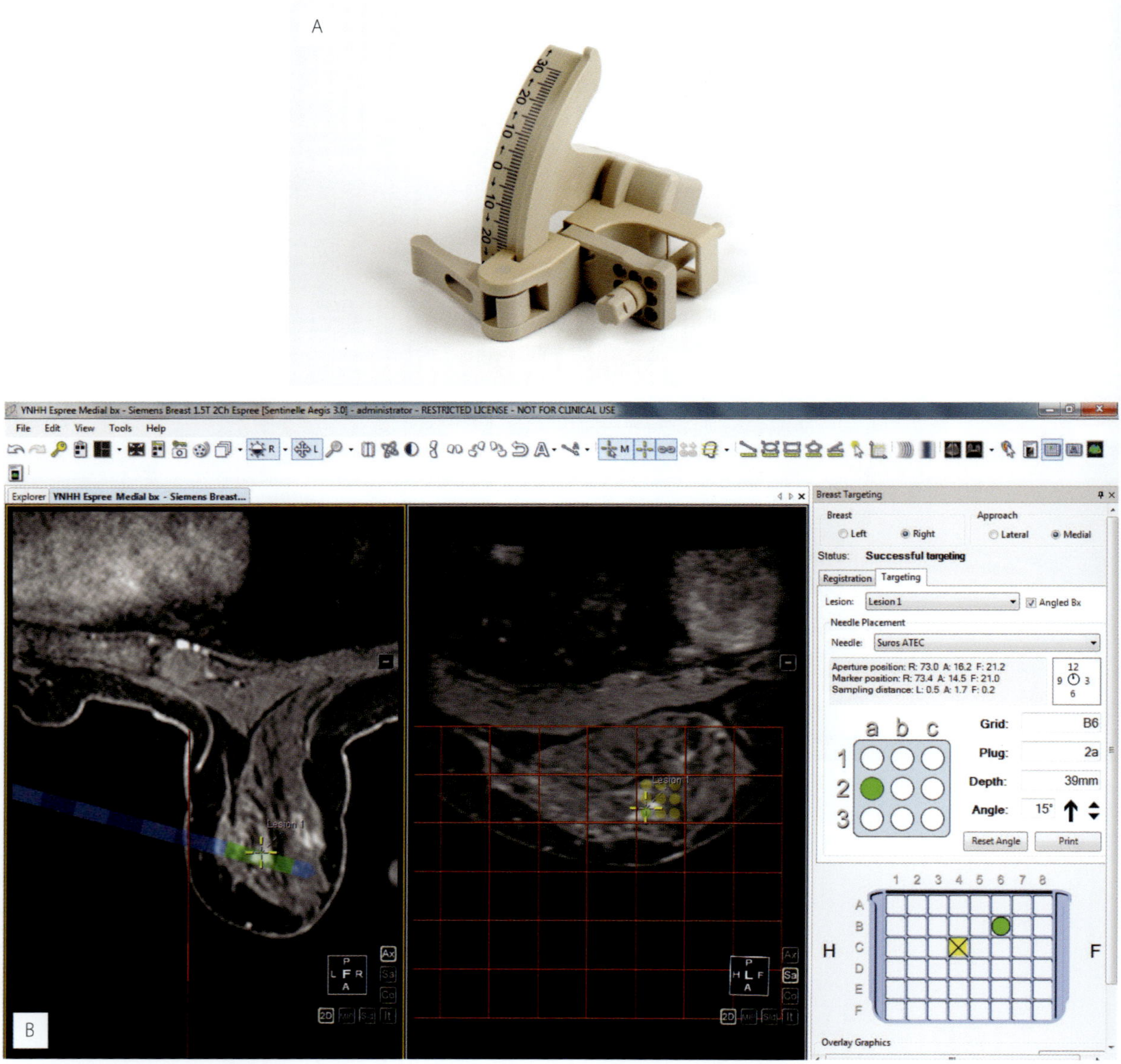

Plate 4 Hybrid grid plus pillar-and-post system for VAB: (A) The Sentinelle Verity device plugs into the grid like a needle-block guidance system, but has pillar-and-post flexibility to choose any angled approach. (B) Sophisticated Aegis guidance software facilitates targeting by projecting the biopsy aperture position relative to the lesion, and ensures the approach does not impinge on the grid. See chapter 4.

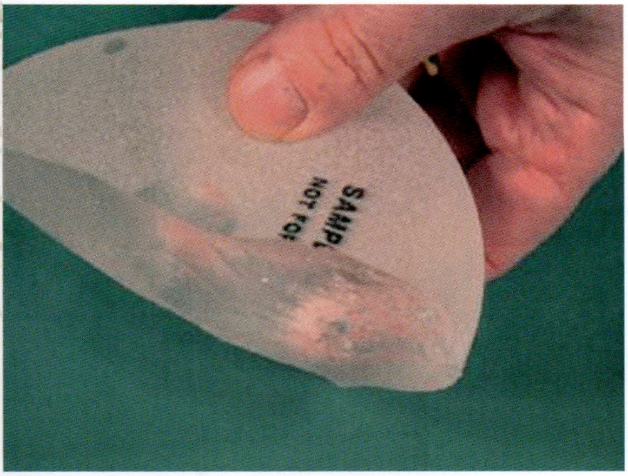

Plate 5 **Gummy bear implant:** Cut surface of fifth generation silicone breast implant showing highly cohesive gel structure which minimizes risk of leakage. (Photograph by kind permission of Associate Professor Bruno Giuffre, Royal North Shore Hospital, Sydney). See chapter 8.

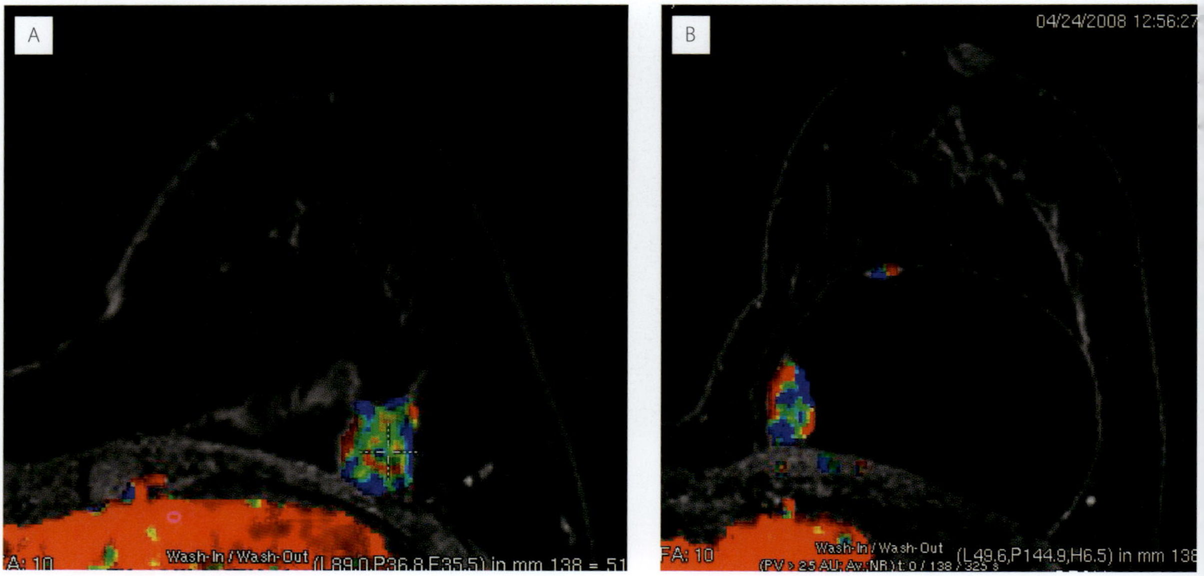

Plate 6 **Silicone granulomas:** Screening MRI in woman with implants from late 1970s shows new finding of heterogeneously enhancing masses adjacent to left implant at (A) 4 o'clock and (B) 9 o'clock which were due to silicone granulomas. (see also Fig. 8.9). See chapter 8.

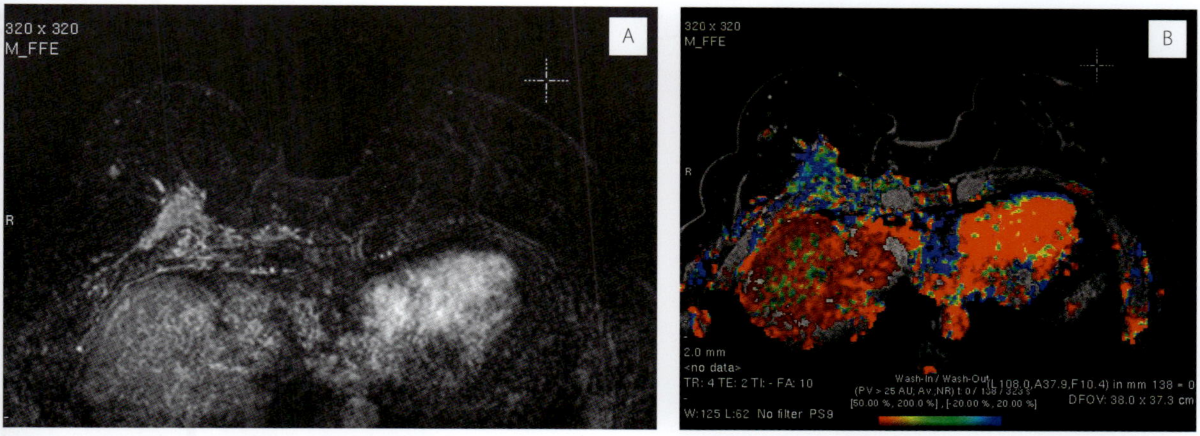

Plate 7 **Recurrence after TRAM flap reconstruction:** 59-year-old woman with right mastectomy and TRAM flap performed 5 years earlier, now feels discomfort at inferior margin, difficult to assess clinically. (A) Subtracted axial scan and (B) T1-weighted image with color-mapping shows heterogeneous enhancement with chest wall invasion. Biopsy confirmed recurrent invasive carcinoma. See chapter 8.

level I lymph node, so the search for abnormal nodes at TUS should begin in the axillary tail [48].

As mentioned, involved lymph nodes in the IMC can also be detected by MRI. Enlarged nodes are well seen on axial and coronal images, parasternally located in the second to fourth intercostal spaces adjacent to the internal thoracic vessels. Normal internal mammary nodes are seldom visible, so any MRI-detected node in this group is regarded as suspicious.

An alternative MRI technique for axillary staging uses the specific contrast agent USPIO, with reported 80–100% sensitivity and 98–100% specificity [49, 50]. If this high level of accuracy can be confirmed in larger studies, it could become possible to dispense with SLNB in the presence of a positive USPIO result. The main disadvantage is that an additional MRI examination is required because USPIO is not a general intravascular contrast agent. There is a moderate incidence of side effects, and USPIO needs to be administered by slow drip infusion [49].

Identifying distant metastases

Discussion of the indications and possible techniques for breast cancer staging are outside the scope of this text. Currently there is no routine role for breast MRI in tumor staging beyond the detection of locoregional disease. However, because much of the chest wall, mediastinum, liver, lungs and pleura are included in the FOV at breast MRI, distant metastatic disease is occasionally detected. All protocols should include a fat-suppressed IR T2-weighted sequence which is highly water-sensitive, and accordingly it is important to carefully review these images for unsuspected metastases, even in presumed EBC cases (Figs. 6.5 and 6.6). Some centers now routinely add a coronal STIR sequence of chest and upper abdomen to "screen" for metastases.

Note that, in the prone position, even very small quantities of pleural fluid collect anteriorly and are evident on T2-weighted images. Small unilateral or bilateral effusions are then extremely common on breast MRI, even in asymptomatic young women. Kaiser has suggested a cutoff depth of 7 mm above which the possibility of a pathologic cause might be considered [51].

The controversy over routine preoperative MRI

Many published articles have shown that breast MRI reveals additional multifocal, multicentric and contralateral disease. Meta-analysis suggests that overall, MRI can be expected to demonstrate additional malignant disease in about 20% of patients (16% ipsilateral, 4% contralateral) and about half of those (11%) undergo more extensive surgery than originally anticipated as a result [26, 29]. In most of these cases, additional ipsilateral disease results in conversion from WLE to mastectomy (~8%), while for the remainder (~3%), wider local excision is performed [26]. The main controversy is whether those extra mastectomies represent correct management or inappropriate overtreatment.

Opponents of routine breast MRI argue that the extra mastectomies can only be overtreatment because (i) mastectomy for EBC offers no survival benefit over BCT, and (ii) the current paradigm for BCT with ALND and RT provides good locoregional control, so there can be no benefit from adding MRI. Therefore, in effect, the claim is that MRI can only show clinically irrelevant disease that would have been successfully treated by existing protocols. Where local control does fail, the recurrence can be treated by completion mastectomy, with no apparent reduction in survival. In these circumstances, additional mastectomies could only be justified by reduced recurrence rates.

So are these valid arguments against using the most accurate available imaging technique to map disease extent prior to surgery? Table 6.5 outlines some of the expected benefits which argue the case for adopting MRI as a preoperative standard, while Table 6.6 summarizes the case against. To better understand the controversy, let us consider some of the points of argument:

1. Is there any reason at all to believe that additional disease shown by MRI is not as biologically important as that shown by conventional imaging? The answer is, of course, no. If anything, the opposite is probably true as low-grade disease is more often missed by MRI because of the lack of enhancement. Any inherent bias would be towards MRI depicting more rather than less aggressive disease.
2. Women with disease in multiple quadrants are not candidates for BCT. How can the desire for obtaining clear surgical margins be reconciled with the refusal to perform an imaging technique which reveals otherwise occult multicentric disease in the ipsilateral breast in up to 15% of cases? While it can be argued that the additional disease might have responded to standard treatment, given that MRI-detected cancer is no

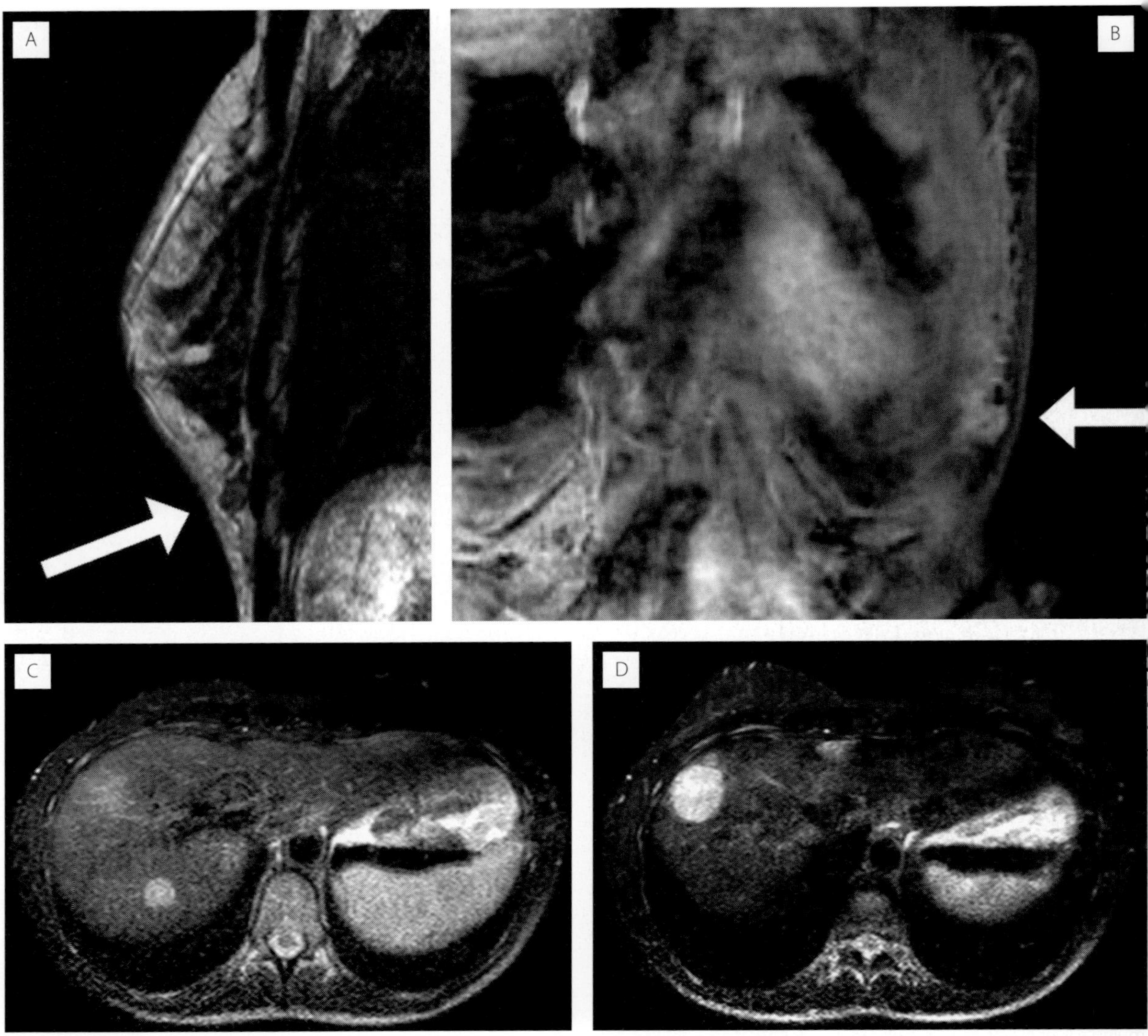

Fig. 6.5 Distant metastatic disease: MRI in a 35-year-old woman with self-detected small palpable lump peripherally in LOQ of left breast, malignant on biopsy (grade 3 IDC, ER/PR +ve, HER2 –ve). Sagittal FSE T2-weighted image (A) and coronal post-contrast fat-suppressed T1-weighted image (B) show ~10 mm circumscribed mass inferiorly protruding into subcutaneous fat (arrows). Routine IR T2-weighted images (C and D) reveal unsuspected liver masses with adenocarcinoma shown on US-guided FNAB.

less biologically important than disease shown by XRM or US, then it is not rational to ignore this MRI-detected disease in surgical planning.

3. The yield of contralateral breast cancer revealed only by MRI is ~4%, and these are of equal or higher stage in ~50% of cases. By existing treatment paradigms, such contralateral cancers would require local excision and RT. While it can be argued that systemic therapy given for the index lesion might reduce the likelihood that the contralateral cancer would actually present clinically, it is illogical to dismiss these cancers which would have been separately treated had they been found by any other means. If the patient does not undergo systemic therapy for the index cancer, then the contralateral cancer would receive no treatment at all.
4. The aim of BCT for EBC is curative treatment. Obtaining surgically clear margins is emphasized as a prerequisite for success, even if a second or third surgical procedure is required to achieve this, because obtaining final negative margins is essential to preventing local recurrence. Is it not then better to aim for a single surgical procedure

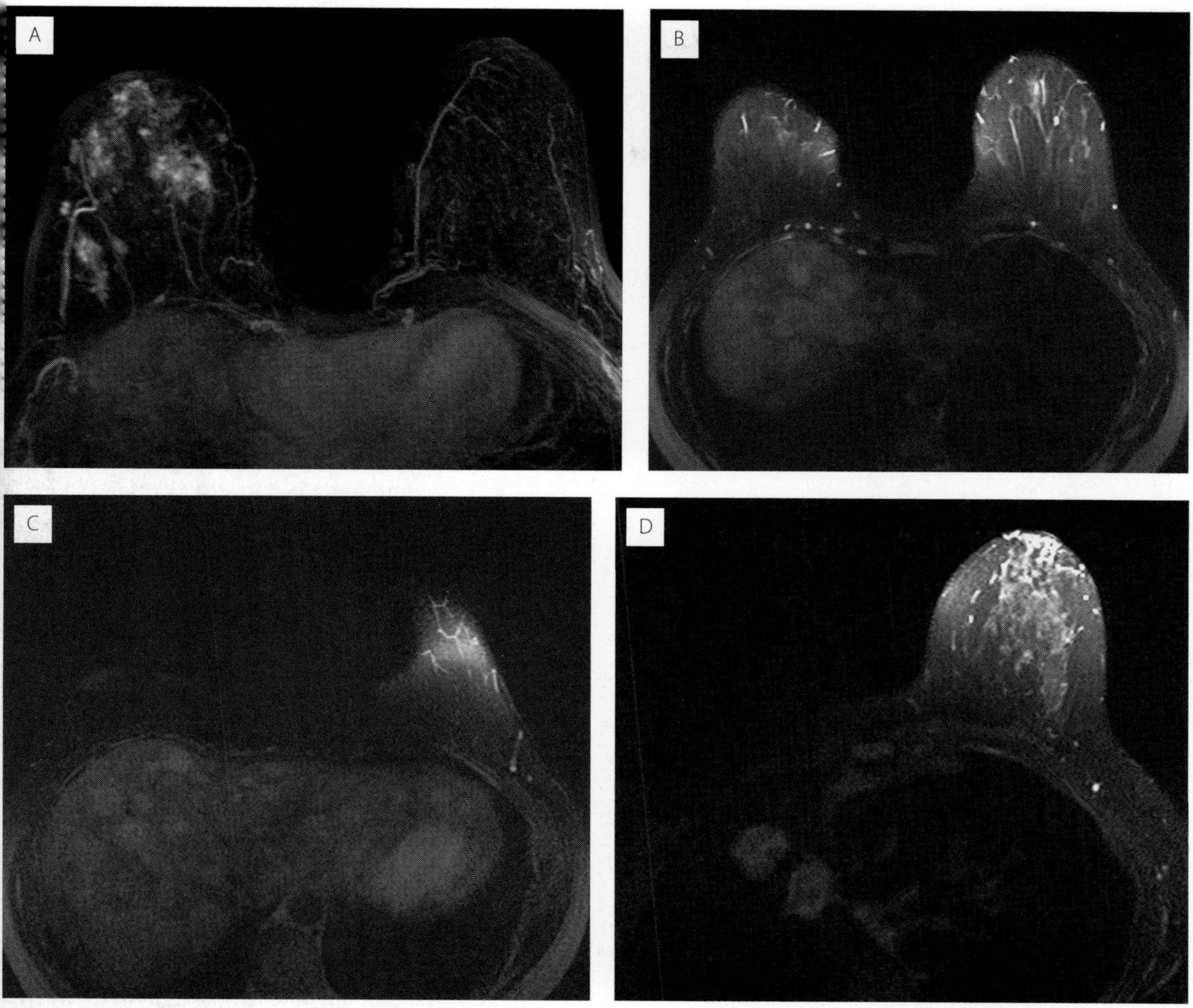

Fig. 6.6 **Distant metastatic disease:** MRI in a 45-year-old woman with self-detected 3–4 cm IDC at 4:00 in right breast and further 12 mm IDC at 9:00 shown by US. (A) MIP image confirms grossly multicentric disease. Routine IR T2-weighted images (B and C) show unsuspected multiple liver metastases. In a different patient with previous right mastectomy, MRI was requested to exclude contralateral cancer prior to breast reconstruction. Routine IR T2-weighted image (D) shows two unsuspected right lung metastases, confirmed by CT-guided biopsy.

by using an imaging technique which frequently reveals more extensive ipsilateral disease than is shown by XRM or US? If mapping of local disease extent allowed the surgeon to correctly triage patients to mastectomy where this was clearly inevitable and yet allowed for a more frequent complete excision of disease which was still amenable to BCT, this would have compelling advantages. In theory, this should be reflected in lower re-excision rates in the short term (because positive margins and re-excisions are avoided by dealing with the disease in a single operation) and lower local recurrence rates in the long term.

5. Local recurrence rates after BCT are variable. Even in the best modern series, reported rates are 5–10% at 10 years. Clearly, where specialized centers have very low recurrence rates (< 5%), the additional absolute benefit from MRI is likely to be small. However, in centers experiencing recurrence rates at the upper end of the accepted range, a correspondingly more significant benefit from MRI might be achieved. If an additional 8% of women appropriately had a mastectomy, and this reduced recurrence rates by only 50%, this could still be considered a worthwhile trade-off.

Table 6.5 Arguments in favor of routine preoperative breast MRI

Shows additional ipsilateral disease in ~16% of patients of which about half is multicentric
Additional disease shown by MRI is biologically important and should not be dismissed
An additional 8% of women having mastectomy is appropriate and could improve outcomes
More accurate delineation of disease extent could reduce re-excision rates required for BCT
Overall fewer surgical episodes required to achieve correct result, either BCT or mastectomy
Shows contralateral cancer in ~4%, of which ~50% are equal or higher stage than index lesion
Assists staging by accurately sizing invasive cancer or showing axillary/IMC nodal disease
Potential for metastatic screening by adding routine coronal STIR sequence to staging MRI

Table 6.6 Arguments against routine preoperative breast MRI

Additional disease shown by MRI is not clinically relevant to outcomes
Additional mastectomies or wider excisions represent overtreatment
Recurrence rates of standard BCT with RT benchmarked at ~10% at 10 years are acceptable
Additional cost, anxiety, false-positive biopsy procedures and delayed surgery not justified
COMICE trial showed no reduction in number of surgical episodes after preoperative MRI
No long-term prospective trial evidence of reduced recurrence rates or survival benefit

6. Assumptions regarding outcomes after local recurrence may be flawed. Is it really correct that adopting a "wait and see" approach to local recurrence after BCT does not affect survival? Despite the conclusions from the trials of mastectomy versus BCT that survival was not affected, there have been many reports in the literature to the contrary. A large meta-analysis of outcomes at 15 years estimated that one breast cancer death is prevented for every four local recurrences avoided [52]. Therefore, if using MRI to more accurately delineate disease extent prior to surgery could help to minimize local recurrence, this could also improve long-term overall survival.

Does preoperative MRI reduce re-operation rates?

There is rather little evidence in the recent literature regarding the impact of preoperative MRI on short-term reduction in re-excision rates. One single-center study of 349 consecutive women eligible for BCT (173 women with MRI workup and 176 without) found a lower re-excision rate of 13.8% in the MRI group compared with 19.4% in the non-MRI group, although this was not statistically significant [53]. As a result of the MRI, 19 women (11%) had more extensive surgery, with mastectomy performed in 15 (8.7)%.

Another single-center review of 79 consecutive women who underwent preoperative MRI over a 30-month period found a low re-excision rate of 10% (versus 20% in prior published data from the same institution) [43]. The authors attributed the reduction to improved local staging, allowing better selection of patients for neoadjuvant chemotherapy prior to BCT and guiding the surgeon as to the extent of partial mastectomy required. Similarly, Harms also attributed a low 10% re-excision rate to preoperative MRI in an editorial with regard to treatment of DCIS [44].

Recently, Mann *et al.* published their experience in relation to ILC, and reported a 9% re-excision rate in 99 women who had preoperative MRI compared with 27% in the non-MRI group [36]. Therefore, it appears that in some experienced centers at least, and in some patient subgroups, preoperative MRI can have a favorable impact on operation rates.

On the other hand, the prospective UK COMICE trial, in which 1623 women across 45 centers were randomly assigned to groups with and without preoperative MRI, showed similar re-excision rates of ~11% and identical total re-operation rates of 19% in both groups [54]. However, with 1623 women recruited across 45 centers, (a mean of only 7 patients per center per year), the authors acknowledged that level of experience of the participating radiologists was a limitation of the study. Moreover, many women in the study proceeded to mastectomy without pathologic verification of the MRI findings due to a lack of biopsy capability, which is contrary to standard recommendations.

The COMICE trial authors also observed that the failure of MRI to improve surgical treatment could relate to "mode of presentation of imaging data to the surgeon," and specifically cited difficulties in lesion palpation, differences in position at imaging versus surgery and the potential for inadequate tumor delineation when only a single hookwire is used [54].

The MONET trial is another recent prospective study, conducted at 3T across three centers in the Netherlands. In this study, over 400 women with non-palpable cancers were randomly assigned to MRI and non-MRI groups [55]. Somewhat paradoxically, there was a higher re-excision rate of 18/53 (34%) in the MRI group versus 6/50 (12%) in the non-MRI group, while mastectomy rates were not significantly different. However, due to the selection criteria requiring non-palpable cancers, there was an unusually high proportion (60%) of DCIS cases appearing as microcalcification alone, over-representing a subset where MRI is known to have difficulty in accurately determining extent. This could have translated into surgeons being misled into attempting smaller initial lumpectomies. As in the COMICE trial, the MONET authors also commented on the difficulty of effectively conveying the MRI data to the operating room.

Does preoperative MRI influence long-term outcomes?

To date, there are just two published trials which address the influence of preoperative MRI on local recurrence rates, with conflicting conclusions. In a retrospective review of 346 women (121 with MRI, 225 without) with a minimum 20-month follow-up (mean 40 months), Fischer *et al.* found a significantly lower local recurrence rate of 1.2% (1/86) in the MRI group versus 6.8% (9/133) in the non-MRI group [56]. Among patients in the MRI group, 71% had BCT and 29% had mastectomy, versus 61% and 39% for the non-MRI group, while the incidence of contralateral breast cancer was also lower in the MRI group (1.6% versus 4% in the non-MRI group).

In another retrospective study, Solin *et al.* reviewed 8-year outcome data for 756 women with EBC (215 with MRI, 541 without) and found no significant difference in recurrence rates (3% for the MRI group, and 4% for the non-MRI group) or in contralateral breast cancer incidence [57]. While this study is frequently quoted by opponents of routine breast MRI as evidence of no long-term benefit, several flaws in the study design limit the conclusions which can be drawn:

(i) The study took no account of the potential benefit to an unspecified number of women who had a mastectomy because extensive disease was shown by MRI, and who were then excluded. The low recurrence rates that these women could be expected to experience were then disregarded, a point of difference compared with the study by Fischer *et al.* [56].

(ii) The study was non-randomized, with ~40% of women in the MRI group being aged < 50 years compared with only ~30% in the non-MRI group, suggesting selection bias towards more aggressive disease and therefore potentially poorer outcomes in the MRI group.

(iii) Most importantly, a full 50% of the MRI studies were not preoperative staging examinations because they were performed after at least one surgical excision had been undertaken. In these circumstances, MRI is less reliable due to the presence of post-surgical changes with sensitivity of only around 60% [58]. This reduced sensitivity of MRI to additional disease may well have been enough to mask any benefit in this study.

(iv) Finally, as the authors observed, given the very low local recurrence rates of less than 5% in both groups, demonstrating any statistically significant improvement in the MRI group "would be extremely difficult in a retrospective cohort study."

Another argument used against preoperative MRI is that the rate at which additional disease is detected by MRI (~16%) is 2- to 3-fold higher than observed recurrence rates after BCT, implying that this disease is often not clinically relevant [3, 59–61]. However, of this total 16% additional ipsilateral disease shown by MRI about half (the multifocal disease) would probably have manifested as positive margins and been dealt with by re-excision. Only the multicentric disease (shown by MRI in ~8%) would be expected to escape detection with the risk of later recurrence. Dealing with these cases at the first operation (usually by mastectomy) is where the most benefit can be expected in a cohort undergoing routine MRI assessment, by triaging them out from the BCT group. While this effect helps to explain the findings in the study by Solin *et al.* [57], the argument seems entirely fallacious as evidence against the value of routine preoperative MRI. An ~8% rate of multifocal disease seen only by MRI is consistent with observed rates of ipsilateral local recurrence.

A similar argument is sometimes also used in relation to contralateral disease, i.e., that the observed incidence is lower than would be expected from the reported prevalence of synchronous disease at MRI

(~4%). However, a 4% upfront detection rate is consistent with the cumulative rates of 3% by 5 years and 6% by 10 years reported by Gao *et al.* [62], particularly if the protective effects of adjuvant systemic therapy are taken into account.

Based on limited evidence, how should we proceed?

Currently, while some centers embrace routine preoperative breast MRI for all newly diagnosed breast cancer cases, others reject it entirely. So the great news is that if you are just starting up your MRI service and are already having trouble keeping up with demand for high-risk screening, you don't have to feel under pressure to offer routine preoperative staging!

With regard to the potential for MRI to improve management, it seems perfectly reasonable that this should be possible, at least for some patient subgroups. As the COMICE trial suggests though, local factors are likely to influence how well breast MRI findings translate into better surgical results, and it should not be assumed that the experience of small, highly experienced centers is readily transferable to the wider medical community.

Probably the most logical approach is to start by using MRI in selected women who are at highest risk of local treatment failure [63]. Young women, who tend to have more aggressive disease, are prime candidates, particularly when combined with dense breast tissue or other factors which may make it more difficult to define extent. Women with familial breast cancer may also be more likely to have multifocal or multicentric disease. Suggested selection criteria for preoperative MRI are summarized in Table 6.7. Equally important are establishing exclusion criteria. In the older patient with a fatty breast and an ER-positive stellate invasive cancer, or with a small mammographic area of low-grade DCIS on biopsy, any potential survival benefit from adding MRI is likely to be minimal.

Table 6.7 Suggested candidates for selective preoperative breast MRI

Young patients
High risk of heritable breast cancer (up to 50% multifocal or multicentric)
Patients with dense breasts (BI-RADS Class 3–4)
Infiltrating lobular carcinoma
Extensive DCIS component
Multifocal, multicentric or contralateral tumor on conventional workup
Large tumor of > 3 cm or difficult to define extent conventionally
Potential candidate for partial breast irradiation
Personal preference of patient for breast MRI

A point of note from the meta-analysis by Houssami *et al.* is that while < 5% of patients incorrectly had more extensive lumpectomy for benign changes, 1% had inappropriate mastectomy rate as a result of false-positive MRI findings [26]. This underscores the need for MRI-guided biopsy whenever a reported MRI abnormality could alter surgical management. The surgical dilemma of the trade-off between resecting a smaller tissue volume and risking positive margins should also be kept in mind. Close cooperation between surgeon, radiologist and pathologist is likely to yield the best results.

Given the logistical difficulties involved in developing a trial of sufficient power, it is doubtful whether an adequate prospective randomized trial will ever be undertaken to resolve questions in relation to long-term outcomes observed in altered recurrence rates or even a possible survival benefit [3, 57, 60]. In any event, conclusive data are not expected any time soon.

The impact of accelerated partial breast irradiation

A further point to consider is the increasing trend towards partial breast irradiation in its several different forms (Appendix 5). With ABPI, the treatment effect is limited to a small tissue of 1–2 cm around the index tumor. The benefit of whole breast irradiation in addressing any occult disease in other quadrants of the breast is lost completely. To be eligible for ABPI, disease must therefore be localized to a single quadrant on clinical evaluation and conventional imaging. The upper limit of total tumor size for ABPI (both IDC and DCIS) is usually taken as 3 cm and with negative axillary lymph nodes. Invasive lobular carcinoma is usually considered a contraindication as it is frequently multifocal and may be underestimated by conventional imaging. There is clearly a strong case for adding MRI to the workup of any patient where ABPI is planned [27, 64–66].

It is also possible that, in the future, RT as a local control measure might be omitted in selected patients if MRI can be safely used to infer that no significant residual disease is present. This may ultimately be a more important issue for clinical trials to address than whether MRI can marginally reduce local recurrence rates [67].

The element of personal choice

Last but not least, we should not forget that the owner of the disease must be the major stakeholder in how her disease is managed [68]. The need for re-excision after initial lumpectomy not only entails increased expense but also anxiety, the risk of a poorer cosmesis and delay in beginning adjuvant therapy. The news of late recurrence can also be a huge emotional blow for some women who had believed they had "beaten" breast cancer. So there is every reason to let the women decide if they would prefer to have a staging MRI study.

Women who are of a mind-set such that they would prefer to minimize the chance of any future events by having more extensive surgery or even mastectomy (with the option of reconstruction) may well elect to know the full extent of their disease. On the other hand, other women who are strongly motivated towards BCT and RT may be comfortable in the knowledge that there is a risk of future local recurrence and later mastectomy. Furthermore, women in the "undecided" group may find it easier to accept initial mastectomy where MRI clearly shows very extensive disease. As a profession, we should not be paternalistic in making recommendations for or against preoperative MRI in individual cases. Rather we should ensure that women are fully aware of both the potential benefits and the downsides of undergoing the most accurate available imaging test for defining the extent of their newly diagnosed breast cancer.

MULTIPLE CHOICE QUESTIONS

6.1 Answer true or false to the following statements

A. Pleural effusions over 20 mm in depth are a frequent normal finding on breast MRI.
B. MRI staging detects a contralateral mammographically occult cancer in ~3–5% cases.
C. Patients with multicentric invasive disease or extensive DCIS usually require mastectomy.
D. Early-stage breast cancer (EBC) always means only DCIS or Stage I invasive breast cancer.
E. Overestimation of DCIS extent by MRI is more common with low-grade than high-grade disease.

6.2 Answer true or false to the following statements

A. A 30 mm invasive cancer with skin nodules and ulceration is within the definition of EBC.
B. An invasive cancer > 5 cm diameter is an absolute contraindication to BCT.
C. Involvement of level 3 (infraclavicular) nodes is associated with generally poorer prognosis.
D. Routine preoperative MRI can reveal ipsilateral multicentric disease in over 50% of cases.
E. Routine axillary lymph node dissection includes the removal of level III (infraclavicular) nodes.

See page 189 for answers.

References

1. Morrow M, Strom EA, Bassett LW, *et al.* Standard for breast conservation in the management of invasive breast carcinoma. *CA Cancer J Clin* 2002; **52**: 277–300.
2. Fisher B, Anderson S, Bryant J, *et al.* Twenty-year follow-up of a randomized trial comparing total mastectomy, lumpectomy, and lumpectomy plus irradiation for the treatment of invasive breast cancer. *N Engl J Med* 2002; **347**: 1233–41.
3. Houssami N, Hayes DF. Review of preoperative magnetic resonance imaging (MRI) in breast cancer. Should MRI be performed on all women with newly diagnosed, early stage breast cancer? *CA Cancer J Clin* 2009; **59**: 290–302.
4. Houghton J, George WD, Cuzick J, *et al.* RT and tamoxifen in women with completely excised ductal carcinoma in situ of the breast in the UK, Australia, and New Zealand: randomised controlled trial. *Lancet* 2003; **362**: 95–102.
5. Bijker N, Meijnen P, Peterse JL, *et al.* Breast-conserving treatment with or without RT in ductal carcinoma-in-situ: ten-year results of European Organisation for Research and Treatment of Cancer Randomized Phase III Trial 10853 – a study by the EORTC Breast Cancer Cooperative Group and EORTC RT Group. *J Clin Oncol* 2006; **24**: 3381–7.
6. Solin LJ. Is excision alone adequate treatment for low-risk ductal carcinoma-in-situ of the breast? *J Clin Oncol* 2006; **24**: 1017–19.
7. Sakorafas GH, Farley DR, Peros G. Recent advances and current controversies in the management of DCIS of the breast. *Cancer Treat Rev* 2008; **34**: 483–97.
8. Boughey JC, Gonzalez RJ, Bonner E, *et al.* Current treatment and clinical trial developments for ductal carcinoma in situ of the breast. *The Oncologist* 2007; **12**: 1276–87.
9. Kuerer HM, Albarracin CT, Yang WT, *et al.* Ductal carcinoma in situ: state of the science and roadmap to advance the field.

J Clin Oncol 2009; **27**: 279–88.

10. Sanders ME, Schuyler PA, Dupont WD, *et al.* The natural history of low-grade ductal carcinoma in situ of the breast in women treated by biopsy only revealed over 30 years of long-term follow-up. *Cancer* 2005; **103**: 2481–4.
11. Macdonald HR, Silverstein MJ, Lee LA, *et al.* Margin width as the sole determinant of local recurrence after breast conservation in patients with ductal carcinoma in situ of the breast. *Am J Surg* 2006; **192**: 420–2.
12. Guerrieri-Gonzaga A, Botteri E, Rotmensz N, *et al.* Ductal intraepithelial neoplasia: postsurgical outcome for 1,267 women cared for in one single institution over 10 years. *The Oncologist* 2009; **14**: 201–12.
13. Fisher B, Dignam J, Wolmark N, *et al.* Tamoxifen in treatment of intraductal breast cancer: National Surgical Adjuvant Breast and Bowel Project B-24 randomised controlled trial. *Lancet* 1999; **353**: 1993–2000.
14. Jatoi I, Proschan MA. Randomized trials of breast-conserving therapy versus mastectomy for primary breast cancer: a pooled analysis of updated results. *Am J Clin Oncol* 2005; **28**: 289–94.
15. Kettritz U. Modern concepts of ductal carcinoma in situ (DCIS) and its diagnosis through percutaneous biopsy. *Eur Radiol* 2008; **18**: 343–50.
16. Leonard GD, Swain SM. Ductal carcinoma in situ, complexities and challenges. *J Natl Cancer Inst* 2004; **96**: 906–20.
17. Singletary SE, Connolly JL. Breast cancer staging: working with the sixth edition of the AJCC Cancer Staging Manual. *CA Cancer J Clin* 2006; **56**: 37–47.
18. Weir L, Speers C, D'yachkova Y, *et al.* Prognostic significance of the number of axillary lymph nodes removed in patients with node-negative breast cancer. *J Clin Oncol* 2002; **20**: 1793–9.
19. Mansel RE, Fallowfield L, Kissin M, *et al.* Randomized multicenter trial of sentinel node biopsy versus standard axillary treatment in operable breast cancer: the ALMANAC trial. *J Natl Cancer Inst* 2006; **98**: 599–609.
20. Ciocchetti JM, Joy N, Staller S, *et al.* The effect of magnetic resonance imaging in the workup of breast cancer. *Am J Surg* 2009; **198**: 824–8.
21. Liberman L, Morris EA, Dershaw DD, *et al.* MR imaging of the ipsilateral breast in women with percutaneously proven breast cancer. *AJR Am J Roentgenol* 2003; **180**: 901–10.
22. Berg W A, Gutierrez L, NessAiver MS, *et al.* Diagnostic accuracy of mammography, clinical examination, US, and MR imaging in preoperative assessment of breast cancer. *Radiology* 2004; **233**: 830–49.
23. Grimsby GM, Gray R, Dueck A, *et al.* Is there concordance of invasive breast cancer pathologic tumor size with magnetic resonance imaging? *Am J Surg* 2009; **198**: 500–4.
24. Onesti JK, Mangus BE, Helmer SD, *et al.* Breast cancer tumor size: correlation between magnetic resonance imaging and pathology measurements. *Am J Surg* 2008; **196**: 844–50.
25. van Goethem M, Schelfout K, Kersschot E, *et al.* Enhancing area surrounding breast carcinoma on MR mammography: comparison with pathologic examination. *Eur Radiol* 2004; **14**: 1363–70.
26. Houssami N, Ciatto S, Macaskill P, *et al.* Accuracy and surgical impact of magnetic resonance imaging in breast cancer staging: systematic review and meta-analysis in detection of multifocal and multicentric cancer. *J Clin Oncol* 2008; **26**: 3248–58.
27. Hollingsworth AB, Stough RG, O'Dell CA, *et al.* Breast magnetic resonance imaging for preoperative locoregional staging. *Am J Surg* 2008; **196**: 389–97.
28. Schnall MD, Blume J, Bluemke DA, *et al.* MRI detection of distinct incidental cancer in women with primary breast cancer studied in IBMC 6883. *J Surg Oncol* 2005; **92**: 32–8.
29. Brennan ME, Houssami N, Lord S, *et al.* Magnetic resonance imaging screening of the contralateral breast in women with newly diagnosed breast cancer: systematic review and meta-analysis of incremental cancer detection and impact on surgical management. *J Clin Oncol* 2009; **27**: 5640–9.
30. Lehman C, Gatsonis C, Kuhl CK, *et al.* MRI evaluation of the contralateral breast in women with recently diagnosed breast cancer. *N Engl J Med* 2007; **356**: 1295–303.
31. Pestalozzi BC, Zahrieh D, Mallon E, *et al.* Distinct clinical and prognostic features of infiltrating lobular carcinoma of the breast: combined results of 15 International Breast Cancer Study Group clinical trials. *J Clin Oncol* 2008; **26**: 3006–14.
32. Mann RM, Hoogeveen YL, Blickman JG, *et al.* MRI compared to conventional diagnostic workup in the detection and evaluation of invasive lobular carcinoma of the breast: a review of existing literature. *Breast Cancer Res Treat* 2008; **107**: 1–14.
33. Marcotte-Bloch C, Balu-Maestro C, Chamorey E, *et al.* MRI for the size assessment of pure ductal carcinoma in situ (DCIS): a prospective study of 33 patients. *Eur J Radiol* 2011; **77**: 462–7.
34. Mann RM, Veltman J, Barentsz JO, *et al.* The value of MRI compared to mammography in

the assessment of tumor extent in invasive lobular carcinoma of the breast. *Eur J Surg Oncol* 2008; **34**: 135–42.

35. McGhan LJ, Wasif N, Gray RJ, *et al.* Use of preoperative magnetic resonance imaging for invasive lobular cancer: good, better, but maybe not the best? *Ann Surg Oncol* 2010; **17**: 255–62.
36. Mann RM, Loo CE, Wobbes T, *et al.* The impact of preoperative breast MRI on the re-excision rate in invasive lobular carcinoma of the breast. *Breast Cancer Res Treat* 2010; **119**: 415–22.
37. Kuhl CK, Schrading S, Bieling HB, *et al.* MRI for diagnosis of pure ductal carcinoma in situ: a prospective observational study. *Lancet* 2007; **370**: 485–92.
38. Kumar AS, Chen DF, Au A, *et al.* Biologic significance of false-positive magnetic resonance imaging enhancement in the setting of ductal carcinoma in situ. *Am J Surg* 2006; **192**: 520–4.
39. Schouten van der Velden AP, Schlooz-Vries MS, Boetes C, *et al.* Magnetic resonance imaging of ductal carcinoma in situ: what is its clinical application? A review. *Am J Surg* 2009; **198**: 262–9.
40. Schouten van der Velden AP, Boetes C, Bult P, *et al.* The value of magnetic resonance imaging in diagnosis and size assessment of in situ and small invasive breast carcinoma. *Am J Surg* 2006; **192**: 172–8.
41. Shiraishi A, Kurosaki Y, Maehara T, *et al.* Extension of ductal carcinoma in situ: histopathological association with MR imaging and mammography. *Magn Reson Med Sci* 2003; **2**: 159–63.
42. Santamaria G, Velasco M, Farrus B, *et al.* Preoperative MRI of pure intraductal breast carcinoma – a valuable adjunct to mammography in assessing cancer extent. *The Breast* 2008; **17**: 186–94.
43. Grobmyer SR, Mortellaro VE, Marshall J, *et al.* Is there a role for routine use of MRI in selection of patients for breast-conserving cancer therapy? *J Am Coll Surg* 2008; **206**: 1045–52.
44. Harms SE. The use of breast magnetic resonance imaging in ductal carcinoma in situ. *Breast J* 2005; **11**: 379–81.
45. Kvistad KA, Rydland J, Smethurst HB, *et al.* Axillary lymph node metastases in breast cancer: preoperative detection with dynamic contrast-enhanced MRI. *Eur Radiol* 2000; **10**: 1464–71.
46. Luciani A, Dao TH, Lapeyre M, *et al.* Simultaneous bilateral breast and high-resolution axillary MRI of patients with breast cancer: preliminary results. *AJR Am J Roentgenol* 2004; **182**: 1059–67.
47. Luciani A, Pigneur F, Ghozali F, *et al.* Ex vivo MRI of axillary lymph nodes in breast cancer. *Eur J Radiol* 2009; **69**: 59–66.
48. Britton P, Moyle P, Benson JR, *et al.* Ultrasound of the axilla: where to look for the sentinel lymph node. *Clin Radiol* 2010; **65**: 373–6.
49. Michel SCA, Keller TM, Frohlich JM, *et al.* Preoperative breast cancer staging: MR imaging of the axilla with ultrasmall superparamagnetic iron oxide enhancement. *Radiology* 2002; **225**: 527–36.
50. Memarsadeghi M, Riedl CC, Kaneider A, *et al.* Axillary lymph node metastases in patients with breast carcinomas: assessment with nonenhanced versus USPIO-enhanced MR imaging. *Radiology* 2006; **241**: 367–77.
51. Kaiser WA. *Signs in MR-Mammography*. Berlin Heidelberg, Springer-Verlag, 2009.
52. Early Breast Cancer Trialists' Collaborative Group (EBCTCG). Effects of RT and of differences in the extent of surgery for early breast cancer on local recurrence and 15-year survival: an overview of the randomised trials. *Lancet* 2005; **366**: 2087–106.
53. Pengel KE, Loo CE, Teerstra HJ, *et al.* The impact of preoperative MRI on breast-conserving surgery of invasive cancer: a comparative cohort study. *Breast Cancer Res Treat* 2009; **116**: 161–9.
54. Turnbull L, Brown S, Harvey I, *et al.* Comparative effectiveness of MRI in breast cancer (COMICE) trial: a randomised controlled trial. *Lancet* 2010; **375**: 563–71.
55. Peters NHGM, Van Esser S, van den Bosch MAAJ, *et al.* Preoperative MRI and surgical management in patients with nonpalpable breast cancer: the MONET – randomised controlled trial. *Eur J Cancer* 2011; **47**: 879–86.
56. Fischer U, Zachariae O, Baum F, *et al.* The influence of preoperative MRI of the breasts on recurrence rate in patients with breast cancer. *Eur Radiol* 2004; **14**: 1725–31.
57. Solin LJ, Orel SG, Hwange W-T, *et al.* Relationship of breast magnetic resonance imaging to outcome after breast-conservation treatment with radiation for women with early-stage invasive breast carcinoma or ductal carcinoma in situ. *J Clin Oncol* 2008; **26**: 386–91.
58. Lee JM, Orel SG, Czerniecki BJ, *et al.* MRI before reexcision surgery in patients with breast cancer. *AJR Am J Roentgenol* 2004; **182**: 473–80.
59. Morrow M. Magnetic resonance imaging in the breast cancer patient: curb your enthusiasm. *J Clin Oncol* 2008; **26**: 352–3.
60. Houssami N, Morrow M. Preoperative breast MRI in women with recently diagnosed breast cancer – where to next? *The Breast* 2010; **19**: 1–2.
61. Solin LJ. Counterview: preoperative breast MRI (magnetic resonance imaging) is not recommended for all patients with newly diagnosed breast cancer. *The Breast* 2010; **19**: 7–9.
62. Gao X, Fisher SG, Emami B. Risk of second primary cancer in the

contralateral breast in women treated for early-stage breast cancer: a population-based study. *Int J Radiat Oncol Biol Phys* 2003; **56**: 1038–45.

63. Sardanelli F. Overview of the role of preoperative breast MRI in the absence of evidence on patient outcomes. *The Breast* 2010; **19**: 3–6.

64. Godinez J, Gombos EC, Devlin PM, *et al.* Breast MRI in evaluation of eligibility for partial breast irradiation. *AJR Am J Roentgenol* 2008; **191**: 272–7.

65. Al-Hallaq HA, Mell LK, Bradley JA, *et al.* Magnetic resonance imaging identifies multifocal and multicentric disease in breast cancer patients who are eligible for partial breast irradiation. *Cancer* 2008; **113**: 2408–14.

66. Tendulkar RD, Chellman-Jeffers M, Rybicki LA, *et al.* Preoperative breast magnetic resonance imaging in early breast cancer. Implications for partial breast irradiation. *Cancer* 2009; **115**: 1621–30.

67. Morrow M. Magnetic resonance imaging in breast cancer: one step forward, two steps back? *JAMA* 2004; **292**: 2779–80.

68. Ciatto S. Preoperative breast MRI: what do women want? *The Breast* 2010; **19**: 435–6.

Chapter 7

Problem-solving applications of breast MRI

Chapter outline

- Introduction
- Three ground rules for problem-solving MRI
- Evaluating equivocal mammographic lesions
- Evaluating residual disease after surgical excision
- Investigating nipple changes and discharge
- Malignant axillary lymph node with occult breast primary
- Role of MRI in neoadjuvant systemic therapy

Introduction

Problem-solving applications cover a diverse range of clinical situations, and here this category is taken to include anything which is not either (i) screening of asymptomatic women or (ii) staging or mapping the extent of known cancer for treatment planning. Important attributes of MRI in problem-solving are the combination of high sensitivity and high NPV. However, it is also important to minimize false-positive results in the problem-solving setting, where the aim of MRI is to solve a diagnostic dilemma, not create a new one. Used judiciously, MRI can reduce clinical uncertainty in several scenarios, provided its limitations are clearly understood by both radiologist and referring clinician. The various problem-solving applications of MRI mentioned in this chapter are listed in Table 7.1.

Table 7.1 Problem-solving applications of breast MRI

Equivocal conventional imaging
Vague asymmetric density and/or architectural disturbance on XRM
Multiple circumscribed masses on XRM and US
Scar versus tumor recurrence after lumpectomy
Scar versus tumor at site of previous benign biopsy
Adjunct to difficult clinical or conventional imaging assessment
Vague palpable abnormality in complex breast
New unilateral nipple retraction, normal XRM and US
Pathologic nipple discharge with normal XRM and US
Recurrent subareolar breast abscess to define disease extent
Suspected occult malignant disease
Involved or close margins after surgical excision
Malignant axillary lymph node with occult breast primary
Nipple discharge with positive fluid cytology, normal XRM and US
Paget's disease of the nipple with normal XRM and US
Monitoring of neoadjuvant systemic therapy
Early identification of non-responders after 1–2 cycles
Define extent of residual disease for surgery after completion

Three ground rules for problem-solving MRI

So, when can MRI be expected to perform well in a problem-solving role? One important principle derives from the IBMC multicenter trial, in which the study population comprised over 1000 women who were candidates for biopsy of a known abnormality found either on XRM, US or clinical examination. A major conclusion of the study was that the overall NPV for malignancy of 85% (based on lesions given a BI-RADS final assessment score of 1–3) meant that a so-called "benign" MRI result could never substitute for biopsy in the case of an already suspicious lesion [1].

When to avoid MRI: microcalcification and masses

Essentially, MRI detection of cancer relies on showing enhancement, and exclusion of malignancy relies on its absence. In the IBMC study, absence of enhancement had an NPV for invasive cancer of 94% but for DCIS the false-negative rate was higher, with 16% showing absent enhancement [2]. In a more recent single-center study, < 2% of the invasive cancers but 10% of all DCIS lesions failed to enhance [3].

Low-grade DCIS is particularly likely to be occult on MRI and yet may be evident as mammographic microcalcification. In fact, while MRI sensitivity of up to 98% is reported for high-grade DCIS, some 20% of low-grade DCIS cases are occult to MRI [4, 5]. Furthermore, some benign lesions which are known to enhance and cause false-positive MRI findings (fibroadenoma, papilloma and spectrum of fibrocystic changes) may also show mammographic calcification. Consequently, the ability of MRI to exclude DCIS in the presence of microcalcification on XRM is limited.

In an Italian multicenter trial, Bazzocchi and coworkers evaluated MRI in 112 patients with suspicious microcalcifications on XRM [6]. They reported an 87% overall sensitivity of MRI for malignancy associated with microcalcifications, but the NPV was only 70%, and it was concluded that breast MRI did not help in presurgical evaluation. However, a more recent UK single-center study using MRI in 88 women with screen-detected microcalcifications reported an NPV of over 90% and suggested that MRI could offer an alternative to open surgical biopsy in selected cases, e.g., technical failure of stereotactic biopsy [7]. While this seems not unreasonable, these cases should be regarded as the exceptions that prove the rule. In general, for a cluster of suspicious microcalcification seen on XRM, there is little to be gained from performing MRI and a significant risk of offering false reassurance. Even with a complete absence of MRI enhancement, biopsy is still required to establish a pathologic diagnosis, which can usually be achieved using conventional x-ray stereotactic guidance.

Despite the higher NPV for invasive cancer, the same principle applies to a suspicious mass lesion which is clearly present on XRM, US or even clinically. If the findings are deemed to warrant biopsy, this should be carried out even if an MRI scan shows absent enhancement, because the lesion could still be malignant. So, **Rule 1** in problem-solving applications of MRI is that it should be avoided when there are already findings for which biopsy is mandated.

> Rule 1 of problem-solving MRI: If a lesion seen on conventional imaging is suspicious (BI-RADS 4), biopsy should be performed using conventional imaging-guided methods. MRI should not be used to try and exclude cancer in this setting.

The next rule we can derive follows from this first principle that a negative MRI should not negate an already suspicious clinical or conventional imaging finding warranting biopsy. **Rule 2** in problem-solving is that MRI should never be a substitute for performing proper conventional mammographic workup and careful US evaluation of a suspected abnormality. Otherwise, lesions which could be confirmed and biopsied by conventional means will be undergoing MRI unnecessarily and potentially misleadingly.

> Rule 2 of problem-solving MRI: If a lesion seen on XRM appears equivocal, MRI should never be used as a substitute for thorough conventional workup including TUS. However, MRI may be preferable to attempting x-ray stereotactic biopsy.

So then, when is the use of MRI appropriate? The answer is in circumstances where the suspicion of malignancy is already low because a full conventional workup of an already equivocal abnormality has shown no evidence of cancer. Usually, there is no clear target on which to perform a biopsy. Prior to the availability of MRI, many such cases would have simply been followed, but the high sensitivity and NPV, at least for invasive cancer, mean MRI can be a valuable addition to management. So **Rule 3** is that where a negative MRI result will allow more confident follow-up without attempting biopsy, MRI has a potentially useful role. For practical purposes, this means that assigning a BI-RADS 3 category becomes possible. The corollary is that if an MRI abnormality is revealed which correlates with the lesion in question, biopsy will usually be required and probably with MRI-guided intervention.

> Rule 3 of problem-solving MRI: If after thorough workup, a lesion seen on conventional imaging remains equivocal, MRI may have a role where a negative result will avoid biopsy. A positive result will usually prompt biopsy, often requiring MRI-guided intervention.

Evaluating equivocal mammographic lesions

Vague asymmetric density or architectural distortion

Most frequently, MRI is used to elucidate a questionable asymmetric density or area of architectural disturbance on XRM [8, 9]. Often the abnormality is only visible on one view and there may be doubt as to whether a real lesion is present at all [8–10]. The probability of cancer is then relatively low, because conventional workup has failed to reveal a definite abnormality. Nevertheless, the concern is that malignancy could be missed, particularly in a dense breast.

Invasive lobular cancer is a particular important consideration in this setting, as it often presents subtle XRM findings which may be seen in only one projection. Although ILC is occasionally missed by MRI, the sensitivity for pure ILC is only slightly lower than for other invasive cancers, reported at 93% in a recent meta-analysis [11]. Meanwhile, in the IBMC study, among 422 invasive cancers, a single ILC case presented as architectural distortion with absence of enhancement [2, 12]. Therefore, the NPV of MRI in this problem-solving role is acceptable as an adjunctive test to increase confidence that there is no lesion present. Applying Rule 3, if MRI is normal, follow-up is adequate, while if a lesion is shown, biopsy is indicated (Fig. 7.1).

In one study, Lee *et al.* used MRI in 86 patients with problematic mammograms, finding an MRI correlate in 26 (30%) of which 9 (10%) were malignant (6 IDC, 2 mixed ductal lobular and 1 DCIS) [8]. There were 12 incidental lesions found of which only 1 was malignant. In a more recent study Moy *et al.* used MRI in 115 women with inconclusive findings on XRM, over 70% of whom also had dense breasts (BI-RADS 3 or 4) [9]. Most of the lesions were asymmetric densities (85%) and the remainder were either architectural distortions (10%) or focal scars. A suspicious MRI correlate was found in 15/115 women (13%) of which 6 (5%) were found to be IDC. Incidental lesions were found on MRI in 18 cases (16%), all of which proved to be benign. In both these studies, about half of all equivocal XRM lesions were seen in only one plane of view. Furthermore, Moy *et al.* noted that over 20% of such women had unsuccessful attempts at either stereotactic biopsy or hook-wire localization [9]. This last observation makes a strong case for favoring MRI over attempting invasive stereotactic biopsy, particularly for lesions seen on only one mammographic view.

So, while most MRI studies for this application will be normal, the yield of otherwise occult cancers is 5–10%. An approximately 15% rate of finding incidental lesions can be expected, with a low yield of additional malignancies.

Vague clinical abnormality with equivocal conventional imaging

A further potential role for MRI is in the context of a vague clinically palpable mass, particularly in a dense or complex post-surgical or reconstructed breast (Fig. 7.2). Where both the clinical assessment and conventional imaging methods are compromised, it may be impossible to define any potential biopsy target. In this setting, MRI offers a reliable alternative to either confirm or exclude malignancy.

Multiple circumscribed masses

For a solitary suspicious mass on conventional imaging, MRI usually has little to contribute, as the lesion requires biopsy (Rule 1). However, most circumscribed masses on XRM or US ultimately prove to be benign, and when multiple lesions are present, it is impractical to perform CNB of every one and difficult to decide which might require biopsy. In this setting, MRI can add lesion specificity by using signal characteristics, morphologic features and enhancement patterns to confidently diagnose cysts, lymph nodes and most fibroadenomas. If there is a particular lesion which displays suspicious features on MRI, it is then singled out for biopsy.

Distinguishing scar from recurrence after lumpectomy

During long-term follow-up after breast-conserving surgery, stellate scarring on XRM and US can make exclusion of recurrence problematic. Differentiating recurrent tumor from scarring at the site of previous lumpectomy was one of the first established indications for breast MRI, which is very accurate in this role. In contrast, the sensitivity of XRM in detecting local recurrence is reported to be in the range of only 55–70% [10].

In the absence of RT, post-surgical sites seldom enhance beyond about 6 months, by which time the fibrotic tissue is mature. Post-traumatic fat necrosis is an exception to this rule, where enhancement can persist for a number of years, although morphologic features usually allow differentiation and enhancement reduces over time. After RT, potentially confusing enhancement can be prolonged for 18 months or even longer.

A scar can also persist on XRM after a benign excisional biopsy, and can result in cancer subsequently being missed at the biopsy site [13]. Rarely, scarring

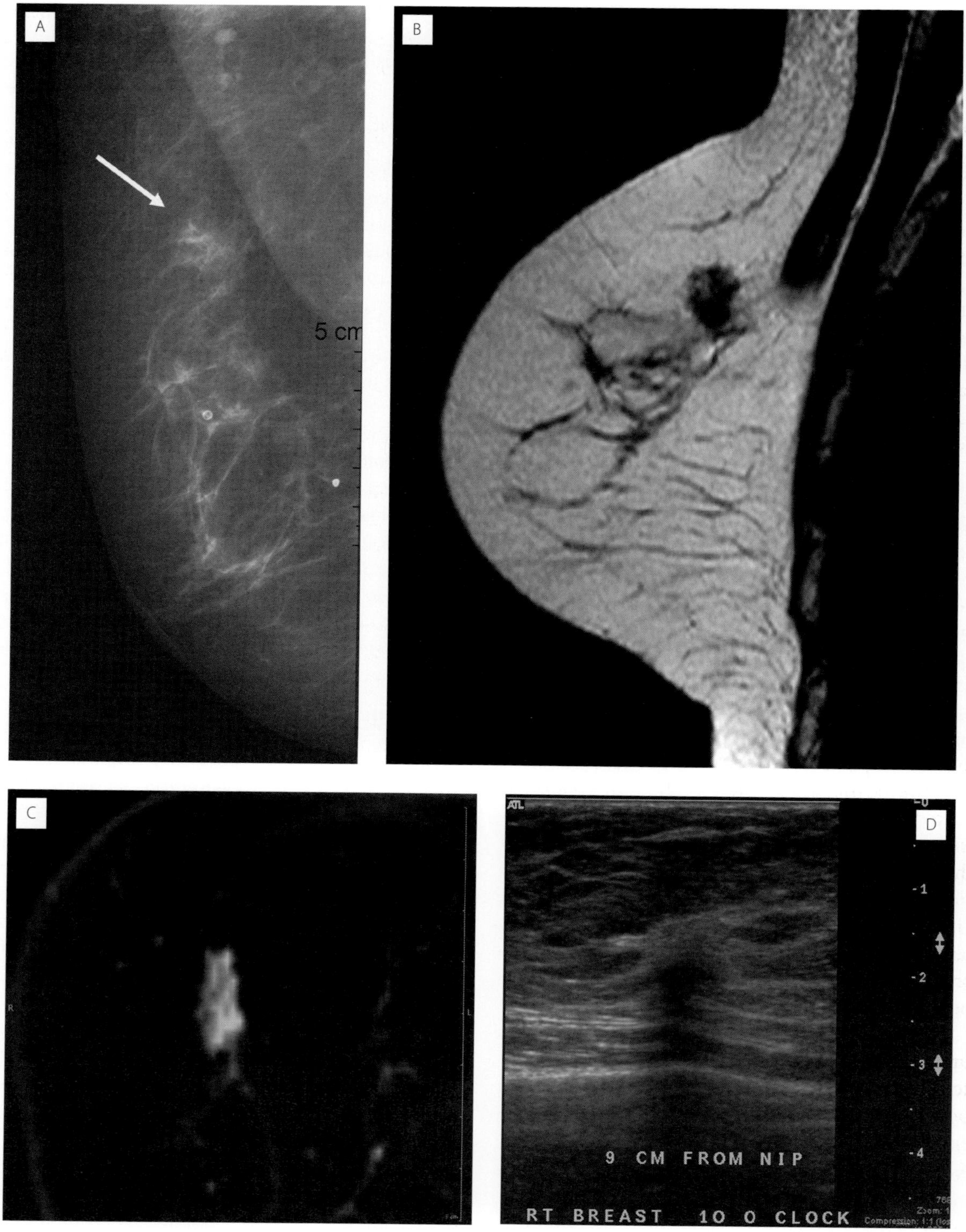

Fig. 7.1 Vague asymmetric density in a single plane of view: A 61-year-old woman with past history of previous left lumpectomy for invasive cribriform cancer 15 years ago. (A) Routine XRM revealed asymmetric density in right breast on MLO view only (arrow), which resolved on spot compression, with no abnormality found on US. (B) Sagittal FSE T2-weighted image confirms corresponding density with architectural distortion. (C) Coronal fat-suppressed T1-weighted image shows 25 × 10 mm mass. Using knowledge of exact lesion location, TUS (D) revealed subtle echogenic lesion with acoustic shadowing found to be invasive cancer on 14-gauge CNB. Surgical pathology showed two distinct cancers (15 mm mixed ILC/IDC and 10 mm IDC).

can even occur after imaging-guided VAB [14]. A change in appearance at the site of a previous benign biopsy is therefore another indication for MRI.

Evaluating residual disease after surgical excision

Residual disease is known to adversely affect recurrence rates after breast-conserving surgery, which is why obtaining negative margins is a fundamental objective. Commonly the unexcised tissue is DCIS which cannot be seen with the naked eye at surgery and is mammographically occult in the absence of microcalcification. In many instances where more than just focal microscopic disease is left behind after BCT, later local recurrence in reality reflects inadequate primary excision.

When histopathology after initial surgery shows either involved or close margins, MRI can help in determining whether re-excision will suffice, or if mastectomy is required. Ideally it is recommended that MRI be deferred for at least 1 month to maximize sensitivity and minimize false-positive findings due to granulation tissue [15]. A smooth uniform <5 mm enhancing rim seen around the surgical cavity is a normal reparative response after BCT which gradually diminishes over 6 months, to often no more than 1–2 mm [16]. Focally thick, irregular or nodular enhancement >5 mm in depth is typical of residual disease [15, 16].

However, the rind of reactive enhancement around a seroma does not interfere with the detection of bulky residual tumor or remote multicentric disease which would dictate that only a mastectomy would be adequate treatment (Fig. 7.2). In these circumstances, if it is accepted that minor focal disease in the wall of the surgical cavity is not an issue, MRI can be performed even within a few days of initial surgery, as soon as the patient is able to lie prone comfortably.

The sensitivity of MRI for residual disease at the surgical site after excision or biopsy is only moderate, and reported to be in the range of 60–95%, with specificity of 50–75% [15–17]. However, MRI demonstrates unsuspected multicentric disease in a significant number of patients. It is important to obtain histologic confirmation of an additional suspicious lesion prior to surgical re-excision, because benign changes may produce false-positive results. Lee *et al.* reported the PPV for an additional suspicious finding at 33% (benign to malignant ratio of 2:1), and the outcome of MRI altered the surgical approach in 30% of cases [16]. Causes of false-positive results include fibrocystic change, fibroadenomas, foreign body reaction and fat necrosis [15, 16].

Investigating nipple changes and discharge

Normal MRI appearances

The surface of the nipple usually shows at least moderate, and sometimes intense, enhancement on MRI, so an inverted but otherwise normal nipple may then mimic a subareolar mass [18]. A normal boundary line at the base of the nipple is described, with disruption of the nipple line signifying malignant infiltration [19].

Nipple retraction and inversion

While bilateral nipple retraction is usually benign, imaging is recommended for acquired unilateral nipple retraction or inversion to exclude subareolar malignancy, although a majority of cases relate to duct ectasia or periductal mastitis [18]. Retroareolar cancers can be missed by XRM, particularly in dense breast tissue [20]. Where XRM and US are normal or equivocal, MRI can be added in order to more reliably exclude malignancy.

Benign and pathologic duct discharge

Bilateral duct discharge with green milky fluid is almost invariably due to benign duct ectasia, but spontaneous unilateral or solitary duct discharge (typically with dark, blood-stained or even straw-colored serous fluid) should be further evaluated. Cytologic examination tends to be relatively unreliable with one study finding a sensitivity of 27% and an NPV of about 80% [21]. The commonest cause of pathologic duct discharge is an intraduct papilloma, accounting for two-thirds of cases in one series while about 20% of cases were due to malignancy [21]. In that study, the value of conventional contrast ductography was highlighted, demonstrating otherwise occult benign intraduct papillomas in about 50% of patients, and malignancy in about 15% [21].

Orel and colleagues used MRI in 23 patients with nipple discharge and normal or non-specific mammographic, ductographic or US findings [22]. The findings on MRI correlated with histopathology in 11/15 (73%) of patients, with 6/7 malignant cases identified (in the remaining case excision of a benign papilloma showed an adjacent focus of

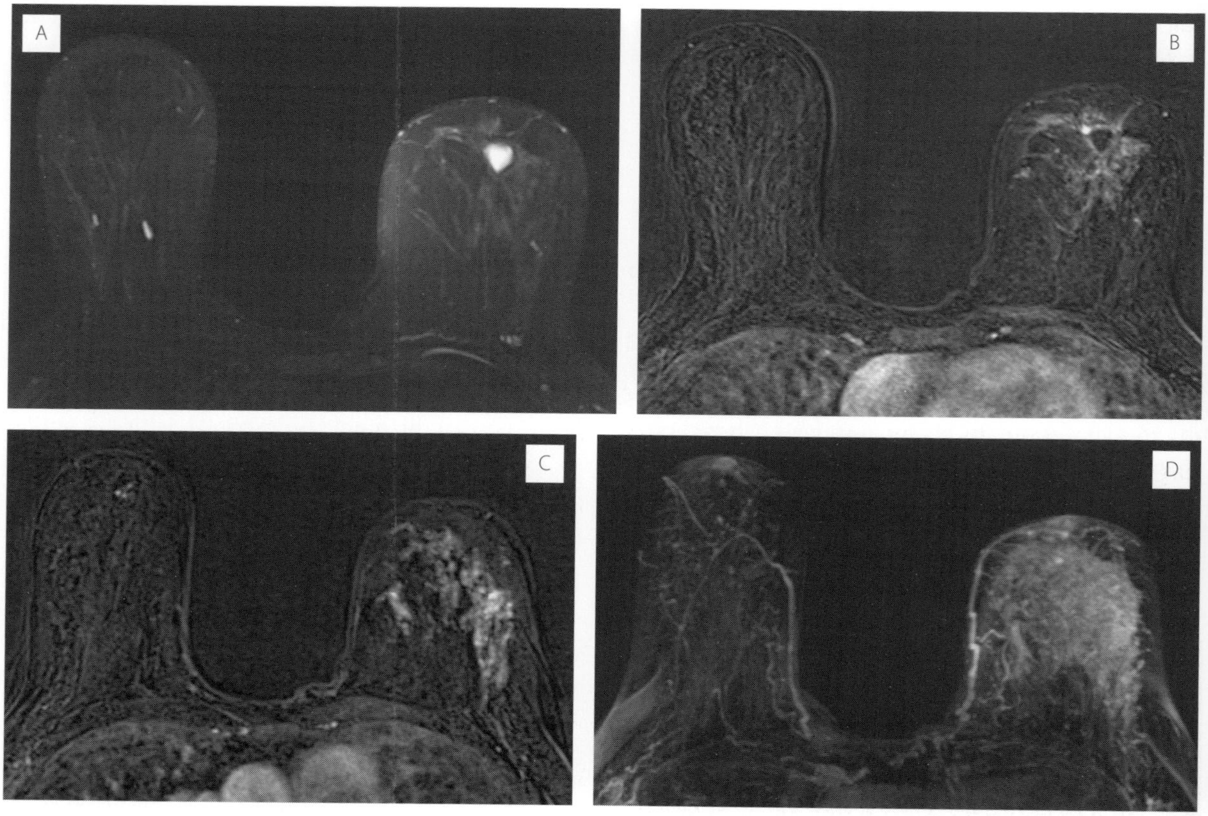

Fig. 7.2 Involved margins after surgical excision: A 57-year-old woman with bloody left nipple discharge, normal XRM, US and cytology. Microductectomy was performed with histopathology revealing low-grade micropapillary DCIS extending to all margins of the excision specimen. MRI scan was performed at 6 weeks to determine residual disease extent. Axial SPAIR image (A) shows post-surgical seroma cavity anteriorly. Subtracted post-contrast image (B) shows normal thin rim of enhancement in the cavity wall with extensive surrounding non-mass enhancement. (C) Subtracted image further cephalad shows contiguous segmental distribution of enhancement extending far posteriorly with anteroposterior extent of 10 cm. (D) axial MIP image shows diffuse nature of disease. Mastectomy was performed with histology confirming 100 mm of micropapillary DCIS.

DCIS). The authors concluded that MRI was a helpful adjunctive method and a potential alternative to conventional ductography. Nakahara *et al.* compared MRI, US and ductography in 55 patients with bloody nipple discharge and a proven histopathologic diagnosis [23]. In that study, MRI correctly identified all malignant lesions and a high NPV of 88% was observed for the finding of a focal mass with smooth borders.

Therefore, MRI is indicated for pathologic discharge where conventional methods fail to show the cause, and may be preferred to conventional ductography (Fig. 7.3).

Techniques for MRI ductography have also been explored. In *indirect MRI ductography* native intraductal fluid is exploited using T1- and T2-weighted images as part of a standard breast MRI study. Meanwhile, *direct MRI ductography* involves cannulating a discharging duct to inject dilute gadolinium. The direct method appears to be feasible to perform and may show additional intraductal disease, but has a technical failure rate of about 10% [24]. The addition of surface *microscopy coils* (e.g., finger coil) has also been used to obtain high-resolution images of the NAC, a technique also advocated for preoperative assessment of recurrent subareolar breast abscess [24, 25].

Paget's disease of the nipple

Paget's disease is characterized by the presence of neoplastic cells in the skin of the NAC and typically presents with unilateral eczema or nipple discharge. Skin at the surface of the nipple is in continuity with ductal epithelium and underlying DCIS is frequently present [18]. When a diagnosis of Paget's disease is confirmed, conventional workup with

XRM and US should first be performed. If these are negative, MRI can then be helpful to increase sensitivity by detecting additional underlying malignant lesions, either non-calcified DCIS or invasive cancer (Fig. 7.4).

On MRI, abnormal enhancement of the NAC is a feature of Paget's disease which may be seen in disease confined to the nipple even without underlying malignancy [26]. In one series, 32/34 (94%) of patients with Paget's disease had underlying malignancy of which almost 80% were DCIS [27]. With negative XRM, MRI revealed otherwise occult disease in 50% patients, although overall MRI was positive for only 7/12 (58%) cancers shown by final surgical pathology [27]. More than half the cancers in that series were unifocal and confined to the central quadrant.

Malignant axillary lymph node with occult breast primary

About 0.3% of all breast cancer present as adenocarcinoma in an axillary lymph node, and are usually due to Stage II disease (about 70%), with only about 5% having distant metastases [28]. While mastectomy was once standard treatment, recent evidence suggests that breast conservation does not adversely affect local control or survival compared with mastectomy [29, 30].

In a recent review of eight studies with a total of 220 patients, MRI revealed an ipsilateral primary invasive breast cancer in about 70% [31]. The primary tumor is IDC in 70–90% of cases, ILC in about 10%, and usually measures < 20 mm in diameter. The primary lesion is identified on TUS in about 80% of cases

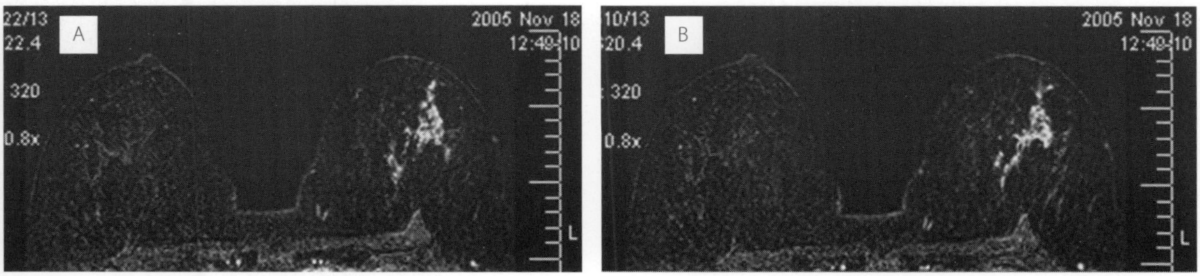

Fig. 7.3 Nipple discharge: A 49-year-old woman with bloody left nipple discharge and positive cytology, but normal XRM and US. Axial post-contrast subtracted images (A and B) show segmental distribution of non-mass enhancement involving UOQ and central left breast with architectural pattern of clustered rings. Mastectomy was performed, with final pathology confirming 80 mm of high-grade DCIS.

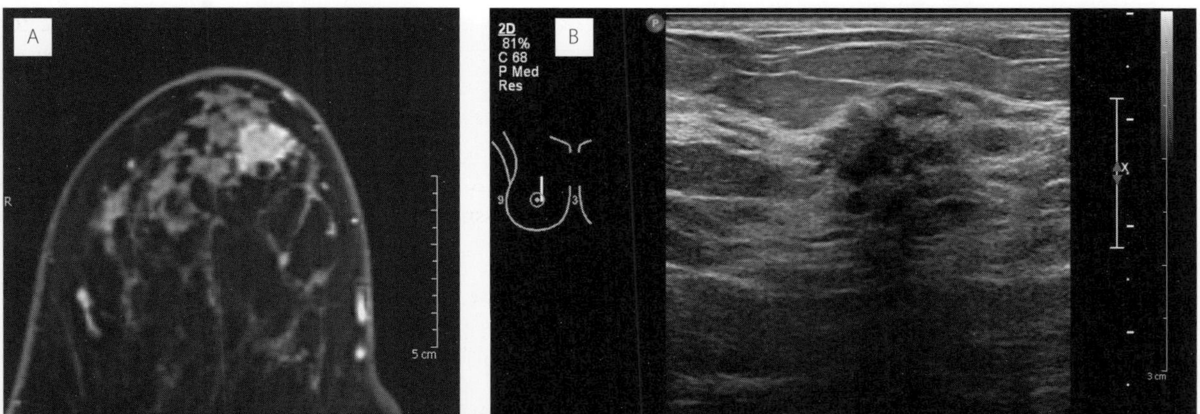

Fig. 7.4 Paget's disease: A 48-year-old woman with Paget's disease on punch biopsy but normal XRM. Post-contrast fat-suppressed axial T1-weighted image (A) shows 18 mm mass with rapid initial-phase enhancement. TUS image (B) shows hypoechoic mass with high-grade DCIS and IDC found on 14-gauge CNB.

[31–36]. In a few patients (< 5%), only DCIS is found on biopsy of a suspicious MRI lesion, attributable to focal microinvasion being overlooked on histology [31, 35]. About 50–60% of patients are suitable for BCT with ALND, and where MRI and subsequent biopsy identify extensive disease, mastectomy is appropriate. For this small group of patients, MRI has a key role in management (Fig. 7.5).

When MRI is normal, while it is still possible that a small primary cancer is present, it is now usual to perform no surgery other than ALND, although whole breast irradiation is usually recommended [30, 33]. Subcutaneous mastectomy is another option, removing most of the breast tissue while providing an excellent cosmetic result. The possibility that lymphadenopathy might relate to a remote primary such as lung, ovary or stomach should also be considered [30].

Role of MRI in neoadjuvant systemic therapy

The original aim of preoperative or NST (as distinct from conventional post-operative or adjuvant therapy) was to deal more effectively with inoperable LABC (locally advanced breast cancer = tumor > 5 cm diameter or involving skin/chest wall or with fixed axillary lymph nodes). By using chemotherapy to shrink these extensive tumors prior to surgery, many cases could be converted to operable disease with improved survival outcomes. Accordingly, neoadjuvant chemotherapy has become standard treatment for patients with LABC.

Furthermore, NST can also be used to downstage large operable cancers for which mastectomy would generally be required, so that BCT becomes a possibility. This is an attractive option for women who are not initially BCT candidates but are strongly motivated towards conservation. Solitary large tumors, [37] particularly high-grade IDCs which are hormone receptor negative, are most likely to respond well.

In many centers, the use of NST has then been widely adopted even in patients who are already candidates for BCT at presentation, although the role of NST in this group of women has been more controversial. Despite potential advantages of evaluating tumor response in vivo (Table 7.2), NST offers no clear benefit for local control when compared to standard adjuvant therapy [38]. A concern has been that the trade-off for more women being able to undergo BCT could be a higher risk of local recurrence, with some trials suggesting this might be the case. Nevertheless, a recent meta-analysis concluded that NST is now an established treatment option for EBC, "reducing mastectomy rates but without hampering local control when compared with conventional adjuvant therapy" [39].

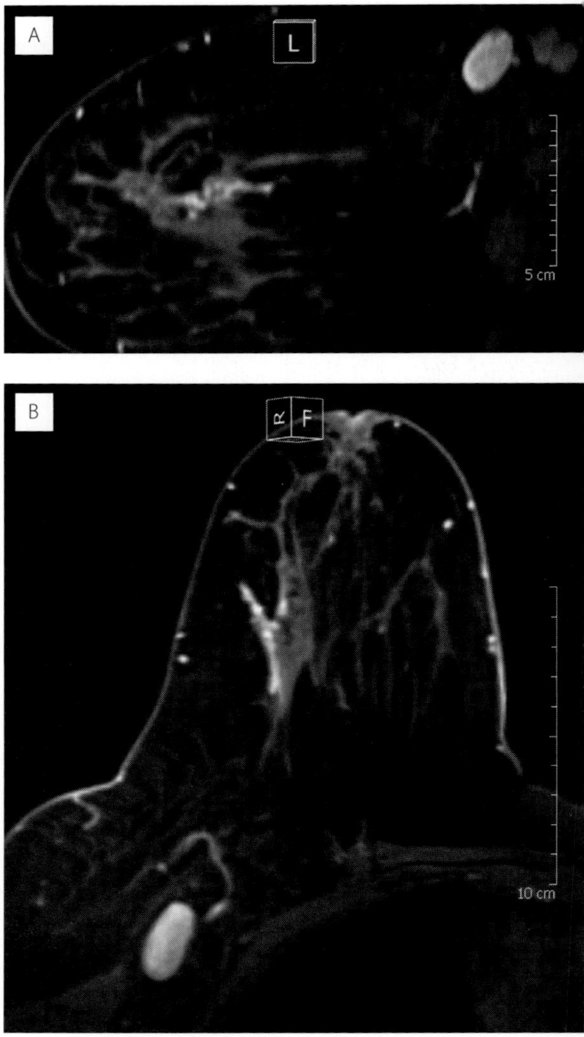

Fig. 7.5 Malignant axillary nodes with occult breast primary: A 45-year-old woman with right axillary nodes positive for adenocarcinoma. (A) Sagittal post-contrast fat-suppressed T1-weighted image shows abnormal nodes and focal area of non-mass enhancement. Oblique axial reformatted image (B) shows linear-ductal distribution with branching pattern and clumped architecture typical of DCIS. Pathology confirmed high-grade DCIS with microinvasive foci treated with oncoplastic reduction mammoplasty, ALND and RT.

Table 7.2 Potential advantages of NST

Reduced extent of surgery and better survival in patients with locally advanced breast cancer
Successfully converts some women with large invasive cancers from mastectomy to BCT
Preserved neoangiogenesis may improve penetration of therapeutic agent in primary tumor
Presence of intact primary tumor acts as in vivo "experiment" for tumor response
Non-responders identified early – switching may also benefit any systemic disease
No delay in commencing systemic chemotherapy for possible distant metastatic disease
Prognostic value of response determined as indicator of disease-free and overall survival
Response may help guide choice of further chemotherapy or radiation treatment

Classifying tumor response to treatment

For clinical purposes, patients are divided into non-responders, those with a partial response and those with a complete response. If no residual viable tumor is found on histopathology at surgical removal after NST, this confirms a *pathologic complete response* (pCR), which is a well-established and reliable predictor of reduced risk of recurrence and improved overall survival rates. Reported rates for achieving pCR range from 10% to 25% for most chemotherapy regimens [40, 41]. A *partial response* indicates significant reduction in tumor burden by predefined criteria, as discussed later.

Non-responders include those with tumors which enlarge (progressive disease) and those with stable disease (unchanged, or change in size not fulfilling criteria for either progression or partial response). A major aim of treatment monitoring is to identify non-responders early, ideally after 1–2 cycles of treatment, to prevent further pointless toxic therapy and instead allow switching to an alternative, hopefully more effective regime.

Role of MRI in monitoring NST

Prior to commencing NST, the pre-treatment extent of disease is established by a baseline staging MRI study. This defines tumor morphology as solitary unifocal or grossly multicentric and excludes the possibility of a contralateral primary. There are then essentially two problem-solving roles for MRI as an adjunct to clinical assessment (i) monitoring response to treatment including early identification of non-responders and (ii) delineating residual disease after completion of treatment to determine appropriate extent of surgical resection. This then requires that a second MRI scan be performed after 1–2 cycles of chemotherapy, with a third MRI examination prior to surgery.

Several studies have shown that MRI is superior to both clinical assessment and to conventional imaging methods in determining initial tumor response to NST [42–45]. Non-responders are the group most easily identified by MRI, because of the lack of interval change. It is also clear that patients who go on to a pCR almost invariably show a good initial response by MRI assessment. Although evaluating residual disease extent has proved more challenging, with both overestimation and underestimation reported, MRI still provides the best imaging correlation with final pathology, and assists in defining patients who are suitable for BCT [46–51].

An important practical consideration prior to MRI monitoring of NST is the possibility that treatment could be so effective that no mass remains at the time of surgery. Therefore, prior to commencing NST and ideally at the time of the initial core biopsy diagnosis, a marker clip is inserted under US guidance, as close as possible to the center of the tumor mass. This serves to identify the location for lumpectomy and to help guide the pathologist in looking for residual tumor in the excision specimen. Additional clips can be used for multicentric disease if required.

At present, even when there is no apparent residual disease after NST, surgery is still an essential part of management, and the success of BCT (with acceptably low recurrence rates) remains heavily reliant on achieving negative surgical margins [52, 53].

Defining tumor response criteria

Intuitively, change in volume might be considered the best indicator of tumor response because of the close correlation between mass and volume. However, when criteria for assessing tumor response were first introduced over 30 years ago, imaging technology had limited ability to measure three-dimensionally. As a result, WHO response criteria used the 2D product of the longest diameter and its perpendicular to approximate tumor volume, with a partial response defined as a 50% or greater reduction in this number.

Theoretically though, a 1D measurement has been shown to have a more direct linear relationship to "cell kill," leading to a simple 1D measurement being adopted in the RECIST system in 2000 [54]. Using RECIST, the single longest diameter of a mass is measured with a 30% decrease as the threshold for partial response. This 30% reduction in longest diameter is equivalent to a 50% reduction in the WHO 2D product and represents a 65% reduction in volume [54, 55]. Although there are no universally agreed tumor response criteria for NST monitoring by MRI, most recent studies have adopted either the 1D RECIST system [42, 44, 48, 56, 57] or 3D volumetric measurements [45, 47, 49, 58, 59].

So is using longest diameter (RECIST) or volumetric MRI measurement likely to be more valid? With modern near-isotropic 3D acquisition and multiplanar reformatting, MRI is certainly ideally suited to the use of 3D measurements. Furthermore, using a single linear measurement to approximate volume may be unreliable with irregularly shaped masses or multifocal tumors, and in such circumstances direct volumetric measurements appear to more accurately capture disease extent [58].

Another important question is to what extent assessment of response by MRI may be able to predict the risk of future recurrence, thereby allowing individually tailored therapy. One study, at least, suggests that change in tumor volume is better than linear measurement in predicting recurrence-free survival [58]. The ongoing ACRIN 6657 multicenter trial is addressing both these questions in LABC, with preliminary data indicating that volumetric MRI is superior to linear measurement when correlated with residual pathologic size after completion of NST. Reduction in measured volume by MRI was also the only variable predictive of pCR after only one cycle of treatment [60].

Based on the available evidence then, it appears that volumetric MRI measurements should be favored over RECIST criteria, with 65% estimated tumor volume reduction defining a partial response.

Pitfalls in evaluating tumor response/residual disease extent by lesion size

For the most part, enhancement on MRI during NST correlates with viable tumor. Therefore, the simplest means to determine if chemotherapy is working would be to measure reduction in overall size of enhancement after 1–2 cycles and at completion of treatment (Fig. 7.6). However, tumor size estimation by measuring extent of enhancement is imperfect due to several interrelated confounding factors (Table 7.3).

1. *Enhancing reparative reaction*: In a typical good response to chemotherapy, there is a reduction in vascularity in association with tumor necrosis, accompanied by reparative changes

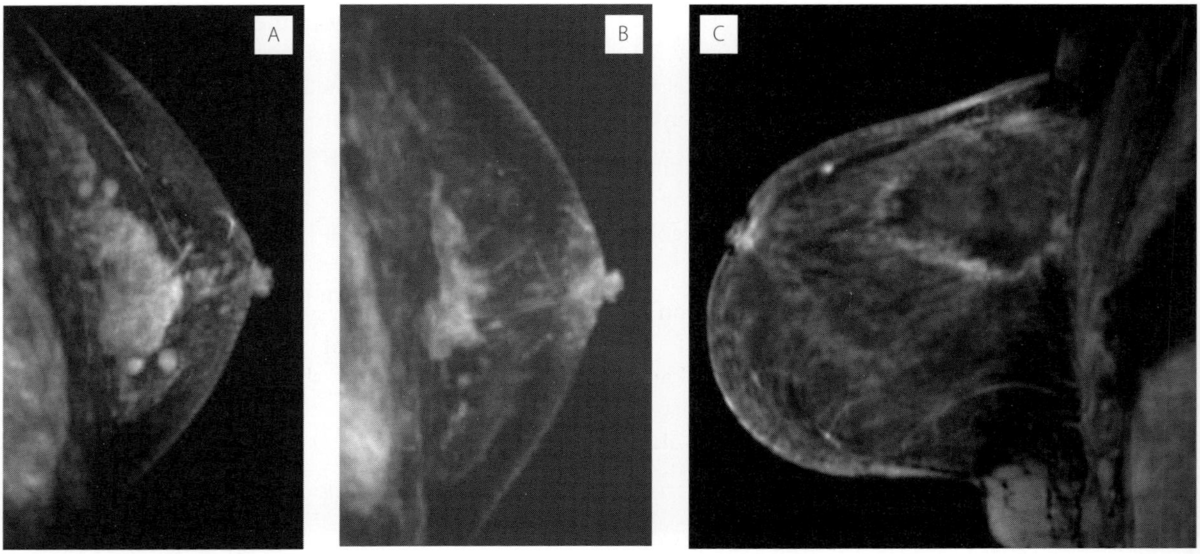

Fig. 7.6 Monitoring response to neoadjuvant chemotherapy: Contrast-enhanced T1-weighted images (A) before and (B) after NST show marked reduction in tumor volume consistent with a partial response. (C) In another patient, following treatment of a solitary large tumor there is persisting rim enhancement around a necrotic cavity, but with pCR found on histopathology. Images from both cases by kind permission of Professor Shih-chang (Ming) Wang, Westmead Hospital, Sydney.

Table 7.3 Confounding factors affecting MRI interpretation in NST

Enhancing reparative changes, e.g., residual rim-enhancing mass may persist despite pCR
Hypovascularity and reduced enhancement may occur without commensurate tumor necrosis
"Break-up" pattern with scattered foci – reparative changes or residual tumor nests?
Tumor growth pattern and histologic type, e.g. grossly multicentric ILC more difficult than solitary mass
Chemotherapeutic agent, e.g., can underestimate residual tumor with taxane regimens

of granulation tissue formation and reactive fibrosis. As tumor enhancement reduces, however, the reparative reaction may itself show significant enhancement. In the case of a solitary mass, concentric shrinkage usually occurs, but the residual lesion may continue to exhibit rim enhancement even though no viable tumor is found on pathology. Furthermore, size reduction is variable, and it is possible for a mass to persist unchanged in overall diameter despite necrosis of the entire tumor and pCR (Fig. 7.6). Persisting rim enhancement is easily mistaken as indicating viable tumor, leading to overestimation of residual disease if the possibility of a normal host reaction around a necrotic mass is not considered.

2. *Reduced vascularity without tumor necrosis*: In some cases, reduction in vascularity may occur in response to chemotherapy without the usually commensurate degree of tumor necrosis. Chemotherapeutic agents have a direct effect on angiogenesis, and in some cases this may be sufficient to reduce blood flow and enhancement, but not to cause widespread tumor cell death. This is an important consideration when a tumor shows clearly reduced enhancement during NST, but without reduction in size, potentially leading to underestimation of residual disease.
3. *Break-up pattern of extensive tumors*: Large multifocal or multicentric tumors may further fragment during the course of NST, resulting in scattered patchy enhancement throughout the original location of the mass. It is usually then impossible to distinguish between residual tumor and reparative reaction, so that simple measurements of residual enhancement are unreliable. When viable tumor is present on histology of excision specimens, typically small scattered tumor nests are described, interspersed among areas of necrosis, granuloma formation and fibrosis. After NST, further surgery is the usual recommendation if viable tumor is found throughout an initial excision specimen, even if this does not extend to the margins [61]. Data from the MD Anderson Cancer Center suggest that such residual multifocal disease on pathology is one of four important factors associated with higher local recurrence rates and which in combination may prompt consideration for mastectomy (Tables 7.4) [53, 62].
4. *Pathologic tumor type*: Different types of tumors show different responses to NST, and this can influence the accuracy of MRI. In general, the better the response to NST, the more accurately it can be assessed. Solitary large high-grade IDCs (particularly triple-negative/basal-like subtype), respond well to NST, have high pCR rates and show close correlation between MRI extent and pathologic findings [63, 64]. Cancers which are HER2 positive are also emerging as a group which respond well to regimens which include trastuzumab, and MRI again accurately predicts pCR [65]. Chemotherapy is generally less effective for ER-positive tumors, and ILC is particularly problematic to monitor with MRI because it is frequently multicentric and enhances less intensely than other tumor types. Tumor characteristics associated with a good response to NST are listed in Table 7.5.
5. *Chemotherapeutic agent*: The specific type of chemotherapy used can also affect MRI appearances, e.g., taxane-containing regimens are reportedly more likely to be associated with underestimation of residual tumor burden [66]. This may relate to a tendency towards a fragmented response to treatment, with scattered residual tumor nests rather than concentric mass shrinkage. This interaction between the chemotherapeutic agent and tumor may in turn reflect the anti-angiogenic effects described earlier. This likely also influences tumor response behavior in other cases, e.g., reported greater anti-angiogenic properties for bevacizumab than trastuzumab in treatment of HER2-positive cancers, with corresponding reduction in MRI accuracy [65].

Pitfall 1 of MRI for monitoring NST: Overestimation of residual tumor (false positive) may be due to enhancing granulation tissue and fibrosis in response to tumor necrosis. A persisting rim-enhancing mass after NST does not always imply residual tumor.

Pitfall 2 of MRI for monitoring NST: Underestimation of residual tumor (false negative) may be due to anti-angiogenic properties of the specific chemotherapeutic agent, e.g., taxanes reducing vascularity without commensurate tumor necrosis.

Pitfall 3 of MRI for monitoring NST: In the presence of scattered focal areas of enhancement after NST, distinction between residual tumor nests and reparative changes is usually impossible and should not be attempted. Only surgical pathology is reliable in this situation.

Integrating kinetic information

Several studies have established that there is a reduction in wash-in rate or early-phase peak enhancement (see first formula below) in response to NST [44, 45, 47, 57]. Furthermore, where a type 3 curve is present initially, reduced early-phase peak enhancement is typically accompanied by a corresponding decrease in late-phase washout, flattening the curve to a plateau or persistent type.

Table 7.4 Risk factors for local recurrence with breast conservation after NST

Advanced nodal involvement (clinical N2 or N3 disease) at initial presentation
Residual pathologic tumor size > 2 cm
Multifocal pattern of residual disease on histopathology
Presence of lymphovascular invasion on histopathology

Table 7.5 Tumor characteristics associated with a good response to NST

High nuclear grade
Solitary circumscribed mass
Triple-negative phenotype
High proliferative activity (high Ki-67 index)
HER2-positive status (using trastuzumab)
ER-negative status > ER-positive status

This so-called *dampening effect* in response to treatment can be quantified as a fall in SER (signal enhancement ratio, see second formula below), which compares early- and late-phase enhancement. In one study, median tumor peak enhancement fell from 210% before to 166% after treatment [47]. Similarly, median peak SER dropped from 1.96 before to 1.52 after treatment due to reduced washout in the treated tumors.

$$\text{Early peak enhancement} = \frac{SI_{early} - SI_{baseline}}{SI_{baseline}} \times 100$$

$$\text{Signal enhancement ratio} = \frac{SI_{early} - SI_{baseline}}{SI_{delayed} - SI_{baseline}}$$

In another study, complete disappearance of washout or plateau kinetics was observed in about 25% of tumors after 2 cycles of chemotherapy, and about 70% of these patients went on to pCR [56]. Meanwhile, only 10% of tumors with residual disease at final pathology showed disappearance of type 2 or 3 kinetic curves. Such findings indicate that a shift in kinetic curve towards type 1 is a valid indicator of tumor response and residual disease extent.

Kinetic criteria also offer a means to differentiate or *segment* tumor from surrounding non-involved tissue. Partridge *et al.* described enhancement thresholds of > 70–80% and an SER > 1 as pre-treatment criteria for tumor segmentation, but relaxed the threshold after treatment to compensate for the dampening effect [47, 58]. After NST, taking any tumor bed enhancement to be abnormal (or using a very low early-phase enhancement threshold of only 30–40%) improves the accuracy of residual disease estimation [47, 58, 67].

As explained in Chapter 1, peak enhancement and SER are the kinetic criteria used to derive parametric overlays in CAD systems, with adjustable thresholds for peak early enhancement, and SER defining the color-coding (SER > 1 = washout, coded red and SER < 1 = persistent, coded blue).

Color-mapping then, offers a convenient way to combine kinetic information into the diagnostic algorithm for monitoring NST response. With commercial CAD systems, it is possible to display the kinetics of all voxels in any defined VOI. Furthermore, the percentages of each curve type can be automatically calculated, allowing comparison before and after treatment. El Khoury *et al.* showed that quantifying reduction in the % volume of washout within a tumor in response to therapy may help in predicting responders [68].

Using color-mapping, Chou *et al.* found that pre-treatment tumors had a high proportion of red (washout) and green (plateau) pixels, and used these as criteria to segment viable tumor post-NST with good histopathologic correlation [67]. Blue pixels (persistent kinetics) post-NST were considered to represent non-involved breast tissue, reparative fibrosis or slowly perfused tumor tissue.

The possibility that functional information from quantitative pharmacokinetic analysis could reveal the earliest MRI signs of response, occurring before any measurable change in tumor size, has been the subject of intense research interest. Among the many possible kinetic parameters which can be derived, the *transfer constant* K^{trans} has shown promise. Nevertheless, in one recent study, Padhani *et al.* still found that substantial change in size preceded any change in kinetic parameters (after one cycle), while after two cycles K^{trans} and change in size were equally sensitive in identifying non-responders [69].

Currently, pending the results of further research, semi-quantitative analysis appears adequate for practical purposes. A CAD system with the capability for volumetric analysis and color-mapping provides a useful means of routinely incorporating kinetic information when estimating tumor extent. Reduction in enhancing tissue volume, reduction in peak enhancement and evidence of dampening effect with reduced washout are all valid indicators of a good response (Table 7.6) Nevertheless, CAD should be used to complement but not replace assessment by an experienced radiologist [70, 71]. In one study, absence of significant enhancement on CAD underestimated residual disease in about half of cases, with measurement by an experienced radiologist proving to be more accurate than CAD-generated estimates of tumor size [70].

Table 7.6 MRI parameters for assessing response to chemotherapy

Linear (RECIST) or volumetric reduction in size of enhancing tumor
Kinetic curve – slower rise with delayed and lower peak level of enhancement
Curve type – less washout and plateau, overall shift towards type 1 kinetics
Volumetric measurement combined with color-coded parametric analysis
MRS – drop in choline peak
DWI – cytotoxic effects seen as altered diffusion

Future developments and other techniques

As adjuncts to routine MRI studies for NST monitoring, spectroscopy and DWI both show potential. In the case of MRS, a reduction in the choline peak (characteristic of malignancy) may be able to distinguish responders and non-responders as early as 24 hours after the first cycle of chemotherapy, while the initial intensity of the choline peak may even predict the likelihood of response. Meanwhile, DWI shows cytotoxic effects of chemotherapy as changes in diffusion patterns, with increasing ADC values reflecting tumor necrosis. Even simple visual analysis of non-contrast high b-value DWI appears to have high accuracy in assessing tumor response [72].

Positron emission tomography using FDG can be used to stage breast cancer and monitor treatment. Dedicated positron emission mammography units are now commercially available. In the context of NST monitoring, FDG PET has the potential to depict abnormal metabolic activity before anatomic change occurs [73]. Typically a >50% reduction in FDG uptake is seen in tumors with a good response, and can be detected after one or two cycles of therapy [73]. Combined PET/CT systems, using image fusion for anatomic correlation, are now standard for new PET installations and may increasingly compete with MRI for monitoring NST response and defining residual disease extent [73, 74].

Summary of MRI for NST monitoring

Breast MRI has a well-established role in NST monitoring for LABC and its use in EBC is increasing. Key advantages of monitoring tumor response in vivo are the ability to identify non-responders at an early stage and to assist in predicting prognosis, which may allow a more individually tailored approach to treatment in future.

Non-responders can be identified early in treatment using a combination of size and kinetic changes, with interpretation facilitated by CAD systems which offer volumetric analysis and parametric color-mapping. Solitary large high-grade IDCs (particularly of basal-like molecular subtype), show the best response to NST and the best pathologic correlation with residual disease extent.

Multiple complex factors influence changes in enhancement in response to NST relating to the tumor and even to the specific chemotherapeutic agent. Scattered, patchy patterns of enhancement after treatment are more difficult to measure and to interpret, with resulting poorer histopathologic correlation.

A limitation of MRI is the difficulty in distinguishing multifocal tumor nests from enhancing reparative response when determining residual disease extent. A multidisciplinary team approach involving oncologists, surgeons, radiologists and pathologists is essential to identify patients at high risk of locoregional recurrence and offer them appropriate options.

MULTIPLE CHOICE QUESTIONS

7.1 Answer true or false to the following statements

A. With adenocarcinoma in axillary nodes, MRI reveals a breast primary in about 70% of cases.

B. MRI is widely recommended for evaluation of any equivocal microcalcifications prior to biopsy.

C. Partial tumor response = > 30% reduction in longest diameter or > 65% reduction in volume.

D. A complete pCR after NST predicts improved survival.

E. In general, ER-positive tumors respond well to endocrine therapy but poorly to chemotherapy.

7.2 Answer true or false to the following statements

A. After NST, residual tumor and reparative response are always easily distinguished.

B. Anti-angiogenic properties of taxanes may lead to underestimation of residual tumor.

C. An increase in tumor SER before and after NST is an indicator of a good response.

D. A fall in the proportion of tumor voxels showing washout is an indicator of a good response.

E. Large solitary circumscribed ER-negative invasive cancers are unlikely to respond to NST.

See page 189 for answers.

References

1. Bluemke DA, Gatsonis CA, Chen MH, *et al.* Magnetic resonance imaging of the breast prior to biopsy. *JAMA* 2004; **292**: 2735–42.
2. Schnall MD, Blume J, Bluemke DA, *et al.* Diagnostic architectural and dynamic features at breast MR imaging: multicenter study. *Radiology 2006;* **238**: 42–53.
3. Shimauchi A, Jansen SA, Abe H, *et al.* Breast cancers not detected at MRI: review of false-negative lesions. *AJR Am J Roentgenol* 2010; **194**: 1674–9.
4. Kuhl CK, Schrading S, Wardelmann E, *et al.* Magnetic resonance imaging versus mammography for diagnosing ductal carcinoma in situ. *J Clin Oncol* 2007; **25**: 1504.
5. Kuhl CK. Science to practice: why do purely intraductal cancers enhance on breast MR images? *Radiology* 2009; **253**: 281–3.
6. Bazzocchi M, Zuiani C, Panizza P, *et al.* Contrast-enhanced breast MRI in patients with suspicious microcalcifications on mammography: results of a multicenter trial. *AJR Am J Roentgenol* 2006; **186**: 1723–32.
7. Kneeshaw PJ, Lowry M, Manton D, *et al.* Differentiation of benign from malignant breast disease associated with screening detected microcalcifications using dynamic contrast enhanced magnetic resonance imaging. *The Breast* 2006; **15**: 29–38.
8. Lee CH, Smith RC, Levine JA, *et al.* Clinical usefulness of MR imaging of the breast in the evaluation of the problematic mammogram. *AJR Am J Roentgenol* 1999; **173**: 1323–9.
9. Moy L, Elias K, Patel V, *et al.* Is breast MRI helpful in the evaluation of inconclusive mammographic findings? *AJR Am J Roentgenol* 2009; **193**: 986–93.
10. Lee CH. Problem solving MR imaging of the breast. *Radiol Clin N Am* 2004; **42**: 919–34.
11. Mann RM, Veltman J, Barentsz JO, *et al.* The value of MRI compared to mammography in the assessment of tumor extent in invasive lobular carcinoma of the breast. *Eur J Surg Oncol* 2008; **34**: 135–42.
12. Schnall M, Orel S. Breast MR imaging in the diagnostic setting. *Magn Reson Imaging Clin N Am* 2006; **14**: 329–37.
13. Bird RE, Wallace TW, Yankaskas BC. Analysis of cancers missed at screening mammography. *Radiology* 1992; **184**: 613–17.
14. Yazici B, Sever AR, Mills P, *et al.* Scar formation after stereotactic vacuum-assisted core biopsy of benign breast lesions. *Clin Radiol* 2006; **61**: 619–24.
15. Frei KA, Kinkel K, Bonel HM, *et al.* MR imaging of the breast in patients with positive margins after lumpectomy: influence of the time interval between lumpectomy and MR imaging. *AJR Am J Roentgenol* 2000; **175**: 1577–84.
16. Lee JM, Orel SG, Czerniecki BJ, *et al.* MRI before reexcision surgery in patients with breast

cancer. *AJR Am J Roentgenol* 2004; **182**: 473–80.

17. Hwang ES, Kinkel K, Esserman LJ, *et al.* Magnetic resonance imaging in patients diagnosed with ductal carcinoma-in-situ: value in the diagnosis of residual disease, occult invasion, and multicentricity. *Ann Surg Oncol* 2003; **10**: 381–8.
18. Nicholson BT, Harvey JA, Cohen MA. Nipple-areolar complex: normal anatomy and benign and malignant processes. *RadioGraphics* 2009; **29**: 509–23.
19. Kaiser WA. *Signs in MR-Mammography*. Berlin Heidelberg, Springer-Verlag, 2009.
20. Giess CS, Keating DM, Osborne MP, *et al.* Retroareolar breast carcinoma: clinical, imaging and histopathological features. *Radiology* 1998; **207**: 669–73.
21. Cabioglu N, Hunt KH, Singletary SE, *et al.* Surgical decision making and factors determining a diagnosis of breast carcinoma in women presenting with nipple discharge. *J Am Coll Surg* 2003; **196**: 354–64.
22. Orel SG, Dougherty CS, Reynolds C, *et al.* MR imaging in patients with nipple discharge: initial experience. *Radiology* 2000; **216**: 248–54.
23. Nakahara H, Namba K, Watanabe R, *et al.* A comparison of MR imaging, galactography and ultrasonography in patients with nipple discharge. *Breast Cancer* 2003; **10**: 320–9.
24. Schwab SA, Uder M, Schulz-Wendtland R, *et al.* Direct MR galactography: feasibility study. *Radiology* 2008; **249**: 54–61.
25. Fu P, Kurihara Y, Kanemaki Y, *et al.* High-resolution MRI in detecting subareolar breast abscess. *AJR Am J Roentgenol* 2007; **188**: 1568–72.
26. Echevarria JJ, Lopez-Ruiz JA, Martin D, *et al.* Usefulness of MRI in detecting occult breast cancer associated with Paget's disease of the nipple–areolar complex. *Br J Radiol* 2004; **77**: 1036–9.
27. Morrogh M, Morris EA, Liberman L, *et al.* MRI identifies otherwise occult disease in select patients with Paget disease of the nipple. *J Am Coll Surg* 2008; **206**: 316–21.
28. Pavlidis N, Briasoulis E, Hainsworth J, *et al.* Diagnostic and therapeutic management of cancer of an unknown primary. *Eur J Cancer* 2003; **39**: 1990–2005.
29. Vlastos G, Jean ME, Mirza AN, *et al.* Feasibility of breast preservation in the treatment of occult primary carcinoma presenting with axillary metastases. *Ann Surg Oncol* 2001; **8**: 425–31.
30. Varadarajan R, Edge SB, Yu J, *et al.* Prognosis of occult breast carcinoma presenting as isolated axillary nodal metastasis. *Oncology* 2006; **71**: 456–9.
31. de Bresser J, de Vo B, van der Ent F, *et al.* Breast MRI in clinically and mammographically occult breast cancer presenting with an axillary metastasis: a systematic review. *Eur J Surg Oncol* 2010; **36**: 114–19.
32. Olson JA, Morris EA, Van Zee KJ, *et al.* Magnetic resonance imaging facilitates breast conservation for occult breast cancer. *Ann Surg Oncol* 2000; **7**: 411–15.
33. Galimberti V, Bassani G, Monti S, *et al.* Clinical experience with axillary presentation breast cancer. *Breast Cancer Res Treat* 2004; **88**: 43–7.
34. Morris EA, Schwartz LH, Dershaw DD, *et al.* MR imaging of the breast in patients with occult primary breast carcinoma. *Radiology* 1997; **205**: 437–40.
35. Buchanan CL, Morris EA, Dorn PL, *et al.* Utility of breast magnetic resonance imaging in patients with occult primary breast cancer. *Ann Surg Oncol* 2005; **12**: 1045–53.
36. McMahon K, Medoro L, Kennedy D. Breast magnetic resonance imaging: an essential role in malignant axillary lymphadenopathy of unknown origin. *Australas Radiol* 2005; **49**: 382–9.
37. Esserman L, Kaplan J, Partridge S, *et al.* MRI phenotype Is associated with response to doxorubicin and cyclophosphamide neoadjuvant chemotherapy in stage III breast cancer. *Ann Surg Oncol* 2001; **8**: 549–59.
38. Mauri D, Pavlidis N, Ioannidis JPA. Neoadjuvant versus adjuvant systemic treatment in breast cancer: a meta-analysis. *J Natl Cancer Inst* 2005; **97**: 188–94.
39. Mieog JS, van der Hage JA, van de Velde CJ. Neoadjuvant chemotherapy for operable breast cancer. *Br J Surg* 2007; **94**: 1189–200.
40. Mazouni C, Peintinger F, Wan-Kau S, *et al.* Residual ductal carcinoma in situ in patients with complete eradication of invasive breast cancer after neoadjuvant chemotherapy does not adversely affect patient outcome. *J Clin Oncol* 2007; **25**: 2650–5.
41. Fisher ER, Wang J, Bryant J, *et al.* Pathobiology of preoperative chemotherapy. Findings from the National Surgical Adjuvant Breast and Bowel Project (NSABP) protocol B-18a. *Cancer* 2002; **95**: 681–95.
42. Gilles R, Guinebretiere J, Toussaint C, *et al.* Locally advanced breast cancer: contrast-enhanced subtraction MR imaging of response to preoperative chemotherapy. *Radiology* 1994; **191**: 633–8.
43. Balu-Maestro C, Chapellier C, Bleuse A, *et al.* Imaging in evaluation of reponse to neoadjuvant breast cancer treatment benefits of MRI. *Breast Cancer Res Treat* 2002; **72**: 145–52.
44. Rieber A, Brambs H, Gabelmann A, *et al.* Breast MRI for monitoring response of primary breast cancer

to neo-adjuvant chemotherapy. *Eur Radiol* 2002; **12**: 1711–19.

45. Martincich L, Montemurro F, De Rosa G, *et al.* Monitoring response to primary chemotherapy in breast cancer using dynamic contrast-enhanced magnetic resonance imaging. *Breast Cancer Res Treat* 2004; **83**: 67–76.

46. Belli P, Costantini M, Malaspina C, *et al.* MRI accuracy in residual disease evaluation in breast cancer patients treated with neoadjuvant chemotherapy. *Clin Radiol* 2006; **61**: 946–53.

47. Partridge SC, Gibbs JE, Lu Y, *et al.* Accuracy of MR imaging for revealing residual breast cancer in patients who have undergone neoadjuvant chemotherapy. *AJR Am J Roentgenol* 2002; **179**: 1193–9.

48. Thibault F, Nos C, Meunier M, *et al.* MRI for surgical planning in patients with breast cancer who undergo preoperative chemotherapy. *AJR Am J Roentgenol* 2004; **183**: 1159–68.

49. Yeh E, Slanetz P, Kopans DB, *et al.* Prospective comparison of mammography, sonography, and MRI in patients undergoing neoadjuvant chemotherapy for palpable breast cancer. *AJR Am J Roentgenol* 2005; **184**: 868–77.

50. Julius T, Kemp SEG, Kneeshaw PJ, *et al.* MRI and conservative treatment of locally advanced breast cancer. *Eur J Surg Oncol* 2005; **31**: 1129–34.

51. Stucky C-CH, McLaughlin SA, Dueck AC, *et al.* Does magnetic resonance imaging accurately predict residual disease in breast cancer? *Am J Surg* 2009; **198**: 547–52.

52. Buchholz TA, Lehman CD, Harris JR, *et al.* Statement of the science concerning locoregional treatments after preoperative chemotherapy for breast cancer: a National Cancer Institute Conference. *J Clin Oncol* 2008; **26**: 791–7.

53. Chen AM, Meric-Bernstam F, Hunt KK, *et al.* Breast conservation after neoadjuvant chemotherapy: the M.D. Anderson Cancer Center experience. *J Clin Oncol* 2004; **22**: 2303–12.

54. James K, Eisenhauer E, Christian M, *et al.* Measuring response in solid tumors: unidimensional versus bidimensional measurement. *J Natl Cancer Inst* 1999; **91**: 532–8.

55. Suzuki C, Jacobsson H, Hatschek T, *et al.* Radiologic measurements of tumor response to treatment: practical approaches and limitations. *RadioGraphics* 2008; **28**: 329–44.

56. Loo CE, Teerstra HJ, Rodenhuis S, *et al.* Dynamic contrast-enhanced MRI for prediction of breast cancer response to neoadjuvant chemotherapy: initial results. *AJR Am J Roentgenol* 2008; **191**: 1331–8.

57. Rosen EL, Blackwell KL, Baker JA, *et al.* Accuracy of MRI in the detection of residual breast cancer after neoadjuvant chemotherapy. *AJR Am J Roentgenol* 2003; **181**: 1275–82.

58. Partridge SC, Gibbs JE, Lu Y, *et al.* MRI measurements of breast tumor volume predict response to neoadjuvant chemotherapy and recurrence-free survival. *AJR Am J Roentgenol* 2005; **184**: 1774–81.

59. Lorenzon M, Zuiani C, Londero V, *et al.* Assessment of breast cancer response to neoadjuvant chemotherapy: is volumetric MRI a reliable tool? *Eur J Radiol* 2009; **71**: 82–8.

60. Hylton N, Blume J, Gatsonis C, *et al.* MRI tumor volume for predicting response to neoadjuvant chemotherapy in locally advanced breast cancer: findings from ACRIN 6657/CALGB 150007. *J Clin Oncol, 2009 ASCO Annual Meeting Proceedings (Post-Meeting Edition)* 2009; **27**(15S): 529.

61. Morrow M, Strom EA, Bassett LW, *et al.* Standard for breast conservation in the management of invasive breast carcinoma. *CA Cancer J Clin* 2002; **52**: 277–300.

62. Chen AM, Meric-Bernstam F, Hunt KK, *et al.* Breast conservation after neoadjuvant chemotherapy. A prognostic index for clinical decision-making. *Cancer* 2005; **103**: 689–95.

63. Goldhirsch A, Ingle JN, Gelber RD, *et al.* Thresholds for therapies: highlights of the St Gallen International Expert Consensus on the Primary Therapy of Early Breast Cancer 2009. *Ann Oncol* 2009; **20**: 1319–29.

64. Chen J-H, Mehta RS, Carpenter PM, *et al.* Magnetic resonance imaging in predicting pathologic response of triple negative breast cancer following neoadjuvant chemotherapy. *J Clin Oncol* 2007; **25**: 5667–9.

65. Chen JH, Feig B, Agrawal G, *et al.* MRI evaluation of pathologically complete response and residual tumors in breast cancer after neoadjuvant chemotherapy. *Cancer* 2008; **112**: 17–26.

66. Denis F, Desbiez-Bourcier AV, Chapiron C, *et al.* Contrast enhanced magnetic resonance imaging underestimates residual disease following neoadjuvant docetaxel based chemotherapy for breast cancer. *Eur J Surg Oncol* 2004; **30**: 1069–76.

67. Chou C-P, Wu M-T, Chang H-T, *et al.* Monitoring breast cancer response to neoadjuvant systemic chemotherapy using parametric contrast-enhanced MRI: a pilot study. *Acad Radiol* 2007; **14**: 561–73.

68. El Khoury C, Servois V, Thibault F, *et al.* MR quantification of the washout changes in breast tumors under preoperative chemotherapy: feasibility and preliminary results. *AJR Am J Roentgenol* 2005; **184**: 1499–504.

69. Padhani AR, Hayes C, Assersohn L, *et al.* Prediction of clinicopathologic response of breast cancer to primary chemotherapy at contrast-enhanced MR imaging: initial clinical results. *Radiology* 2006; **239**: 361–74.

70. DeMartini WB, Lehman CD, Peacock S, *et al.* Computer-aided detection applied to breast MRI: assessment of CAD-generated enhancement and tumor sizes in breast cancers before and after neoadjuvant chemotherapy. *Acad Radiol* 2005; **12**: 806–14.

71. Williams TC, Demartini WB, Partridge SC, *et al.* Breast MR imaging: computer-aided evaluation program for discriminating benign from malignant lesions. *Radiology* 2007; **244**: 94–103.

72. Woodhams R, Kakita S, Hata H, *et al.* Identification of residual breast carcinoma following neoadjuvant chemotherapy: diffusion-weighted imaging – comparison with contrast-enhanced MR imaging and pathologic findings. *Radiology* 2010; **254**: 357–66.

73. Rosen EL, Eubank WB, Mankoff DA. FDG PET, PET/CT, and breast cancer imaging. *RadioGraphics* 2007; **27**: S215–29.

74. Lim HS, Yoon W, Chung TW, *et al.* FDG PET/CT for the detection and evaluation of breast diseases: usefulness and limitations. *RadioGraphics* 2007; **27**: S197–213.

Chapter 8

MRI after breast augmentation

Chapter outline

- Historical background
- Implant types and terminology
- Fibrous capsule formation and contracture
- The evolution of silicone implants
- Normal MRI features of silicone implants
- MRI appearances of implant complications
- Cancer incidence and detection in women with implants
- Tissue breast reconstructive surgery
- Augmentation by direct injection procedures

Historical background

Over the last hundred or so years, attempts at breast augmentation have been documented using an astonishing variety of materials including ivory, glass beads, ground rubber, gutta percha and ox cartilage [1]. The range of injectable substances used includes paraffin oil, petroleum jelly, glazier's putty, beeswax, shellac and epoxy resin [1]. Not surprisingly, complications were frequent, often relating to foreign body reactions with tissue necrosis, fistula formation and infection. With the advent of synthetic polymers, new concepts were trialled in the form of polythene chips, polythene tape or strips wound into a ball-shape, polymer sponges, Terylene wool, silastic rubber and polypropylene string, but none of these materials gave a particularly natural cosmetic effect.

In the early 1960s, direct injection of medical-grade *silicone gel* emerged as a promising technique, but although initial results were encouraging, serious delayed complications developed. Of even greater concern, silicone pulmonary embolism was also reported as an acute and sometimes fatal complication of direct injection.

Silicone breast implants were first introduced in 1962, and were considered to be a radical improvement over the practice of direct injection of silicone. By encasing the silicone gel in a durable *elastomer shell* (silicone rubber), it was widely anticipated that implants would avoid local and distant complications.

Free silicone in the breast is associated with a high incidence of granuloma formation, with *siliconomas* often presenting clinically as painful breast lumps. Granulomas can involve the duct system, leading to discharge of gel from the nipple, and free gel often migrates to the axillary nodes, causing adenopathy. Neurologic symptoms may result from involvement of the brachial plexus. Less commonly, free gel can migrate to the chest or abdominal wall, to the arms and other remote sites with various adverse clinical effects reported due to granulomatous reactions [1, 2].

Though initially thought to be uncommon, it became apparent that failure of the elastomer shell (i.e., loss of integrity with escape of gel filler) occurred with increasing frequency beyond around 8 years from implantation.

For implants performed from 1972 up to the mid 1980s, rupture rates as high as 95% at 12 years have been reported [1]. It was estimated that by 1997, in the USA alone, some 2 million women had received silicone implants, either for cosmetic reasons (~70%) or for reconstruction after mastectomy (~30%) [1]. As concern mounted over the potential for silicone gel to escape from implants, a reliable method to detect leakage was needed. From the early 1990s, non-contrast breast MRI became rapidly established as the technique of choice for assessing breast implant integrity.

More frequent than implant leakage was the complication of painful hardening around the implant due to *fibrous contracture*, which sometimes necessitated revision surgery. Silicone implants were also linked to fibromyalgia and other connective tissue disorders, although exhaustive analysis has since concluded that there are no scientific data to suggest a causal relationship. Nevertheless, safety concerns resulted in tight restrictions being placed on the further use of silicone implants by the United States FDA in 1992.

Subsequently, in the mid 1990s, a series of legal class actions totalling some 19 000 claims, led to the largest product liability settlement in the history of the USA and bankrupted the Dow Corning corporation. Following the 1992 moratorium, saline-filled implants became widely used as a substitute for silicone, although the cosmetic results were not as favorable because of the less natural look and feel of saline implants.

The use of silicone implants was again approved by the FDA for reconstructive surgery in 1998 and for cosmetic surgery only as recently as November 2006. The FDA has also endorsed MRI screening for implant failure, recommending an initial scan after 3 years and subsequent scans every 2 years thereafter. This precautionary measure was taken despite an expected low incidence of complications due to improved implant design.

Implant types and terminology

Implants are available in a wide range of sizes (volumes usually from 80 to 800 ml, diameters from 7.5 to 16.8 cm and profiles from 1.5 to 7.5 cm) and a variety of shapes (round, oval, teardrop or contoured) [1]. Numerous designs have been used containing either silicone, saline or in the case of *double-lumen* implants, a combination of both (Fig. 8.1). Single-lumen silicone implants are the most commonly encountered, and were used in 60–80% of implantation procedures in the USA prior to 1992. After the 1992 moratorium until recently, 95% of all new implants in the USA were saline-filled. Some single-lumen saline implants are prefilled, but most have a filler valve through which the implant can be inflated by the surgeon after insertion, allowing a smaller incision to be used. Terminology applied to various implant types and features is given in Table 8.1.

In some cases, implants were filled with other materials such as peanut oil or soya bean oil. The radiolucency of oil-filled implants meant that visualization of adjacent breast tissue was much improved, and in theory the triglyceride oil content was not harmful if leakage occurred. In the UK, around 5000 women received Trilucent soya bean oil-filled implants in the 1990s. A further 4000 women received implants filled with a water-retaining polymer called hydrogel in the same period. By the year 2000, both implant types had been withdrawn due to concern over the safety of these filler materials, with a recommendation that implants already in place be removed.

Table 8.1 Types of implant and common terminology

Single-lumen silicone – most common, 60–80% in USA prior to 1992 FDA moratorium
Single-lumen saline – adjustable through filler valve at time of surgery, 5% in USA prior to 1992
Standard double-lumen – inner silicone, outer saline, 12–15% in USA prior to 1992 (< 1% after)
Reversed double-lumen – outer silicone, inner saline, use limited to tissue-expander designs
Tissue expanders – subcutaneous access port allows saline to be gradually added after surgery
Textured implants – roughened outer surface aims to prevent fibrous contracture
Fixation patches – Dacron patches promoted tissue in growth, intended to stabilize the implants
Stacked implants – refers to the use of more than one implant in the same breast

Tissue expanders, used in reconstruction surgery after mastectomy, have a subcutaneous access port through which saline can be gradually added over some months to form an enlarging cavity. Breast tissue expanders are usually used as temporary devices in preparation for subsequent replacement by another implant, although some designs can be retained permanently.

Although injection ports can usually be identified by palpation, breast tissue expanders often feature magnetic access ports with various ingenious locator devices [3]. These magnetic ports can be problematic when performing MRI, and some devices including the Contour Profile Tissue Expander (Mentor, Santa Barbara, CA, USA) and the McGhan Style 133 Breast Tissue Expanders with Magna-Site injection ports (Allergan, Irvine, CA, USA) are considered unsafe for MRI [4]. Displacement of magnetic infusion ports after MRI has been reported, requiring revision surgery [5]. Magnetic ports also produce relatively large artifacts on breast MRI studies, and may cause local discomfort due to heating effects [6].

Fibrous capsule formation and contracture

No matter what implant type is used, it will have an outer envelope or *shell*. The shell is made from elastomer (silicone rubber), even when it contains saline rather than silicone gel. Once implanted in the breast, the shell excites a foreign body reaction resulting in the formation of a *fibrous capsule*, which may contract

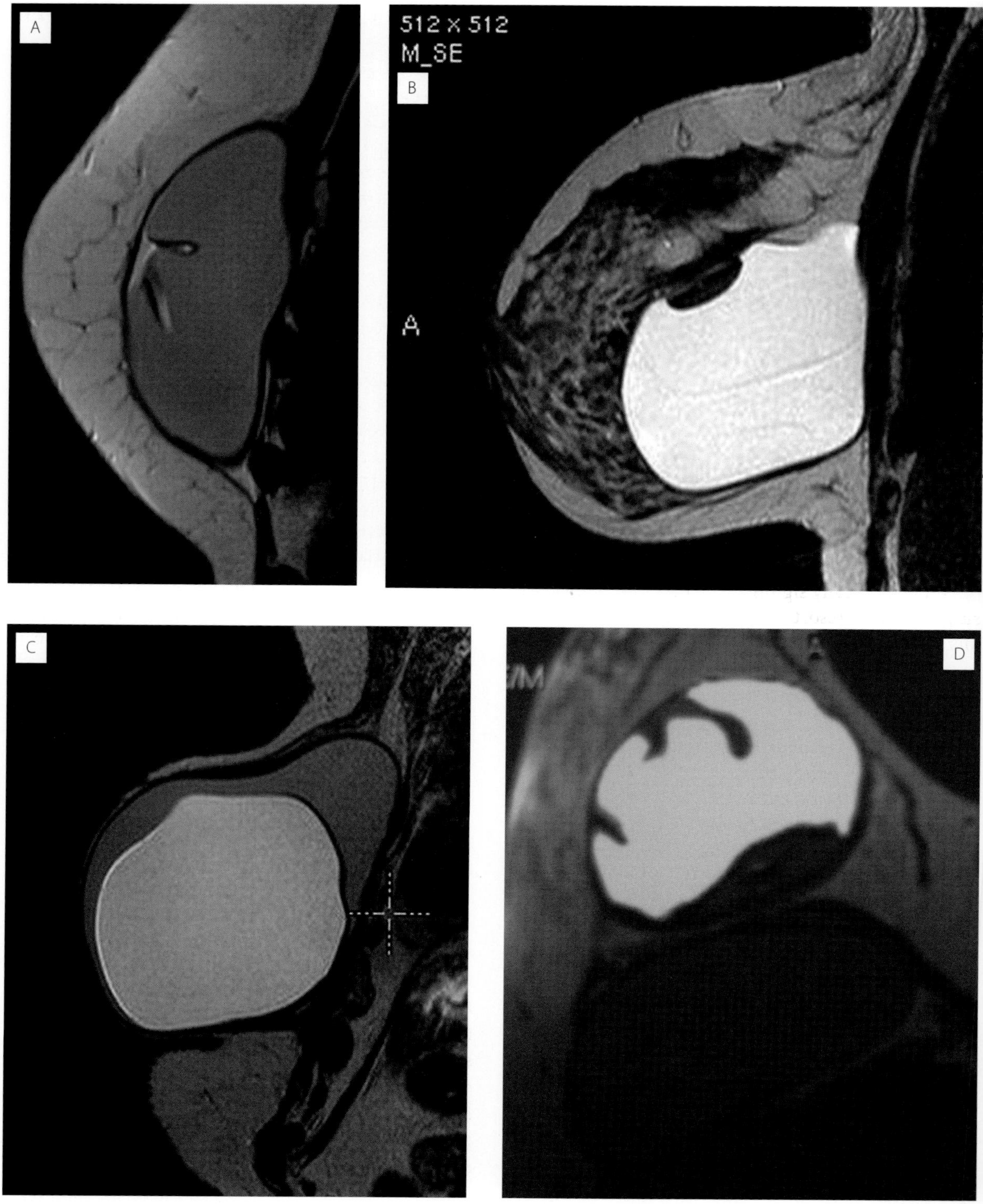

Fig. 8.1 **Normal appearances of implants:** (A) Sagittal T2-weighted image of normal silicone implant with normal trace of fluid at inferior angle, between implant shell and fibrous capsule. Note also peripheral fold with further fluid between the leaves anteriorly. (B) Sagittal T2-weighted image of normal saline implant with filler valve superiorly. Note subglandular location, superficial to pectoral muscle. (C) Tissue-expander type of double-lumen implant used for reconstruction after mastectomy. Sagittal T2-weighted image shows silicone surrounding the saline component. Note subpectoral location of implant. (D) Stacked implants. Silicone implant is deep to pectoral muscle with reversed double-lumen implant in subglandular location.

slightly over time. More excessive fibrous contracture leads to clinical hardening, discomfort and change in shape. The fibrous capsule may even become calcified, a feature visible on XRM.

Various measures to reduce the incidence of fibrous contracture have been tried, notably the use of *textured implants* with a roughened outer surface to the shell. This design emulated earlier implants with a polyurethane foam coating, successful in reducing contracture but withdrawn in the USA because of safety concerns over possible carcinogenic effects. Outside the USA, these implants have continued to be used, with one study reporting a contracture rate of just 1% after 5- to 15-year follow-up in 730 patients [7].

The standard double-lumen implant (saline surrounding silicone) was another strategy aimed at preventing fibrous contracture and gel leakage. There was, however, little evidence to support a reduced risk of contracture, although a lower incidence of implant rupture has been reported with this design [8]. In the USA, the use of standard double-lumen implants fell to less than 1% after the 1992 FDA moratorium [1].

When clinically significant contracture does arise, surgeons may resort to performing *closed capsulotomy*, in which the implant is manipulated externally to break down the hardened capsule. Unfortunately, this procedure can be complicated by rupture of the underlying implant.

Surgeons traditionally placed implants either behind the breast parenchyma (*retromammary* or *subglandular*), or entirely deep to the pectoralis major (*retropectoral, subpectoral* or *submuscular*) (Fig. 8.1). Subpectoral implants are associated with a much lower incidence of fibrous contracture, but are more prone to rupture than subglandular implants. Recently, combined pocket locations have become popular, in which usually the upper part of the implant is behind the pectoralis major while the inferior portion lies in the retromammary pocket (*partial subpectoral). Advantages of *dual-plane mammaplasty* have been reported, including use in revision surgery for fibrous contracture arising in conventional single pocket implants, and new techniques continue to be developed [9, 10].

The evolution of silicone implants

First generation silicone implants, used in the 1960s and 1970s were made with thick elastomer shells and were filled with thick gel. Capsular contracture and calcification were common, but because of the thick shell, leakage was far less frequent than with implants in the next generation designs.

Second generation silicone implants, available in the 1970s and 1980s, were made with thinner shells and much more fluid silicone gel, designed to give a more natural cosmetic effect. Unfortunately, the improved cosmesis was at the expense of mechanical shell strength, resulting in much higher rates of implant rupture. The resulting complications and concerns over silicone leakage led to the FDA's later decision to restrict the use of silicone implants.

Third generation implants, available from the late 1980s, were designed with barrier-coated shells and contained a thicker, more cohesive gel filler giving the implants "low-bleed" characteristics. Nevertheless, an MRI-based study indicated that while third generation implants were relatively durable for the first 6–8 years, it was estimated that a minimum of 15% would rupture by 10 years [8].

Fourth generation implants, which were first used outside the USA from 1993, featured further refinements on third generation designs with stronger shells and the use of "highly cohesive gel fillers." Unfortunately, in the absence of clear industry standards, "highly cohesive" has become a marketing buzzword with almost no meaning [11]. Many implant types produced since the mid 1990s claimed to be highly cohesive but varied widely in their physical characteristics.

The clinical importance of high gel cohesion is its effect on "elastic memory" and shape retention of the implant, allowing good cosmetic contouring while also preventing gel migration in the event of rupture of the shell. The term "form-stable" is often preferred for implants where the design has been shown to fulfill these objectives.

The designation fifth generation is reserved for what are now widely known as "Gummy Bear" implants, the name deriving from Gummy Bear confectionery (Haribo, Bonn, Germany), which has a very similar semi-solid gel consistency. When cut across, like the confectionery, the firm gel in these implants retains its shape, greatly reducing the risk of silicone gel migration (Plate 5). The durable design of fifth generation breast implants is resistant to folding and weakening, with very low rates of rupture expected. Such form-stable implants have been manufactured since 1993, with the McGhan Style 410 and Mentor Memory Gel types now widely considered to qualify as fifth generation (though classed as fourth generation at the time of manufacture).

Table 8.2 Generations in the evolution of silicone implant design

First 1960s–70s	Thick-shell/thick-gel – low rupture but high contracture rates
Second 1970s–80s	Thin-shell/thin-gel – high rupture and high contracture rates
Third late 1980s–	Stronger-shell/textured/low-bleed features added in design
Fourth early 1990s–	Refinements on third generation designs further reduce complications
Fifth 1993–	Gummy Bear semi-solid implants designed to eliminate gel migration

Key features of the different generations of silicone implants are summarized in Table 8.2. Women are still encountered who have retained their second or third generation implants dating back to the 1970–80s, with a high prevalence of rupture in this group. Some fourth generation implants can be expected to show usual MRI signs of rupture, even if claiming to be highly cohesive. It is doubtful if gel migration can occur at all with true form-stable or Gummy Bear fifth generation implants.

Normal MRI features of silicone implants

On MRI, the fibrous capsule is seen as a hypointense line around the implant. The immediately subjacent implant shell is not easily distinguished when it is in contact with the capsule, but there is a potential space at this interface. It is normal to see a small amount of reactive fluid in this space, a finding more frequent where implants with textured surfaces have been used. Such fluid is often most visible at the angled margins of the implant (Fig. 8.1).

Peripheral *radial folds* at the interface where the elastomer shell abuts the fibrous capsule are a normal

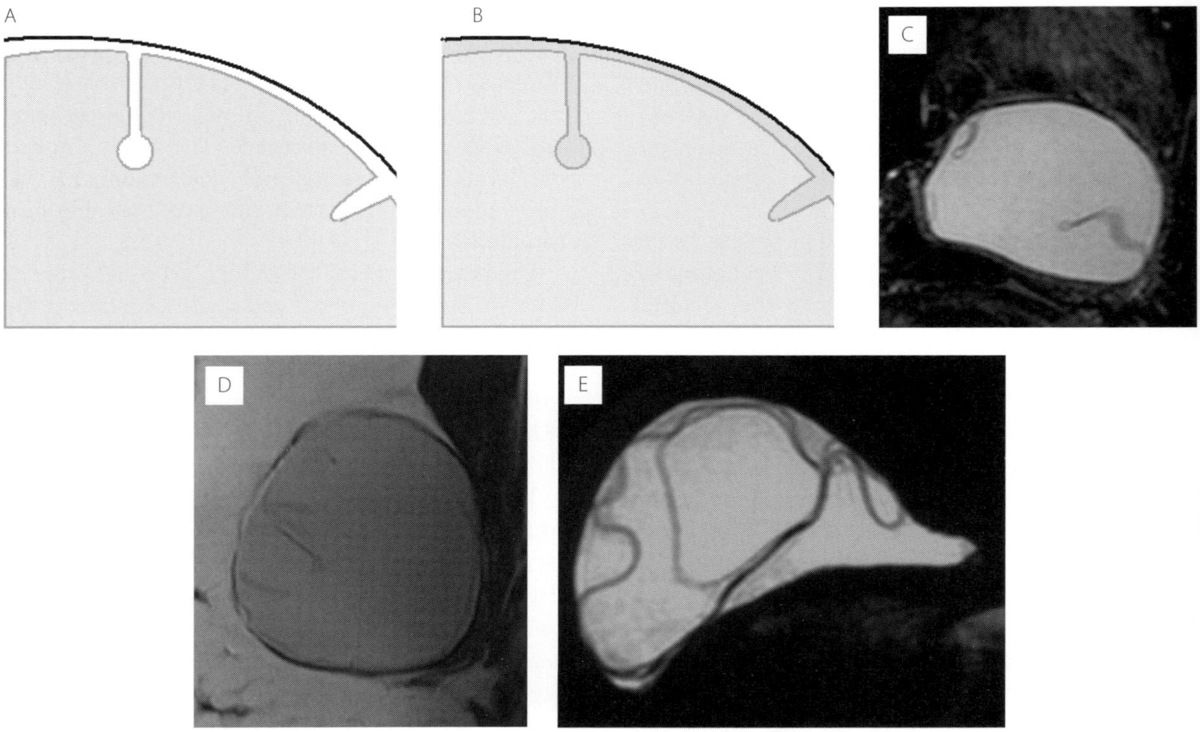

Fig. 8.2 Intracapsular (contained) rupture: (A) Schematic of normal subcapsular fluid signal extending between the leaves of simple radial folds in the implant shell. Normal folds can be traced back to the surface where they abut the fibrous capsule (thick outer line). (B) In the noose sign of silicone implant failure, silicone has filled the potential space between the envelope and fibrous capsule so silicone signal is seen between the leaves of radial folds (due to either gel bleeding from an intact implant or contained rupture). (C) Noose sign of intracapsular rupture. Two radial folds are seen, each with silicone signal in the noose. Circumferential faint line just inside the shell is due to artifact, which can mimic the subcapsular line sign. (D) Subcapsular line sign seen on sagittal T2-weighted image, with developing undulations beginning to form a wavy-line sign. Note also multiple noose signs anteriorly. (E) Linguine sign seen on silicone-only (water-suppressed, T2-weighted IR) image due to intracapsular rupture.

appearance. Such folds can be quite long and sometimes complex, but the margins can always be traced back to the implant surface where it contacts the fibrous capsule [12–14]. Where the fold reflects back on itself within the implant, a trace of water signal may be seen, giving the appearance of a "noose" around a droplet of water. This is also a normal finding, and is to be expected where reactive fluid is present and can extend down between the surfaces of the fold (Figs. 8.1 and 8.2).

Droplets of water are sometimes seen floating free within the silicone gel of an otherwise normal intact implant, presenting a puzzling appearance. This relates to the practice of injecting implants with steroid, betadine or antibiotics at the time of implantation in the hope of preventing complications of infection and fibrous contracture. For this reason, when the *droplet sign* is seen as an isolated finding, it has to be regarded as a normal appearance [15].

Other features can be specific to the type of implant used, such as the filler valves seen in most saline implants. A focally thickened appearance of the elastomer shell posteriorly may be seen if Dacron *fixation patches* have been used to stabilize an implant. Some normal appearances of implants are listed in Table 8.3.

MRI appearances of implant complications

With fibrous contracture, patients notice a change in the feel of the implant and may experience discomfort or pain. Contracture may be correlated on MRI as distortion of the normal smooth contour, sometimes with a serrated appearance to the implant margin [12]. Eventually, spherical deformity results with marked increase in the anteroposterior diameter of the implant relative to the transverse. In general though, such deformity is clinically obvious, and MRI adds little to the standard clinical assessment using the Baker classification (Table 8.4). On contrast-enhanced MRI studies, a thin rim of enhancement of the fibrous capsule can be seen, but this phenomenon of "capsulitis" is usually asymptomatic.

Implant rupture can result from gross trauma, but this is a rare occurrence. In most cases there is no traumatic event, and gradual mechanical weakening of the implant shell with age is the key predisposing factor. It is widely believed that normal peripheral folds may result in lines of weakness developing in the elastomer shell, which can then easily or spontaneously tear. As mentioned earlier, closed capsulotomy can result in implant rupture, and anecdotal cases have been attributed to mammographic compression [1, 16].

In the presence of failure of the elastomer shell, saline and silicone implants behave differently. With silicone implants, the viscous gel oozes out quite slowly, while a ruptured saline implant usually deflates very rapidly. Saline implant failure or *deflation* is then a simple clinical diagnosis with no need for imaging. Gradual saline loss through the envelope can also occur over a period of years as a normal occurrence [12, 13].

It is helpful to know as much as possible about the implant type used before interpreting the MRI study. For example, if the outer saline component of a double-lumen implant has deflated completely, this can mimic a normal silicone implant. Similarly, a standard double-lumen implant could be mistaken for a silicone implant with surrounding reactive fluid unless the surgical history is known.

The major role of MRI is to assess the integrity of silicone implants and, more importantly, of the surrounding biologic fibrous capsule. Two types of *implant rupture* are recognized – *intracapsular* and *extracapsular*. With intracapsular or *contained rupture* silicone gel escapes through the elastomer shell but is confined within the fibrous capsule. This is sometimes termed "silent rupture" because there are

Table 8.3 Normal appearances of breast implants

Reactive fluid between elastomer shell and capsule – particularly textured implants
Radial folds – peripheral folding due to minor capsular contraction is very common
Fluid signal within the "noose" of peripheral radial folds – extension of reactive fluid
Droplet sign – isolated fluid signal droplets may relate to injection of silicone implants
Filler valve or injection port in shell – commonly with adjustable saline implants
Fixation patches – thickened areas usually posterior capsule, common prior to 1980s

Table 8.4 Baker clinical grading of capsular contraction

Grade I	Soft breast which feels and looks normal
Grade II	Slightly firm breast but looks normal
Grade III	Firm breast with visible distortion
Grade IV	Hard, painful breast with marked visible distortion

no associated clinical symptoms despite the implant failure. So long as the fibrous capsule remains intact, shape is preserved and there is no granulomatous reaction to the silicone gel.

In extracapsular rupture, gel escapes beyond the confines of the fibrous capsule into surrounding breast tissue. There is then the likelihood of silicone granuloma formation and the contour of the implant may also be affected by gross gel extrusion. In symptomatic women at least, extracapsular rupture is generally considered to be an indication for explantation, while many surgeons elect to manage intracapsular rupture conservatively.

> In a symptomatic woman, while contained rupture may be managed conservatively, an MRI diagnosis of extracapsular rupture will often prompt surgical explantation.

Intracapsular (contained) rupture of silicone implants

Contained rupture can be thought of as a spectrum of failure of the elastomer shell from *gel bleed*, through pinhole defects allowing gradual gel leakage, to frank tears in which the shell collapses down and is surrounded by leaked gel.

The phenomenon of *gel bleeding* refers to a process in which low molecular weight components in the silicone gel are able to migrate across an intact elastomer shell. This diffusion or slow seepage through a grossly intact shell occurs gradually over time and is therefore frequently seen in older implants. If removed, implants are found to be sticky due to silicone gel spread over the outer surface, and in some cases, perhaps 20–25%, tiny pinhole defects may be found although there is no overt tear. It is very probable that such pinhole tears develop along weakened radial folds in the elastomer shell as described earlier. With either a gel bleed or the early stages of implant failure (referred to as *uncollapsed rupture*) the elastomer shell remains in close contact with the fibrous capsule. Not surprisingly then, early MRI signs of implant rupture can be indistinguishable from a "normal" gel bleed.

On MRI, the earliest sign of implant leak relates to the presence of gel in the potential space between shell and fibrous capsule. Water signal in the noose of a radial fold is normal, as explained earlier. Conversely, if the noose contains silicone signal, the gel must have transgressed the boundary of the elastomer shell. This produces the appearance variously known as the *noose, teardrop, lariat, lasso, keyhole or loop sign* (Fig. 8.2). As an isolated finding this could relate to normal gel bleeding, so that only multiple noose signs are considered diagnostic of intracapsular rupture [13–15].

As more silicone collects outside the shell, a parallel *subcapsular line sign* may be seen as the implant wall retracts slightly, indicating minimal collapse of the shell [13]. This can be mimicked by ghosting artifact from movement, which is a potential pitfall. The subcapsular line becomes more undulating as the shell collapses further and begins to deform, then also termed the *wavy-line* or *fall-away* sign, often seen in combination with the noose sign (Fig. 8.2).

Eventually, as more silicone escapes, the shell retracts further away from the fibrous capsule and becomes grossly collapsed, then appearing as a mass of folded lines giving the classic *linguine* sign, correlating with the *stepladder sign* sonographically.

At the "linguine" stage the diagnosis is easy, but difficulty can be encountered in differentiating lesser degrees of implant collapse from normal complex radial folds. Carefully scrolling through images in at least two planes or in 3D usually allows a clear distinction to be made.

Droplets of water signal intensity suspended in silicone gel may be seen in conjunction with other signs of intracapsular implant rupture. Although not significant as an isolated finding, in the context of other signs of rupture, the droplet sign adds supportive evidence (Fig. 8.3).

Using these signs, the MRI assessment of gross silicone implant failure has been shown to be highly accurate, with reported sensitivity of up to 98%, and specificities of 85–100% in various series [1]. Sensitivity is, however, lower for the earliest stage of uncollapsed rupture. Key signs of intracapsular rupture are summarized in Table 8.5.

Analyzing failure in double-lumen implants can be something of a logic puzzle, and knowledge of the implant type is important. As mentioned, if the outer shell of a standard (water outside silicone) double-lumen implant ruptures, the saline will resorb and the implant comes to resemble a single-lumen silicone implant. In the case of rupture of the inner component shell only, free mixing of water and silicone occur, giving rise to the *salad-oil sign*. However, neither of these findings should be an

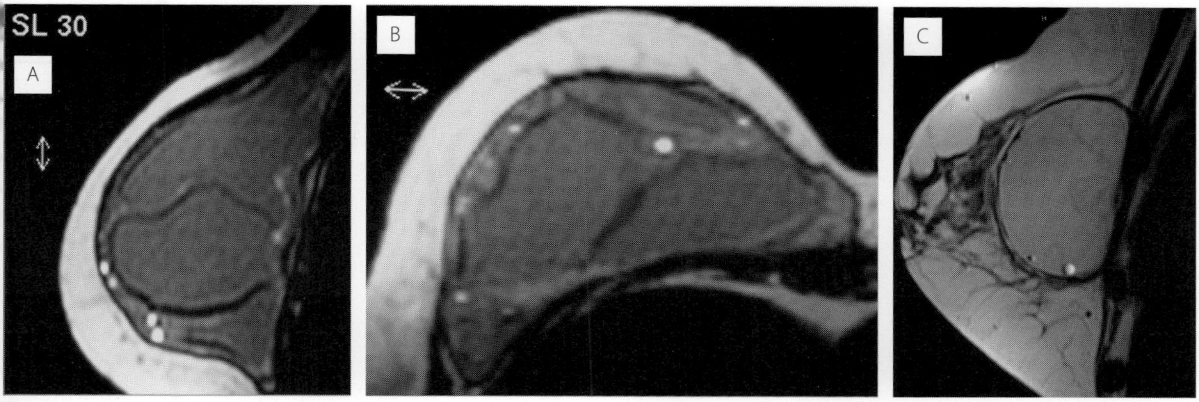

Fig. 8.3 Droplet sign: (A) Sagittal and (B) axial T2-weighted images on background of gross intracapsular rupture with collapsed shell, which has allowed normal reactive subcapsular fluid to mix with silicone gel. (C) Sagittal T2-weighted image showing droplet sign in another patient with signs of implant rupture. Seen in isolation, the droplet sign can be a spurious finding due to injection of the implant at the time of surgery.

Table 8.5 Signs of intracapsular rupture of silicone implant

Linguine sign – grossly collapsed and folded elastomer shell surrounded by silicone
Wavy-line sign – describes appearance between the subcapsular line and linguine stages
Subcapsular line sign – parallel or undulating line with thin layer of gel between shell and capsule Noose, keyhole, lariat, lasso, teardrop sign due to silicone within the noose – diagnostic if multiple
Droplet sign – not significant alone, but supportive when seen with other signs of rupture

indication for implant removal, so long as the fibrous capsule remains intact.

Extracapsular rupture of silicone implants

A recent study of the prevalence of implant failure found that 22% of all ruptured implants on MRI were extracapsular, with silicone gel extending beyond the confines of the fibrous capsule [17]. This may appear as a discrete silicone mass adjacent to the implant, which in the most obvious cases may even be visible on XRM. Silicone may also be seen in axillary lymph nodes. Siliconomas in breast parenchyma remote from the implant are less common.

On MRI, a bulge of the implant contour with loss of the normal hypointense capsular line, focal thinning or irregularity are useful clues. If such an area of capsular deficiency is also associated with a discrete globular or tongue-like extension of silicone signal, the findings are suggestive of a leak [18]. However, it is not uncommon for an intact implant to herniate into a focal weakness in the capsule. Berg *et al.* found that difficulty distinguishing a bulge due to herniation of an intact implant from true extracapsular extrusion of silicone was the most frequent cause for disagreement among experienced readers [18]. As a rule, if there is a bulge of the implant but with no other features of intracapsular implant rupture, the findings favor focal herniation. Where there are signs of implant rupture with a focal capsular defect, extracapsular extrusion of silicone is more likely (Fig. 8.4).

Fortunately, in many instances, the often difficult distinction between focal capsular herniation and true extracapsular leak is probably academic. In cases where there is a circumscribed globule of extracapsular silicone adjacent to the implant, this will trigger a further fibrotic reaction and so become walled-off or "re-encapsulated." If the patient remains asymptomatic, this may be best left alone. Nevertheless any such questionable area needs to be brought to the attention of the surgeon, to minimize the risk that extruded silicone could be overlooked at explantation and retained in the breast.

Often though, when extracapsular silicone results in formation of a granuloma adjacent to the implant, the MRI findings are more subtle. The composite signal of silicone gel with reactive granulomatous tissue can be difficult to distinguish from surrounding fat on FSE T2-weighted images, but may appear slightly hypointense relative to silicone within the implant (Fig. 8.5). When observed, this reduction in T2 signal is considered to be a reliable indicator of extracapsular rupture [18].

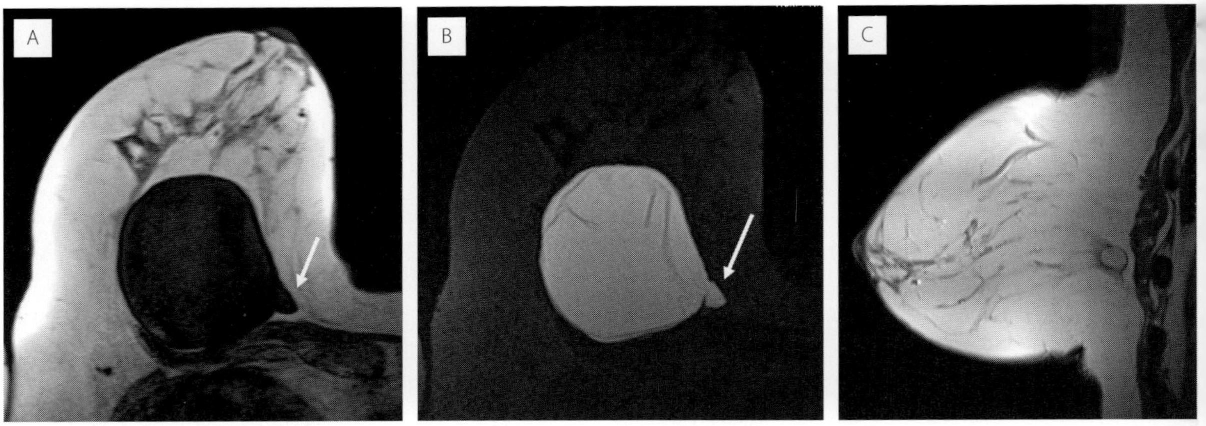

Fig. 8.4 Herniation versus extracapsular rupture: (A) Axial T1-weighted non-fat-suppressed and (B) silicone-only images show focal outpouching of silicone medially (arrows) together with noose, subcapsular line and falling-away signs of implant failure. (C) Circumscribed globular extension of silicone at medial margin of implant on sagittal FSE T2-weighted image. The findings, considered equivocal, were unchanged over a 3-year period. Explantation was not performed as patient was asymptomatic.

When MRI findings of extracapsular rupture are equivocal, TUS may be helpful to confirm extracapsular silicone with the "snowstorm" appearance considered pathognomonic.

While the anatomic detail offered by FSE T2-weighted images is ideal for demonstrating intracapsular rupture, extracapsular silicone can be overlooked because its signal can be indistinguishable from normal fat. Viewing either a fat-suppressed or silicone-suppressed T2-weighted IR sequence can be helpful, since granulomas then show brighter signal than fat, although distinction from normal fibroglandular tissue can be difficult. Accordingly, a water-suppressed T2-weighted IR sequence, in which only silicone is bright (so-called *silicone-only sequence*), is the key to overcoming these difficulties, and readily shows even small amounts of extracapsular silicone (Figs. 8.5–8.7). A potential pitfall of this sequence relates to incomplete water suppression, so that cysts or even normal small pleural effusions can mimic extracapsular silicone [18].

Extracapsular silicone can be overlooked on routine FSE T2-weighted sequences, but is readily seen on a water-suppressed IR T2-weighted "silicone-only" sequence.

Berg *et al.* found that the poor demonstration of extracapsular silicone on FSE T2-weighted images and failure to review the water-suppressed IR sequence were sources of error, even with expert interpretation [18]. Clearly then, sequence selection is important in designing a suitable implant failure protocol, together with a knowledge of which sequences yield the most helpful clues. The silicone-only sequence is an essential addition to FSE T2 and fat-suppressed T2 sequences to detect extracapsular silicone. Key signs of extracapsular rupture are given in Table 8.6 while Table 8.7 lists some of the pitfalls in interpretation.

If MRI signs of extracapsular silicone are equivocal, TUS can be helpful for confirmation, with the *snowstorm* appearance due to reverberation artifact considered pathognomonic, although there can also be acoustic shadowing [2]. Some walled-off silicone gel nodules appear as hypoechoic cystic lesions on US although usually with a distinctive surrounding *white noise* pattern [2]. Intra operative US can also be helpful to locate any areas of retained silicone at explantation which may otherwise be difficult to remove [19].

Complications in form-stable silicone implants

Form-stable implants like the McGhan Style 410 (Allergan, Irvine, CA, USA) and the Mentor MemoryGel (Mentor, Santa Barbara, CA, USA) are associated with low rates of capsular contracture and rupture rates of ~3% or less at 5–8 years on MRI-based follow-up [20–23]. Nevertheless, a study of the McGhan Style 410 implant suggested that MRI signs of rupture were the same as for third generation implants, with a linguine sign observed in one surgically confirmed case [20]. The authors suggested that

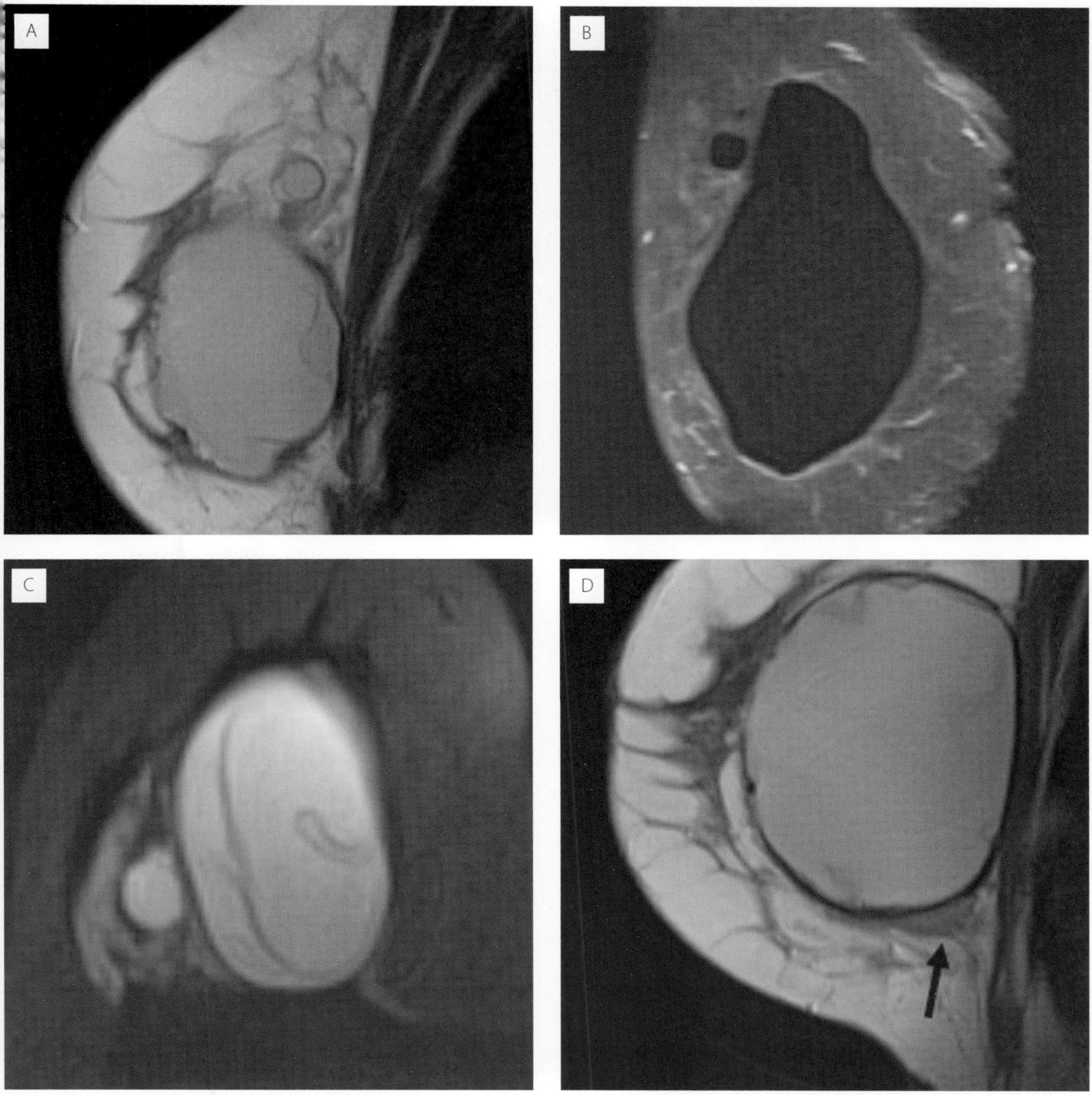

Fig. 8.5 **Extracapsular rupture:** (A) Sagittal FSE T2-weighted image shows wavy-line sign with defect in fibrous capsule superiorly and a globule of free silicone outside. (B) Coronal silicone-suppressed IR image confirms extracapsular silicone mass. (C) Axial silicone-only image shows globule laterally with extensive surrounding free silicone. (D) Sagittal FSE T2-weighted image of left breast in the same patient shows more subtle focal silicone beyond capsule at inferior margin of implant, with reduction in T2 signal compared to silicone contained within the implant (arrow). Extracapsular rupture at this site was also confirmed on silicone-only images.

this was possible because the gel is not a solid but an extremely cohesive liquid.

There are no standards to define whether or not a gel filler is highly cohesive enough to prevent distant gel migration beyond the fibrous capsule in normal circumstances. Extracapsular rupture and gel migration do occur in at least some so-called highly cohesive fourth generation implants, and even silicone lymphadenopathy has been documented [24–26].

With the most durable form-stable "Gummy Bear" implant types now in use, the usual imaging signs of implant rupture may not occur, because it

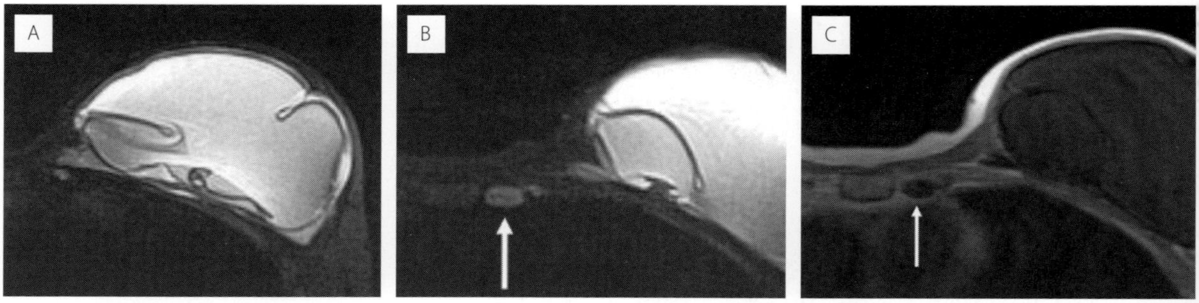

Fig. 8.6 **Extracapsular rupture:** (A) Axial silicone-only image shows intracapsular rupture with medial silicone extrusion and separate globule (arrow) on slightly caudad slice (B). Comparison with corresponding T1-weighted image (C) shows low-signal silicone lateral to sternum, probably in an internal mammary lymph node (arrow).

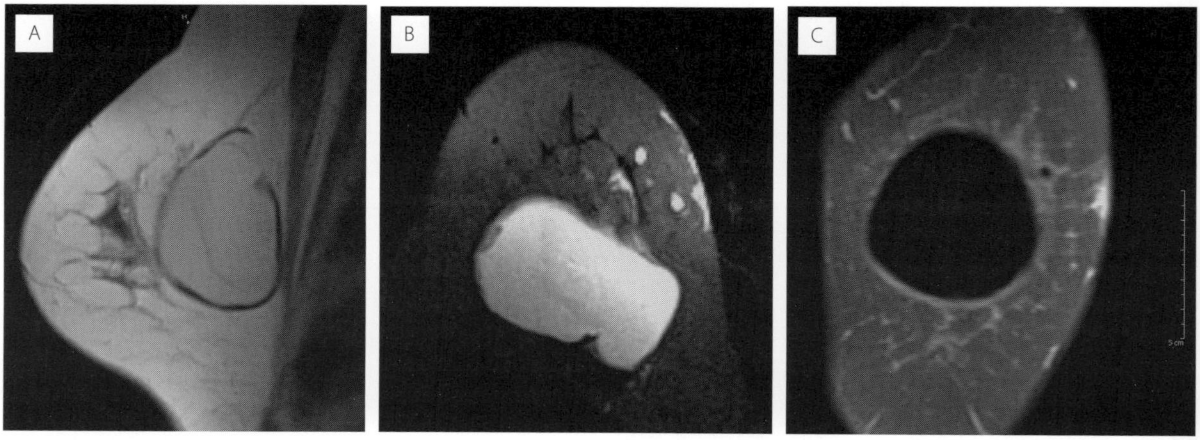

Fig. 8.7 **Extracapsular rupture:** A 63-year-old woman with silicone implants from early 1980s with recent history of acute pain and skin erythema laterally in left breast which subsided with residual nodularity. (A) Sagittal FSE T2-weighted image shows obvious capsular defect with silicone extending into surrounding fatty breast tissue. (B) Axial silicone-only sequence shows misshapen implant and silicone extending to skin due to gross extracapsular rupture, explaining clinical presentation. (C) Coronal post-contrast silicone-suppressed T1-weighted image shows persisting dermal enhancement consistent with granulomatous reaction.

Table 8.6 Signs of extracapsular rupture of silicone implant

Contour bulge with intact implant +/− evidence of focal capsular weakness = probably normal
Signs of intracapsular rupture combined with contour bulge = probable extracapsular rupture
Loss of T2 signal in extracapsular silicone relative to gel within implant = definite
Water-suppressed T2-weighted IR images showing hyperintense masses outside capsule = definite
Distinct foci of silicone signal within extracapsular mass = pathognomonic of silicone granuloma
Free silicone masses in adjacent breast tissue, with no previously ruptured implant = definite

Table 8.7 Pitfalls in MRI interpretation of silicone implant failure

Contour bulge from herniation of intact implant versus extracapsular silicone
Poor T2 FSE demonstration of extracapsular silicone – IR sequences required
Subtle tiny foci of silicone overlooked within granulomas – silicone suppression helps
Ghosting artifact from respiratory motion simulating subcapsular line sign
Cysts or pleural fluid failing to suppress mimicking silicone on water-suppressed T2-weighted IR
Complex radial folds confused with noose or wavy-line signs of intracapsular rupture

is hoped that the semi-solid gel may be unable to extrude outside the elastomer shell or fibrous capsule. Nevertheless, it is possible for such implants to undergo what is termed *gel fracture*, although this appears to be rare in vivo (Fig. 8.8).

Cancer incidence and detection in women with implants

The overall risk of breast malignancy in women with implants appears to be slightly lower than for the

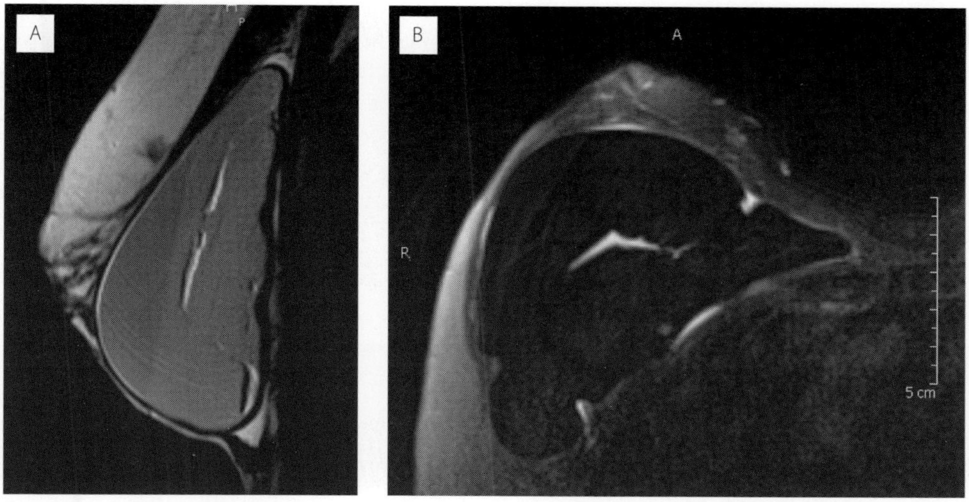

Fig. 8.8 Intrasubstance fracture of fifth generation implant: A 55-year-old woman with McGhan Style 510 Dual Gel implant inserted 9 months earlier following subcutaneous mastectomy for DCIS. This implant features two fused gel components, with the more solid anterior portion designed to improve contouring of the areolar region. (A) Sagittal FSE T2-weighted image shows normal interface between anterior (slightly lower signal) and posterior components. A curvilinear cleft of water signal extends vertically through the posterior component. (B) Axial T2-weighted SPAIR image shows coronal orientation of cleft. On serial images water signal tracked to implant surface in continuity with normal subcapsular fluid. Patient was asymptomatic with no history of trauma.

general population [27]. There have been isolated reports of primary breast lymphoma arising in the fibrous capsule of both silicone and saline implants, presenting as a mass or a periprosthetic fluid collection at a mean of 8 years after insertion [28]. While a true association between ALCL probably exists, the absolute risk of this occurring is exceedingly low [29]. In fact, to put this in perspective, a woman with implants is much more likely to develop a non-specific breast cancer by chance than an implant-associated ALCL [30]. In a series of 53 cases of non-Hodgkin's lymphomas in the breast, only 1 was ALCL presenting 6 years after cosmetic silicone implantation [28]. There have also been anecdotal reports of multifocal ILC associated with breast implants.

While there are no other data to suggest that implants are associated with an increased risk of developing breast cancer, implants do obscure the adjacent parenchyma on XRM, with the potential for a missed cancer diagnosis. As would be expected, this is more problematic with subglandular than with subpectoral implants. In one study, even when Eklund views were used to displace breast tissue away from the implant, there was still an almost 40% decrease in visualized parenchyma for subglandular implants, while the decrease was less than 10% for subpectoral implants [31]. The proportion of adequately visualized tissue is reduced still further in the presence of fibrous contracture [32].

One recent study, over a period when the use of Eklund views was standard practice, analyzed XRM screening data from over 1 000 000 women in the USA, of which over 10 500 had implants (a prevalence of ~1%). Miglioretti *et al.* concluded that XRM screening missed 55% of cancers in women with implants compared with 33% in similarly aged women without breast augmentation [33]. A further concern is that the absorbed radiation dose from XRM is at least doubled with implant studies, and can become unacceptably high unless special measures are taken [34]. Where possible, optimal cancer screening in women with implants should include contrast-enhanced breast MRI. A pitfall with MRI is the potential for a false-positive cancer diagnosis due to enhancing silicone granulomas (Fig. 8.9 and Plate 6).

Tissue breast reconstructive surgery

Breast reconstruction using implants may be *immediate* (performed at the time of mastectomy), or *delayed* using tissue-expander devices to gradually enlarge a cavity over several months. For immediate breast reconstruction, implants are usually avoided if post-mastectomy RT is required due to a high rate of complications, including significant capsular contracture [35, 36].

A range of reconstructive techniques using autologous tissue are available, including TRAM, DIEP and latissimus dorsi flaps. Lower abdominal flaps can only be raised once, but can be used to reconstruct both breasts. Prior to such a reconstruction therefore, MRI has a useful role in excluding contralateral cancer, allowing for the possibility of a bilateral procedure.

A *pedicled TRAM flap* involves harvesting of the entire rectus abdominis muscle and overlying fat and skin, which is tunnelled through to the chest with its own blood supply intact. This has the advantage that specialist microsurgical skills are not required, while the downsides are the considerable donor site trauma (often requiring a mesh repair to reduce the risk of a hernia) and a higher risk of fat necrosis in the reconstructed breast. In a *free TRAM flap*, the graft is completely separated and then reattached to the chest wall, so microvascular surgical expertise is needed. Advantages are that only the lower third of the rectus muscle is required, which reduces donor site

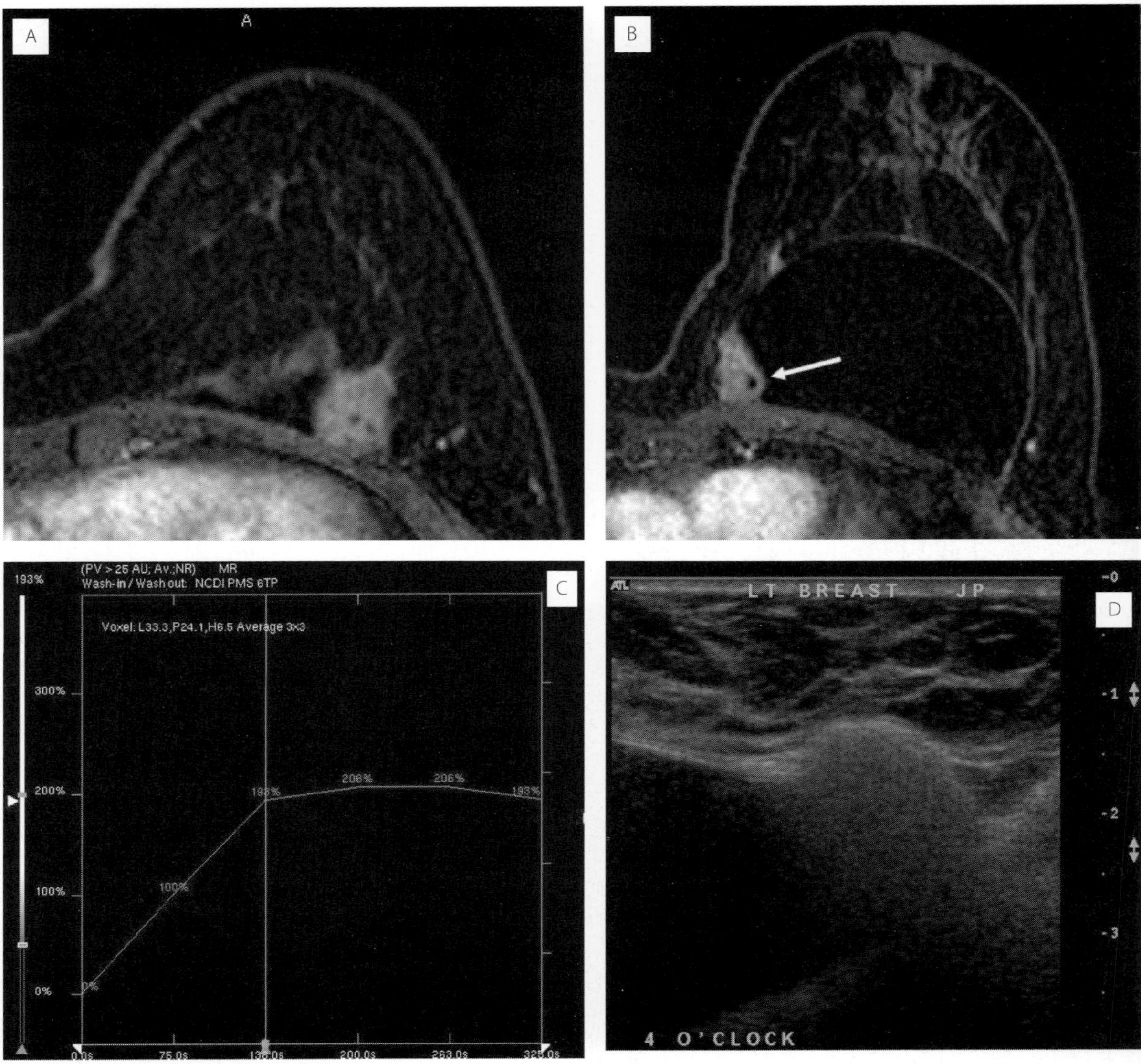

Fig. 8.9 Enhancing silicone granulomas: A 62-year-old asymptomatic women with silicone implants from late 1970s and new findings in left breast since previous normal screening MRI. Early post-contrast axial T1-weighted images (A) showing enhancing mass adjacent to implant at 4:00 and (B) second mass at 9:00. Note dark spot in 9:00 mass consistent with silicone (arrow). (C) Both lesions showed moderate early-phase and late-phase plateau (type 2 kinetic curves). On TUS (D) both masses showed a classical "snowstorm" sign. Silicone granulomas were confirmed at both sites by 14-gauge CNB and appearances remained stable on MRI follow-up. The patient decided against explantation until 3 years later when further MRI revealed gross extracapsular leakage of the contralateral implant. See also Plate 6.

morbidity, [3] and a superior cosmetic result can usually be achieved.

In a DIEP flap, only the branches of the deep inferior epigastric vessels (which perforate the muscle to supply the overlying adipose tissue and the skin) are dissected free and harvested. Since no rectus muscle or fascia is used, there is minimal donor site trauma, [3] and a much lower risk of subsequent hernia.

On MRI, the often triangular-shaped vascular pedicle and muscle of a TRAM flap are seen centrally adjacent to the chest wall and enhance as a normal finding (Fig. 8.10). Tumor recurrence in a reconstructed breast can be difficult to detect clinically and on conventional imaging, and MRI can be helpful for clarification (Plate 7). Caution is needed to avoid mistaking enhancing fat necrosis for recurrence.

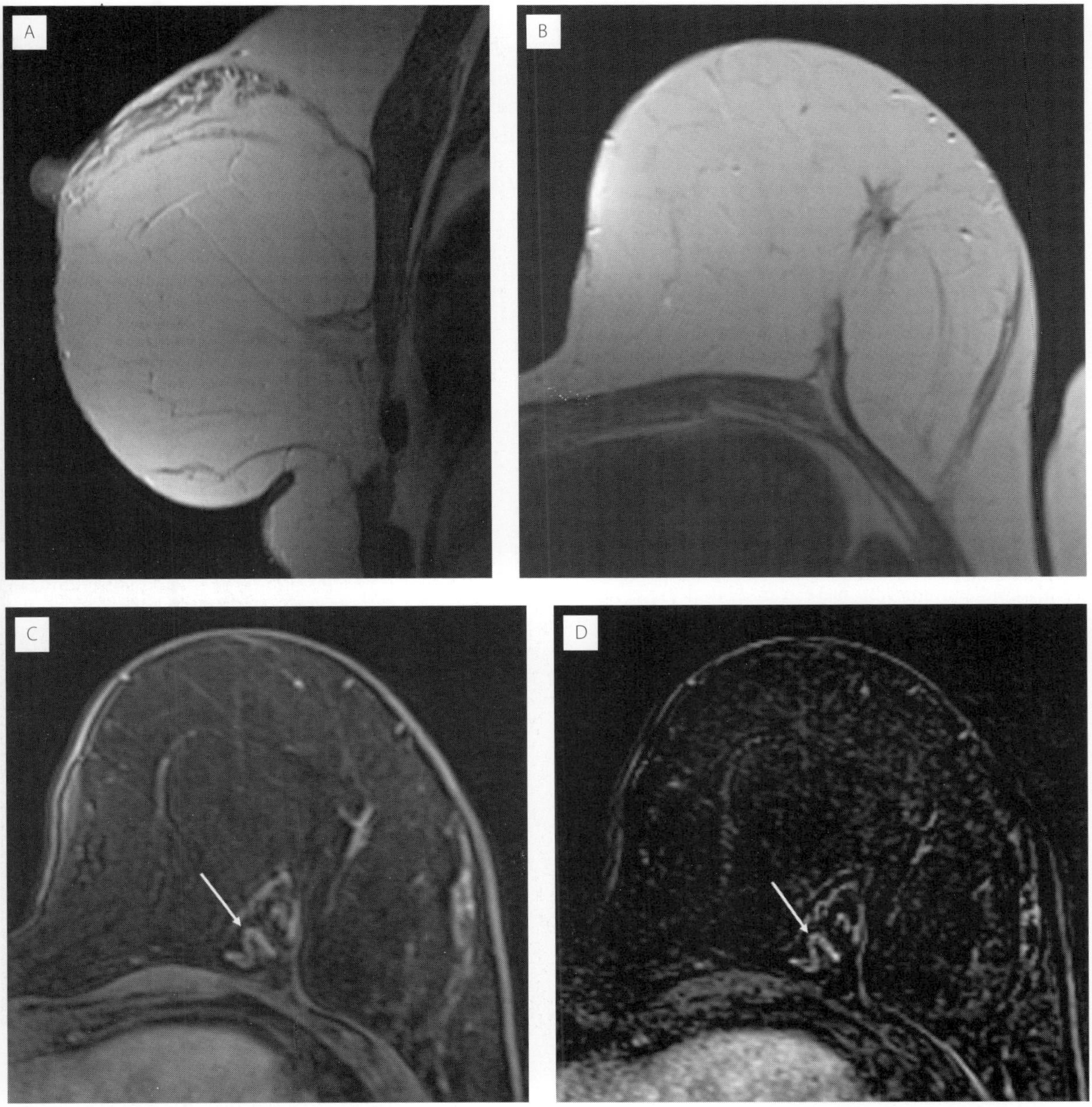

Fig. 8.10 Autologous flap reconstruction: (A) Sagittal and (B) axial FSE T2-weighted images showing left autologous flap reconstruction. Triangular structure close to chest wall represents the vascular pedicle with enhancing vessel seen on (C) axial T1-weighted and (D) subtracted images (arrows). See also plate 7 for example of recurrence in a TRAM flap.

Augmentation by direct injection procedures

Liquid paraffin was used for augmentation worldwide in the early twentieth century but was largely abandoned due to the disastrous complications (granulomas, tissue necrosis, fistulae, pulmonary emboli) [1]. Paraffinomas develop as a delayed complication from 2 years to several decades later, presenting as hard masses which mimic cancer. The procedure continues to be performed by backstreet practitioners in some Asian countries because it is cheap, quick and easy to perform with an immediate, acceptable cosmetic result. A recent report included breast MRI findings in 3 of 16 patients with a history of paraffin augmentation [37]. Recent paraffin injections showed low T1 signal with high signal on T2, even with fat suppression. In a single patient with bilateral hard masses due to injections 30 years before, these showed intermediate signal on T1, low signal on T2 and did not enhance.

After silicone implants were introduced, the practice of direct injection of free silicone into the breasts was discontinued in most western countries, but still persists in some parts of the world. In the USA, direct injection of silicone continues to be performed illicitly, particularly among transsexual males, with injections sometimes administered to multiple recipients at "pumping parties." Consequently, silicone pulmonary embolism also continues to be reported as a potentially fatal complication [38, 39]. In a recent review of 44 affected patients, 25 were transsexual males, with an overall mortality rate of 25% (11/44) [38].

Following direct injection of either silicone or paraffin, clinical, mammographic and sonographic assessment are all severely compromised, and MRI appears to be the method of choice for cancer diagnosis [40]. Using MRI over a 10-year period, Youk and colleagues found 6 cancers in 62 women with previous direct injections, of which 5/6 had palpable lumps [40].

Polyacrylamide hydrogel is a stable, non-toxic, non-resorbable gel, widely used in ophthalmic surgery and in the pharmaceutical, cosmetic and other industries. Since 1997, polyacrylamide gel has been increasingly used for augmentation in the Middle East, Eastern Europe, South America, China and parts of Asia [41, 42]. As a direct injection technique is used, the procedure can be performed in a clinic setting under local anesthesia, contributing to its popularity.

Unfortunately, polyacrylamide gel augmentation has been associated with a range of complications including gel migration, and infection. Lui *et al.* have reported on the MRI appearances in 17 women, in which 5 of 34 breasts were complicated by infection, with one resulting in mastectomy [41]. Uncomplicated polyacrylamide gel augmentations on MRI resemble a subglandular implant, and can be mistaken as such if the correct history is not obtained.

MULTIPLE CHOICE QUESTIONS

8.1 Answer true or false to the following statements

- A. More than 20% of 1970–80s second generation silicone implants had failed after 12 years.
- B. Symptoms of pain, hardening and altered shape are usually due to contained rupture.
- C. Clinically painful lumps can occur due to leakage of silicone outside the fibrous capsule.
- D. Augmentation by direct injection of silicone gel can be life-threatening due to silicone emboli.
- E. On XRM subpectoral implants obscure less parenchyma than do subglandular implants.

8.2 Answer true or false to the following statements

- A. The noose sign is positive if silicone signal is seen between the leaves of a radial fold.
- B. The presence of complex radial folds strongly indicates silicone implant failure.
- C. The subcapsular, wavy-line or falling-away sign strongly indicates fibrous contracture.
- D. Water-suppressed T2-weighted IR images help to detect extracapsular silicone spread.
- E. Screening XRM is less sensitive in women who have silicone breast implants.

See page 189 for answers.

References

1. Bondurant S, Ernster V, Herdman R, editors. *Safety of Silicone Breast Implants*. Washington, National Academy Press, 2000.
2. Caskey CI, Berg WA, Hamper UM, *et al.* Imaging spectrum of extracapsular silicone: correlation of US, MR imaging, mammographic and histopathologic findings. *RadioGraphics* 1999; **19**: S39–51.
3. Klimberg VS. *Atlas of Breast Surgical Techniques*. Philadelphia, PA, Saunders, Elsevier, 2010.
4. Shellock, F. *Reference Manual for Magnetic Resonance Safety, Implants and Devices: 2007 Edition*. Los Angeles, CA, Biomedical Research Publishing Group, 2007.
5. Zegzula HD, Lee WP. Infusion port dislodgment of bilateral

breast tissue expanders after MRI. *Ann Plast Surg* 2001; **46**: 46–8.

6. Duffy FJ, May JW. Tissue expanders and magnetic resonance imaging: the "hot" breast implant. *Ann Plast Surg* 1995; **5**: 647–9.
7. Vazquez G, Pellon A. Polyurethane-coated silicone gel breast implants used for 18 years. *Aesthetic Plast Surg* 2007; **31**: 330–6.
8. Holmich LR, Friis S, Fryzek JP, *et al.* Incidence of silicone breast implant rupture. *Arch Surg* 2003; **138**: 801–6.
9. Tebbetts, J. Dual plane breast augmentation: optimizing implant-soft-tissue relationships in a wide range of breast types. *Plast Reconstr Surg* 2001; **107**: 1255–72.
10. Spear SL, Carter ME, Ganz JC. The correction of capsular contracture by conversion to "dual-plane" positioning: technique and outcomes. *Plast Reconstr Surg* 2003; **112**: 456–66.
11. Tebbetts J. Failure of a "highly cohesive implant": what does it really mean? *Plast Reconstr Surg* 2009; **124**: 323–5.
12. Morgan DE, Kenney PJ, Meeks MC, *et al.* MR imaging of breast implants and their complications. *AJR Am J Roentgenol* 1996; **167**: 1271–5.
13. Soo MS, Kornguth PJ, Walsh R, *et al.* Complex radial folds versus subtle signs of intracapsular rupture of breast implants: MR findings with surgical correlation. *AJR Am J Roentgenol* 1996; **166**: 1421–7.
14. Holmich LR, Vejborg I, Conrad C, *et al.* The diagnosis of breast implant rupture: MRI findings compared with findings at explantation. *Eur J Radiol* 2005; **53**: 213–25.
15. Berg WA, Caskey CI, Hamper UM, *et al.* Single- and double-lumen silicone breast implant integrity: prospective evaluation of MR and US criteria. *Radiology* 1995; **197**: 45–52.
16. Brown SL, Silverman BG, Berg WA. Rupture of silicone-gel breast implants: causes, sequelae, and diagnosis. *Lancet* 1997; **350**: 1531–7.
17. Brown SL, Middleton MS, Berg WA, *et al.* Prevalence of rupture of silicone gel breast implants revealed on MR imaging in a population of women in Birmingham, Alabama. *AJR Am J Roentgenol* 2000; **175**: 1057–64.
18. Berg WA, Nguyen TK, Middleton MS, *et al.* MR imaging of extracapsular silicone from breast implants: diagnostic pitfalls. *AJR Am J Roentgenol* 2002; **178**: 465–72.
19. Conant EF, Forsberg F, Moore JH, *et al.* Surgical removal of ruptured breast implants: the use of intraoperative sonography in localizing free silicone. *AJR Am J Roentgenol* 1994; **165**: 1378–9.
20. Heden P, Bone B, Murphy DK, *et al.* Style 410 cohesive silicone breast implants: safety and effectiveness at 5 to 9 years after implantation. *Plast Reconstr Surg* 2006; **118**: 1281–7.
21. Stevens W, Pacella S, Gear A, *et al.* Clinical experience with a fourth-generation textured silicone gel breast implant: a review of 1012 Mentor MemoryGel breast implants. *Aesthetic Surg J* 2008; **28**: 642–7.
22. Heden P, Bronz G, Elberg JJ, *et al.* Long-term safety and effectiveness of Style 410 highly cohesive silicone breast implants. *Aesthetic Plast Surg* 2009; **33**: 430–6.
23. Cunningham B, McCue J. Safety and effectiveness of Mentor's MemoryGel implants at 6 years. *Aesthetic Plast Surg* 2009; **33**: 440–4.
24. Shaaban H, Jmor S, Alvi R. Leakage and silicone lymphadenopathy with cohesive gel implants. *Br J Plast Surg* 2003; **56**: 518–19.
25. Lahiri A, Waters R. Locoregional silicone spread after high cohesive gel silicone implant rupture. *J Plast Reconstr Aesthetic Surg* 2006; **59**: 885–6.
26. Kaufman GJ, Sakr RA, Inguenault C, *et al.* Silicone migration to the contralateral axillary lymph nodes and breast after highly cohesive silicone gel implant failure: a case report. *Cases J* 2009; **2**: 6420.
27. McLaughlin JK, Lipworth L, Fryzek JP, *et al.* Long-term cancer risk among Swedish women with cosmetic breast implants: an update of a nationwide study. *J Natl Cancer Inst* 2006; **98**: 557–60.
28. Gualco G, Bacchi CE. B-cell and T-cell lymphomas of the breast: clinical pathologic features of 53 cases. *Int J Surg Pathol* 2008; **16**: 407–13.
29. Travis LB, Hill D, Dores GM, *et al.* Cumulative absolute breast cancer risk for young women treated for Hodgkin lymphoma. *J Natl Cancer Inst* 2005; **97**: 1428–37.
30. de Jong D, Vasmel WLE, de Boer JP, *et al.* Anaplastic large-cell lymphoma in women with breast implants. *JAMA* 2008; **300**: 2030–5.
31. Silverstein MJ, Handel N, Gamagami P, *et al.* Mammographic measurements before and after augmentation mammaplasty. *Plast Reconstr Surg* 1989; **86**: 1126–30.
32. Handel N, Silverstein MJ, Gamagami P, *et al.* Factors affecting mammographic visualization of the breast after augmentation mammaplasty. *JAMA* 1992; **268**: 1913–17.
33. Miglioretti DL, Rutter CM, Geller BM, *et al.* Effect of breast augmentation on the accuracy of mammography and cancer characteristics. *JAMA* 2004; **291**: 442–50.
34. Smathers SL, Boone JM, Lee LJ, *et al.* Radiation dose reduction for augmentation mammography. *AJR Am J Roentgenol* 2007; **188**: 1414–21.

35. Buchholz TA, Lehman CD, Harris JR, *et al.* Statement of the science concerning locoregional treatments after preoperative chemotherapy for breast cancer: a National Cancer Institute Conference. *J Clin Oncol* 2008; **26**: 791–7.
36. Behranwala KA, Dua RS, Ross GM, *et al.* The influence of RT on capsule formation and aesthetic outcome after immediate breast reconstruction using biodimensional anatomic expander implants. *J Plast Reconstr Aesthetic Surg* 2006; **59**: 1043–51.
37. Erguvan-Dogan B, Yang WT. Direct injection of paraffin into the breast: mammographic, sonographic, and MRI features of early complications. *AJR Am J Roentgenol* 2006; **186**: 888–94.
38. Restrepo CS, Artunduaga M, Carrillo JA, *et al.* Silicone pulmonary embolism: report of 10 cases and review of the literature. *J Comput Assist Tomogr* 2009; **33**: 233–7.
39. Schmid A, Tzur A, Leshko L, *et al.* Silicone embolism syndrome. *Chest* 2005; **127**: 2276–81.
40. Youk JH, Son EJ, Kim E-K, *et al.* Diagnosis of breast cancer at dynamic MRI in patients with breast augmentation by paraffin or silicone injection. *Clin Radiol* 2009; **64**: 1175–80.
41. Lui CY, Ho CM, Lu PP, *et al.* Evaluation of MRI findings after polyacrylamide gel injection for breast augmentation. *AJR Am J Roentgenol* 2008; **191**: 677–88.
42. Teo SY, Wang SC. Radiologic features of polyacrylamide gel mammoplasty. *AJR Am J Roentgenol* 2008; **191**: W89–95.

Answers to multiple choice questions

Chapter 1

1.1	A. T	B. F	C. T	D. T	E. F
1.2	A. F	B. F	C. F	D. F	E. T

Chapter 2

2.1	A. T	B. F	C. F	D. T	E. F
2.2	A. T	B. T	C. F	D. T	E. T

Chapter 3

3.1	A. T	B. T	C. F	D. F	E. T
3.2	A. F	B. F	C. F	D. T	E. T

Chapter 4

4.1	A. T	B. T	C. F	D. F	E. F
4.2	A. F	B. F	C. F	D. T	E. F

Chapter 5

5.1	A. F	B. T	C. T	D. T	E. F
5.2	A. F	B. F	C. T	D. F	E. T

Chapter 6

6.1	A. F	B. T	C. T	D. F	E. T
6.2	A. F	B. F	C. T	D. F	E. F

Chapter 7

7.1	A. T	B. F	C. T	D. T	E. T
7.2	A. F	B. T	C. F	D. T	E. F

Chapter 8

8.1	A. T	B. F	C. T	D. T	E. T
8.2	A. T	B. F	C. F	D. T	E. T

Appendix 1: Nephrogenic systemic fibrosis

In the last decade, a rare but severe and sometimes fatal adverse effect of gadolinium chelates has emerged in the form of a new disease, known as nephrogenic systemic fibrosis (NSF). Initially thought to be confined to the skin, the condition was at first termed nephrogenic fibrosing dermatopathy, and was originally described in 15 patients with either acute or severe chronic renal failure in 2000 [1]. The designation NSF is preferred because it has become apparent that the fibrosing process can involve a wide variety of tissues in multiple systems (please see table below). That gadolinium was the "trigger" for NSF was first proposed by Grobner in 2006, who observed that five patients with end-stage renal failure had become symptomatic 2–4 weeks after receiving an injection of contrast for an MRI scan [2].

In a 2008 analysis of 190 cases of biopsy-proven NSF identified worldwide, 157 (82%) were related to gadodiamide (Omniscan, GE Healthcare, Chalfont St. Giles, UK) [3]. Gadopentetate (Magnevist, Bayer Schering Pharma, AG, Berlin, Germany) and gadoversetamide (Optimark, Covidien, St. Louis, USA) have also both been implicated in a relatively small number of cases. More recent data on over 600 NSF cases have shown an incidence of almost 30/million doses for Omniscan but < 10 cases/million doses for Magnevist and Optimark. To date, very few if any cases have been substantiated from sole use of either gadobenate (MultiHance, Bracco Diagnostics, Milan, Italy) or gadoteridol (ProHance, Bracco Diagnostics, Milan, Italy) despite their widespread use.

Prevention of NSF relies on identifying those at risk. In the USA, the FDA has determined that prior to receiving any gadolinium chelate, all patients should be screened for renal insufficiency with a GFR of less than 30 mL/min/1.73m^2 to be taken as a contraindication. If it is decided that a gadolinium-enhanced study cannot be avoided in an at-risk patient, a contrast agent other than Omniscan, Magnevist or Optimark is selected at a dose not exceeding the standard of 0.1 mmol/kg and with dialysis often performed immediately afterwards [4].

Sites of involvement and clinical manifestations of NSF

Skin – itching, swelling, tightening, thickening, transient alopecia, persistent brawny induration, hyperpigmentation, maculopapular rash
Typically affects distal extremities +/– trunk, spares face
GI – nausea, vomiting, abdominal pain, diarrhea
Sclera – yellow plaques
MSK – joint stiffness, contractures, bone pain, myalgia, muscle weakness
Liver
Lungs and pleura
Heart muscle and pericardium
Dura, nerves
Testes
Breast (single case report)

Appendix 2: Sensitivity and specificity

A number of useful statistics can be derived from a matrix table which shows the performance of a diagnostic test compared to a defined reference or "gold" standard.

	Disease present	Disease absent
+ve test	True positive (TP)	False positive (FP)
−ve test	False negative (FN)	True negative (TN)

Total subjects tested = TP + FN + FP + TN
Number of subjects with disease = TP + FN
Number of subjects without disease = TN + FP

Sensitivity = percentage correctly identified by the test = TP / (TP + FN)
Specificity = TN / (TN + FP)
PPV = TP / (TP + FP)
NPV = TN / (TN + FN)
Accuracy = percentage of correct results in all tests = (TP + TN) / TOTAL

Note that the prevalence of the target disease in the study population (or pre-test probability) has a significant effect on both PPV and NPV. For example, the PPV of an abnormal MRI finding is greater in a high-risk population than it is in the general population at average risk [5].

Appendix 3: TNM classification

The following tables are used with the permission of the American Joint Committee on Cancer (AJCC), Chicago, Illinois. The original source for this material is the *AJCC Cancer Staging Manual*, Seventh Edition (2010) published by Springer Science and Business Media LLC, www.springerlink.com.

Primary tumor (T)

The T classification of the primary tumor is the same regardless of whether it is based on clinical or pathologic criteria, or both. Size should be measured to the nearest millimeter. If the tumor size is slightly less than or greater than a cutoff for a given T classification, it is recommended that the size be rounded to the millimeter reading that is closest to the cutoff. For example, a reported size of 1.1 mm is reported as 1 mm, or a size of 2.01 cm is reported as 2.0 cm. Designation should be made with the subscript "c" or "p" modifier to indicate whether the T classification was determined by clinical (physical examination or radiologic) or pathologic measurements, respectively. In general, pathologic determination should take precedence over clinical determination of T size.

TX	Primary tumor cannot be assessed
T0	No evidence of primary tumor
Tis	Carcinoma in situ
Tis (DCIS)	Ductal carcinoma in situ
Tis (LCIS)	Lobular carcinoma in situ
Tis (Paget's)	Paget's disease of the nipple NOT associated with invasive carcinoma and/or carcinoma in situ (DCIS and/or LCIS) in the underlying breast parenchyma. Carcinomas in the breast parenchyma associated with Paget's disease are categorized based on the size and characteristics of the parenchymal disease, although the presence of Paget's disease should still be noted
T1	Tumor ≤ 20 mm in greatest dimension
T1mi	Tumor ≤ 1 mm in greatest dimension
T1a	Tumor > 1 mm but ≤ 5 mm in greatest dimension
T1b	Tumor > 5 mm but ≤ 10 mm in greatest dimension
T1c	Tumor > 10 mm but ≤ 20 mm in greatest dimension
T2	Tumor > 20 mm but ≤ 50 mm in greatest dimension
T3	Tumor > 50 mm in greatest dimension
T4	Tumor of any size with direct extension to the chest wall and/or to the skin (ulceration or skin nodules)

Note: Invasion of the dermis alone does not qualify as T4.

T4a	Extension to the chest wall, not including only pectoralis muscle adherence/invasion
T4b	Ulceration and/or ipsilateral satellite nodules and/or edema (including peau d'orange) of the skin, which do not meet the criteria for inflammatory carcinoma
T4c	Both T4a and T4b
T4d	Inflammatory carcinoma

Regional lymph nodes (N)	
Clinical	
NX	Regional lymph nodes cannot be assessed (e.g., previously removed)
N0	No regional lymph node metastases
N1	Metastases to movable ipsilateral level I, II axillary lymph node(s)
N2	Metastases in ipsilateral level I, II axillary lymph nodes that are clinically fixed or matted; or in clinically detected* ipsilateral internal mammary nodes in the absence of clinically evident axillary lymph node metastases
N2a	Metastases in ipsilateral level I, II axillary lymph nodes fixed to one another (matted) or to other structures
N2b	Metastases only in clinically detected* ipsilateral internal mammary nodes and in the absence of clinically evident axillary lymph node metastases
N3	Metastases in ipsilateral infraclavicular (level III axillary) lymph node(s) with or without level I, II axillary lymph node involvement; or in clinically detected* ipsilateral internal mammary lymph node(s) with clinically evident level I, II axillary lymph node metastases; or metastases in ipsilateral supraclavicular lymph node(s) with or without axillary or internal mammary lymph node involvement
N3a	Metastases in ipsilateral infraclavicular lymph node(s)
N3b	Metastases in ipsilateral internal mammary lymph node(s) and axillary lymph node(s)
N3c	Metastases in ipsilateral supraclavicular lymph node(s)

*Note: Clinically detected is defined as detected by imaging studies (excluding lymphoscintigraphy) or by clinical examination and having characteristics highly suspicious for malignancy or a presumed pathologic macrometastasis based on fine needle aspiration biopsy with cytologic examination. Confirmation of clinically detected metastatic disease by fine needle aspiration without excision biopsy is designated with an (f) suffix, for example, cN3a(f). Excisional biopsy of a lymph node or biopsy of a sentinel node, in the absence of assignment of a pT, is classified as a clinical N, for example, cN1. Information regarding the confirmation of the nodal status will be designated in site-specific factors as clinical, fine needle aspiration, core biopsy, or sentinel lymph node biopsy. Pathologic classification (pN) is used for excision or sentinel lymph node biopsy only in conjunction with a pathologic T assignment.

Regional lymph nodes (N)	
Pathologic (pN)*	
pNX	Regional lymph nodes cannot be assessed (e.g., previously removed, or not removed for pathologic study)
pN0	No regional lymph node metastasis identified histologically

Note: Isolated tumor cell clusters (ITC) are defined as small clusters of cells not greater than 0.2 mm, or single tumor cells, or a cluster of fewer than 200 cells in a single histologic cross-section. ITCs may be detected by routine histology or by immunohistochemical (IHC) methods. Nodes containing only ITCs are excluded from the total positive node count for purposes of N classification but should be included in the total number of nodes evaluated.

pN0(i–)	No regional lymph node metastases histologically, negative IHC
pN0(i+)	Malignant cells in regional lymph node(s) no greater than 0.2 mm (detected by H&E or IHC including ITC)
pN0(mol–)	No regional lymph node metastases histologically, negative molecular findings (RT-PCR)
pN0(mol+)	Positive molecular findings (RT-PCR)** but no regional lymph node metastases detected by histology or IHC
pN1	Micrometastases; or metastases in 1–3 axillary lymph nodes; and/or in internal mammary nodes with metastases detected by sentinel lymph node biopsy but not clinically detected***
pN1mi	Micrometastases (greater than 0.2 mm and/or more than 200 cells, but none greater than 2.0 mm)
pN1a	Metastases in 1–3 axillary lymph nodes, at least one metastasis greater than 2.0 mm

Regional lymph nodes (N) (*continued*)	
Pathologic (pN)*	
pN1b	Metastases in internal mammary nodes with micrometastases or macrometastases detected by sentinel lymph node biopsy but not clinically detected***
pN1c	Metastases in 1–3 axillary lymph nodes and in internal mammary lymph nodes with micrometastases or macrometastases detected by sentinel lymph node biopsy but not clinically detected
pN2	Metastases in 4–9 axillary lymph nodes; or in clinically detected**** internal mammary lymph nodes in the absence of axillary lymph node metastases
pN2a	Metastases in 4–9 axillary lymph nodes (at least one tumor deposit greater than 2.0 mm)
pN2b	Metastases in clinically detected**** internal mammary lymph nodes in the absence of axillary lymph node metastases
pN3	Metastases in ten or more axillary lymph nodes; or in infraclavicular (level III axillary) lymph nodes; or in clinically detected**** ipsilateral internal mammary lymph nodes in the presence of one or more positive level I, II axillary lymph nodes; or in more than three axillary lymph nodes and in internal mammary lymph nodes with micrometastases or macrometastases detected by sentinel lymph node biopsy but not clinically detected*** ; or in ipsilateral supraclavicular lymph nodes
pN3a	Metastases in ten or more axillary lymph nodes (at least one tumor deposit greater than 2.0 mm); or metastases to the infraclavicular (level III axillary lymph) nodes
pN3b	Metastases in clinically detected**** ipsilateral internal mammary lymph nodes in the presence of one or more positive axillary lymph nodes; or in more than three axillary lymph nodes and in internal mammary lymph nodes with micrometastases or macrometastases detected by sentinel lymph node biopsy but not clinically detected***
pN3c	Metastases in ipsilateral supraclavicular lymph nodes

Notes:

*Classification is based on axillary lymph node dissection with or without sentinel lymph node biopsy. Classification based solely on sentinel lymph node biopsy without subsequent axillary lymph node dissection is designated (sn) for "sentinel node," for example, pN0(sn).

**RT-PCR: reverse transcriptase/polymerase chain reaction.

***"Not clinically detected" is defined as not detected by imaging studies (excluding lymphoscintigraphy) or not detected by clinical examination.

****"Clinically detected" is defined as detected by imaging studies (excluding lymphoscintigraphy) or by clinical examination and having characteristics highly suspicious for malignancy or a presumed pathologic macrometastasis based on fine needle aspiration biopsy with cytologic examination.

Distant metastases (M)	
M0	No clinical or radiographic evidence of distant metastases
cM0(i+)	No clinical or radiographic evidence of distant metastases, but deposits of molecularly or microscopically detected tumor cells in circulating blood, bone marrow, or other nonregional nodal tissue that are no larger than 0.2 mm in a patient without symptoms or signs of metastases
M1	Distant detectable metastases as determined by classic clinical and radiographic means and/or histologically proven larger than 0.2 mm

Anatomic Stage / Prognostic Groups			
Stage 0	Tis	N0	M0
Stage IA	T1*	N0	M0
Stage IB	T0	N1mi	M0
	T1*	N1mi	M0
Stage IIA	T0	N1**	M0
	T1*	N1**	M0
	T2	N0	M0
Stage IIB	T2	N1	M0
	T3	N0	M0
Stage IIIA	T0	N2	M0
	T1*	N2	M0
	T2	N2	M0
	T3	N1	M0
	T3	N2	M0
Stage IIIB	T4	N0	M0
	T4	N1	M0
	T4	N2	M0
Stage IIIC	Any T	N3	M0
Stage IV	Any T	Any N	M1

Notes:

*T1 includes T1mi.

**T0 and T1 tumors with nodal micrometastases only are excluded from Stage IIA and are classified Stage IB.

M0 includes M0(i+).

The designation pM0 is not valid; any M0 should be clinical.

If a patient presents with M1 prior to neoadjuvant systemic therapy, the stage is considered Stage IV and remains Stage IV regardless of response to neoadjuvant therapy.

Stage designation may be changed if postsurgical imaging studies reveal the presence of distant metastases, provided that the studies are carried out within 4 months of diagnosis in the absence of disease progression and provided that the patient has not received neoadjuvant therapy.

Postneoadjuvant therapy is designated with "yc" or "yp" prefix. Of note, no stage group is assigned if there is a complete pathologic response (CR) to neoadjuvant therapy, for example, ypT0ypN0cM0.

Appendix 4: Overview of surgical procedures

Traditional types of mastectomy

Radical mastectomy (Halsted procedure)

Now rarely performed, radical mastectomy entails removal of the whole breast, the pectoralis major and minor muscles and the entire axillary contents *en bloc*, including the apical (level III) axillary lymph nodes.

Modified radical mastectomy

This procedure is now also uncommon but may be indicated for some very large tumors with palpable axillary nodes or inflammatory breast cancers. The whole breast is removed together with the underlying pectoral fascia. This preserves pectoral muscles and some skin, but the NAC and surrounding skin is excised, together with lymph nodes at least from the lower axilla (level I and II nodes) in an *en bloc* dissection.

Simple mastectomy (total mastectomy)

This is the standard procedure for EBC when breast conservation is not possible. Simple mastectomy is appropriate for large tumors, those with extensive DCIS or where there is skin or nipple involvement. All apparent mammary tissue is removed with the pectoral fascia, the NAC and a variable amount of adjacent skin. The axilla is not dissected unless indicated based on a known positive node or after SLNB. Simple mastectomy is the usual procedure for completion mastectomy after repeatedly positive margins in attempting BCT, or after failure of BCT due to locoregional recurrence. Simple mastectomy is also the standard for prophylactic risk-reducing surgery, because it is the most effective technique for removing as much potential tumor-bearing tissue as possible.

Modern variants of simple mastectomy

Skin-sparing mastectomy

In skin-sparing mastectomy, most of the breast tissue is removed together with the NAC and often any biopsy scar, but the remaining skin is preserved to allow for immediate breast reconstruction, either with an implant or with autologous tissue (TRAM flap or latissimus dorsi flap). Where used for cancer treatment, reported recurrence rates for skin-sparing mastectomy are similar to standard mastectomy in the most recent literature. However, skin-sparing mastectomy is not appropriate for large tumors or those with extensive skin involvement. Skin-sparing mastectomy is a popular option for prophylactic risk-reducing mastectomy and appears to be equally as effective as total mastectomy [6].

Nipple-sparing mastectomy

A skin-sparing procedure is performed but the subareolar tissue is removed from the undersurface of the nipple. The nipple tissue is sampled by intraoperative core biopsy to exclude possible malignant involvement. If clear at frozen section, the NAC is then replaced as a graft, combined with immediate breast reconstruction. An areolar-sparing procedure is now also technically possible.

Subcutaneous mastectomy

Also termed total skin-sparing mastectomy, subcutaneous mastectomy is an alternative technique used for prophylactic mastectomy followed by immediate reconstruction. Tissue is removed through an incision under the breast which leaves the skin, areola and nipple all intact. Women who have prophylactic mastectomy may prefer the subcutaneous procedure, because it retains their nipples (although sensation is usually lost) and offers a very good cosmetic result. In addition to the NAC, some subareolar tissue is also retained, while further breast tissue may be left behind in the axillary tail and close to the pectoral fascia. While considered appropriate as a prophylactic measure (breast cancer risk reduction of ~90%) it is important to recognize that malignancy can still arise in residual tissue.

Breast-conserving surgery

Partial mastectomy

Lumpectomy, partial mastectomy, wide local excision, complete local excision, segmentectomy and tylectomy are synonymous terms used to describe the standard procedure for BCT. Only the tumor is removed with a margin of surrounding tissue wide enough that the resected specimen is free of tumor. Strictly speaking, quadrantectomy (the resection of an entire breast quadrant) is distinct from lumpectomy, although the term is often loosely used as equivalent. Partial mastectomy is appropriate for unicentric tumors which are relatively small compared to the breast size, such that an acceptable cosmesis can be achieved. Nipple involvement generally precludes conservation therapy (although not absolutely, as in some instances excision of the NAC and subareolar tissue may be feasible).

Other oncoplastic surgical techniques

Various other oncoplastic surgical techniques can also be employed in breast conservation, aiming to combine wide surgical margins with excellent cosmesis. These include batwing, parallelogram, donut and reduction types of mastopexy lumpectomy, with the exact technique applied depending on tumor extent and location [7]. Reduction mammoplasty is a particularly useful option for large or pendulous breasts, with local flaps used to reconstruct the breast shape.

Sentinel lymph node biopsy (SLNB)

Sentinel lymph node biopsy is based on the concept that the lymphatic drainage of the breast leads first to one or more "sentinel" nodes, before the remaining axillary nodes become involved. If SLNB proves to be negative, it is very unlikely that any remaining axillary nodes will be positive, and the morbidity of performing full ALND can be avoided. Where available, the technique is used routinely for invasive cancer and in selected cases of extensive high-grade DCIS which carry a significant risk of microinvasion. Peritumoral or periareolar injection of blue dye is performed, with or without a radioactive tracer. While there is some evidence to suggest that the combined surgical/nuclear medicine method may improve accuracy, this is controversial. There is a small risk of anaphylaxis with patent blue. Methylene blue can be used as an alternative, but while allergic reactions are much rarer, staining of lymph nodes is less satisfactory. Injectate tracks to the superficial periareolar (Sappey's) plexus which drains to the axilla. A gamma probe and/or visual inspection are used to identify the sentinel nodes and 1–3 hot and/or blue nodes are retrieved for frozen section. The false-negative rate for SLNB is 8–10%.

Axillary lymph node dissection (ALND)

Axillary dissection is routinely performed in cases where involved axillary nodes have been shown to be present (either clinically palpable, by imaging or at pathologic assessment after sentinel node biopsy). Usually the level I and II lymph nodes are removed. The apical nodes (level III) are generally left as there is no clear survival benefit and the limiting dissection to the lower axilla reduces morbidity (particularly lymphedema but also neurologic damage causing shoulder pain and stiffness).

Appendix 5: Overview of radiation therapy

Radiation therapy after breast conservation

Following breast-conserving surgery, whole breast irradiation aims to reduce the risk of local recurrence by dealing with any possible residual DCIS, and it may also deal effectively with additional small invasive foci. However, the use of RT is not considered to be any substitute for obtaining pathologically clear margins. Frequently a "boost" is given to the tumor bed during whole breast irradiation.

RT for invasive cancer after BCT

While surgery followed by RT is currently standard treatment for most cases of invasive cancer, RT may be omitted for some favorable lesions (small grade 1, ER-positive, node-negative tumors with complete excision) particularly when these arise in older women (age >70 years). In such selected cases, the risk of recurrence is probably not more than ~5% at 10 years even without RT. Tamoxifen and/or an aromatase inhibitor are usually then employed.

RT for pure DCIS after BCT

For pure DCIS, RT after BCT reduces the risk of local recurrence by ~50% and is therefore routinely offered. The exception to an RT recommendation may be a small, completely excised, low-grade DCIS in an older patient. Adjunctive therapy with tamoxifen is commonly also used for ER-positive pure DCIS in addition to RT.

Accelerated partial breast irradiation

Techniques in which only the immediate tumor RT bed are treated with radiation are rapidly gaining popularity as a viable alternative to traditional whole breast irradiation after BCT in selected patients. The major advantage of APBI is that, even using post-operative external beam delivery, the course of treatment is much faster (hence accelerated), typically being completed in 5–6 days rather than the 5–6 weeks required for standard whole breast therapy.

Brachytherapy techniques can also be used for partial breast irradiation, e.g., the balloon catheter system developed by Mammosite (Cytyc, Marlborough, MA) and various other devices, usually inserted post-operatively and left in place for 5–6 days [7]. These methods again treat only the tumor bed and a surrounding 1–2 cm margin of tissue.

An even faster approach has been to deliver partial breast irradiation as a single dose intraoperatively [7]. Results from the ongoing TARGIT-A trial suggest that this is as effective as standard therapy in selected cases (node-negative IDC less than 2–3 cm with no significant DCIS component, patient age over 50 years) [8]. Whatever technique is used, there is a strong argument for performing breast MRI prior to undertaking APBI to exclude additional ipsilateral disease remote from the index cancer which would lie outside the planned radiation field.

Axillary radiation therapy

Radiation to the axilla is used selectively when the risk of recurrence is high, e.g., axillary nodal disease not cleared macroscopically or positive margins due to extranodal tumor spread. Usually the chest wall, the supraclavicular region and IMC are included (cardiotoxicity has to be considered for IMC nodes on the left side). Axillary treatment may also be used where many nodes are positive, but available data do not support routine axillary RT for <4 positive nodes.

Post-mastectomy radiation therapy

This is usually recommended only for a selected group of women with invasive cancer who are at elevated risk of locoregional recurrence or distant metastases based on clinical presentation and pathologic features. In such patients, post-mastectomy RT substantially reduces the risk of local recurrence and improves overall survival. Criteria for the use of post-mastectomy RT are still being refined.

Appendix 6: Overview of systemic therapy

Systemic therapies have two main aims – first to reduce the risk of future local recurrence and to treat possible distant metastatic disease. Toxic chemotherapy is not appropriate for pathologically pure DCIS, as there is only a 1–2% rate of subsequent metastases arising. Nevertheless as DCIS becomes more extensive, so the risk increases that pathologically occult microinvasion may be present and surgeons frequently perform SLNB for DCIS cases of > 30–40 mm in extent.

Most young women with invasive cancer are offered chemotherapy, with the Adjuvant! Online algorithm being widely used as a means of taking into account several important variables (tumor size, tumor grade, nodal status, receptor status) to provide an indication of overall % survival benefit. In older patients with EBC, chemotherapy may only offer significant additional survival benefit for ER-negative cancers.

Endocrine (anti-estrogen) therapy

Some 70–80% of invasive breast cancers are hormone receptor-positive (ER, PR or both) making anti-estrogen therapy appropriate. Endocrine therapy reduces the risk of local recurrence and distant metastatic disease, and is generally used after completion of surgery, RT and chemotherapy.

The choice of treatment depends on menopausal status. Prior to menopause, when the ovaries are the source of estrogen production, anti-ovarian therapies are the first line of treatment. After menopause, the main source of estrogen is from conversion of adrenal androgens by fat cells through the action of the enzyme aromatase.

(i) Anti-ovarian therapies work by artificially inducing menopause in premenopausal women. A temporary drug-induced menopause can be achieved using goserelin (Zoladex). Permanent options are bilateral salpingo-oophrectomy or radiation-induced menopause.

(ii) Anti-estrogen drugs: Selective estrogen receptor modulators (SERMs), e.g., tamoxifen and raloxifene, act by blocking ER. Tamoxifen is recommended for most women with ER-positive tumors as it significantly improves survival outcomes and reduces the incidence of developing contralateral breast cancer. The benefits clearly outweigh the risks of side effects for tamoxifen therapy alone, with an additional benefit when used in combination with chemotherapy. Tamoxifen is used in both pre- or postmenopausal women and can be taken for up to 5 years. Side effects: menopausal symptoms, thrombo-embolic disease, uterine cancer. In contrast to aromatase inhibitors, bone density is increased by SERMs. Raloxifene has a reported lower incidence of side effects than tamoxifen. Lasofoxifene is a newer drug in this class.

(iii) Aromatase inhibitors (AIs): anastrozole (Arimidex), letrozole (Femara) and exemestane. The use of AIs is only appropriate after permanent menopause, as they work by blocking conversion of androgen to estrogen by the enzyme aromatase. Like SERMs, they can be taken for up to 5 years, with AIs offering improved disease-free survival in EBC compared to tamoxifen. They can be used as an alternative to tamoxifen, or taken sequentially for a further 5 years after tamoxifen. Side effects: menopausal symptoms, osteoporosis. Long-term effects are not yet known with possible effects on cognitive function suggested in addition to cardiovascular disease.

Common chemotherapy agents and regimens

Combination therapy is usual, using drugs from a number of different classes to concurrently achieve tumor cell death and prevent further cell proliferation.

- Alkylating agents, e.g., cyclophosphamide
- Antimetabolites, e.g., 5-fluorouracil, methotrexate
- Anthracycline, e.g., epirubicin or doxorubicin (Adriamycin)
- Taxanes (mitotic inhibitors), e.g., paclitaxel, docetaxel, abraxane

Typical regimes of three drugs combined are:

- CMF = cyclophosphamide, methotrexate, 5-fluorouracil
- FAC = 5-fluorouracil, anthracycline, cyclophosphamide
- FEC = 5-fluorouracil, epirubicin, cyclophosphamide
- TAC = taxane, anthracycline, cyclophosphamide

The EBCTCG 15-year trial analysis (published in 2005) showed that in the treatment of EBC, 6 months of anthracycline-based chemotherapy (FAC or FEC) reduced the annual breast cancer death rate by 38% for women aged < 50 years and by about 20% for women in the 50–70 age-group, while 5 years of tamoxifen for ER-positive cancers was associated with a 30% reduction across all groups [9]. Both FAC and FEC were shown to be more effective than CMF. Anthracycline regimes therefore confer a survival benefit over CMF, while TAC is also superior to FAC, each at the cost of increased side effects which include cardiotoxicity and neutropenic crises. An anthracycline or taxane is sometimes combined only with cyclophosphamide as AC and TC respectively.

Choice of systemic therapy is closely related to molecular subtypes, and relatively good prognosis ER-positive cancers (particularly luminal A subtype) receive great benefit from endocrine therapy but less from chemotherapy. Conversely, high-risk ER-negative tumor types receive minimal benefit from endocrine therapy but have a substantially improved outlook from using aggressive chemotherapy. The aim is therefore to increasingly tailor therapy according to the molecular profile.

Treatment for HER2-positive breast cancer

Around 20% of breast cancers are positive for HER2 (human epidermal growth factor receptor type 2), which is associated with accelerated tumor growth and a generally poorer prognosis. Trastuzumab (Herceptin) is a monoclonal antibody (hence the –mab suffix) that inhibits growth of HER2-positive cancer cells, by blocking binding of growth factor to cell surface receptors. Trastuzumab may be used in combination with chemotherapy for EBC and for metastatic disease. Herceptin is usually given as a weekly intravenous infusion over 30–90 minutes for up to 1 year in EBC, or several years for metastatic disease. Side effects include histamine-mediated flu-like symptoms, localized pain, myocardial dysfunction.

Treatment of basal-like breast cancer

About 10–15% of breast cancers are of the basal-like molecular subtype, which are typically triple-negative (ER, PR and HER2 negative) and associated with a poorer prognosis. Although no specific therapy is currently available, new agents such as platinum compounds and PARP inhibitors are under development in clinical trials [10].

Appendix 7: Primary prevention strategies for high-risk women

In secondary prevention, or increased surveillance, it is hoped that if cancer does arise it will be detected at an early and curable stage. Primary preventive measures in women at high risk of breast and ovarian cancer are aimed at reducing the risk of cancer ever developing. These strategies fall into two major groups – risk-reducing surgery and chemoprevention (please see table below). Frequently, young women opt to partake in a high-risk surveillance program until after they have had children, and are then prepared to undertake the more radical surgical options of bilateral prophylactic mastectomy (BPM) and risk-reducing salpingo-oophorectomy (RRSO).

Bilateral prophylactic mastectomy

The cosmetic results which can be achieved today through reconstruction techniques are much better than in past decades, making bilateral prophylactic mastectomy an acceptable option even for younger women with a strong desire to maintain body image. A range of different options are available ranging from standard total mastectomy with reconstruction, through skin-sparing procedures to subcutaneous mastectomy (**Appendix 4**). The disadvantage of subcutaneous mastectomy is that significantly more breast tissue is left behind, with an associated risk of subsequent cancer developing. In a large prospective multicenter cohort study of almost 2482 BRCA mutation carriers, no breast cancers were found in the 10% of women who underwent risk-reducing mastectomy [11].

Primary prevention options for high-risk women

Preventive measure	Breast cancer risk reduction achieved
Prophylactic bilateral mastectomy	90%
Risk-reducing salpingo-oophorectomy	50% (80% reduction in ovarian cancer risk)
Chemoprevention with tamoxifen	50% at 5 years
Chemoprevention with aromatase inhibitors	Trials in progress

Risk-reducing salpingo-oophrectomy

A recent meta-analysis concluded that RRSO in BRCA1/2 mutation carriers was associated with ~50% reduction in breast cancer risk and ~80% reduction in ovarian cancer risk [12]. Furthermore, in prospective studies, RRSO reduced cancer-specific mortality by 90% for breast and 95% for gynecologic cancer [11, 12]. The protective effect for breast cancer is greatest when the procedure is performed before age 40 years, with benefit lasting ~15 years [13]. There is no reduction in breast cancer risk in mutation carriers who undergo RRSO after age 50 years, which is not unexpected as ovarian estrogen production ceases at menopause. To prevent gynecologic cancer, it is essential that the tubes are removed together with the ovaries as fallopian cancer is also BRCA-associated. In fact, most "ovarian" cancers in BRCA 1/2 carriers probably originate in the fimbrial end of the fallopian tube rather than the ovary. As the benefits are so substantial, BRCA mutation carriers are encouraged to consider RRSO as soon as childbearing is complete. Radiation-induced oophorectomy and the reversible goserelin therapy are other options, but non-surgical approaches to ovarian ablation do not address the risk of gynecologic cancer.

Chemoprevention

In a large case–control study of BRCA1/2 carriers with an index breast cancer, tamoxifen reduced the incidence of contralateral breast cancer by ~50%, which is about the same as achieved by RRSO [14, 15]. Long-term trials using raloxifene and AIs in a chemopreventive role are currently in progress.

Appendix 8: Breast cancer genes and genetic testing

BRCA1 and BRCA2

These two genes together account for 5–10% of all breast cancer cases in most populations [16]. Both the BRCA1 and BRCA2 gene mutations are autosomal dominant so that any first degree relative (mother, sister, daughter) of an affected individual has a 50% chance of also carrying the mutation. In the presence of a strong family history but no known mutation, genetic testing is usually considered when computer modeling programs such as BCRAPRO or BOADICEA suggest at least a 10–15% chance that a mutation is present. Young women with high-grade triple-negative cancers are often also tested for a possible BRCA1 mutation even in the absence of an extensive family history.

When a suspicious family history is found, the first step in genetic testing is to take blood from an affected family member. This sample is subjected to full genetic testing for all known mutations of the BRCA1 and BRCA2 genes (about 2000 for each). Although expensive and time-consuming, the results often facilitate management of the entire family, because if a pathogenic mutation such as BRCA1 is identified, the remaining members of the family can then be offered *predictive testing* for that specific mutation, which is both quicker and less expensive.

If predictive testing in a close relative of a known carrier excludes the mutation in question, it is usually concluded that the individual is at average population risk (assuming there are no other independent risk factors). However, the situation is different when an individual with a potentially high-risk family history is tested but no mutation has been identified. In this case the negative result is classified as "uninformative" and does not reduce that individual's potential risk status, because they may still be at high risk due to other unidentified genetic factors.

Some ethnic groups have a high prevalence of specific *founder mutations* passed down from a common ancestor, an effect amplified by a combination of cultural and/or geographic isolation. The frequency of a BRCA mutation being present in those of Ashkenazi Jewish ancestry is about 1 in 50, with two mutations in the BRCA1 gene (185delAG and 5382insC) and one in BRCA2 (6174delT) accounting for ~90% of cases [17]. A similar situation exists in an Icelandic population with the BRCA2 999del5 mutation, and in such instances it is only necessary to undertake predictive testing for the specific founder mutations [17].

Where one of a couple are known to harbor a BRCA mutation, preimplantation genetic diagnosis is now possible in combination with IVF, with only normal healthy embryos selected for implantation into the uterus.

Non-BRCA familial breast cancer

Following identification of the BRCA1 gene in 1994 and BRCA2 in 1995, the expectation that most familial breast cancer would soon be explained by the discovery of further BRCA genes did not eventuate. Several other rare genes account for a small proportion of additional cases with all of these together accounting for probably only about 50% of inherited breast

Hereditary breast cancer genes and percentages of all familial cases

Gene	%	Clinical features
BRCA1	20–40%	Very high risk of breast and ovarian cancer
BRCA2	10–30%	Very high risk of breast and ovarian cancer
TP53	< 1%	Li-Fraumeni syndrome, very high breast cancer risk
PTEN	< 1%	Cowden syndrome, very high breast cancer risk
STK11	~1%	Peutz-Jegher's syndrome
ATM	~1%	Fanconi's anemia gene × 2 breast cancer risk
CHEK2	~1%	× 2 breast cancer risk

cancers (please see table below) [18]. A common theme with confirmed breast cancer susceptibility genes is their roles in pathways which preserve genetic integrity, often through DNA-repair mechanisms. In the Li-Fraumeni syndrome (a mutation in the TP53 gene) breast cancer occurs in association with soft tissue and bone sarcomas. Affected individuals appear to be extremely susceptible to the carcinogenic effects of radiation, and XRM screening is not recommended in this group at least until after age 50 years. Penetrance is high with ~90% lifetime risk of developing breast cancer in the absence of primary preventive measures. Recent evidence suggests a triple-positive phenotype may be typical of breast cancers presenting in women with Li-Fraumeni syndrome.

The remaining cases of familial cancer cannot be attributed to any single causative mutation, but likely relate to the action of various polygenes, combinations of which may confer a moderate increase in breast cancer susceptibility across much larger proportions of the general population. Some of these polygenes probably also act through an effect on breast density, which is itself a strong and heritable risk factor for breast cancer [19, 20].

References

1. Cowper SE, Robin HS, Steinberg SM, *et al.* Scleromyxoedema-like cutaneous diseases in renal-dialysis patients. *Lancet* 2000; **356**: 1000–1.
2. Grobner T. Gadolinium: a specific trigger for the development of nephrogenic fibrosing dermatopathy and nephrogenic systemic fibrosis? *Nephrol Dial Transplant* 2006; **21**: 1104–8.
3. Broome DR. Nephrogenic systemic fibrosis associated with gadolinium based contrast agents: a summary of the medical literature reporting. *Eur J Radiol* 2008; **66**: 230–4.
4. Shellock FG, Spinazzi A. MRI safety update 2008: part 1, MRI contrast agents and nephrogenic systemic fibrosis. *AJR Am J Roentgenol* 2008; **191**: 1129–39.
5. Weinstein S, Obuchowski NA, Lieber ML. Fundamentals of clinical research for radiologists. Clinical evaluation of diagnostic tests. *AJR Am J Roentgenol* 2005; **184**: 14–19.
6. Guillem JG, Wood WC, Moley JF, *et al.* ASCO/SSO review of current role of risk-reducing surgery in common hereditary cancer syndromes. *Ann Surg Oncol* 2006; **13**: 1296–321.
7. Klimberg VS. *Atlas of Breast Surgical Techniques*. Philadelphia, PA, Saunders, Elsevier, 2010.
8. Vaidya JS, Joseph DJ, Tobias JS, *et al.* Targeted intraoperative RT versus whole breast RT for breast cancer (TARGIT-A trial): an international, prospective, randomised, non-inferiority phase 3 trial. *Lancet* 2010; **376**: 91–102.
9. Early Breast Cancer Trialists' Collaborative Group (EBCTCG). Effects of chemotherapy and hormonal therapy for early breast cancer on recurrence and 15-year survival: an overview of the randomised trials. *Lancet* 2005; **365**: 1687–717.
10. Goldhirsch A, Ingle JN, Gelber RD, *et al.* Thresholds for therapies: highlights of the St Gallen International Expert Consensus on the Primary Therapy of Early Breast Cancer 2009. *Ann Oncol* 2009; **20**: 1319–29.
11. Domchek SM, Friebel TM, Singer CF. Association of risk-reducing surgery in BRCA1 or BRCA2 mutation carriers with cancer risk and mortality. *JAMA* 2010; **304**: 965–75.
12. Rebbeck T, Kauff N, Domchek S, *et al.* Meta-analysis of risk reduction estimates associated with risk-reducing salpingo-oophorectomy in BRCA1 or BRCA2 mutation carriers. *J Natl Cancer Inst* 2009; **101**: 80–7.
13. Eisen A, Lubinski J, Klijn J, *et al.* Breast cancer risk following bilateral oophorectomy in BRCA1 and BRCA2 mutation carriers: an international case-control study. *J Clin Oncol* 2005; **23**: 7491–6.
14. Mahoney MC, Bevers T, Linos E, *et al.* Opportunities and strategies for breast cancer prevention through risk reduction. *CA Cancer J Clin* 2008; **58**: 347–71.
15. Pruthi S, Brandt KR, Degnim AC, *et al.* A multidisciplinary approach to the management of breast cancer, part 1: prevention and diagnosis. *Mayo Clin Proc* 2007; **82**: 999–1012.
16. Goldhirsch A, Wood WC, Gelber RD, *et al.* Progress and promise: highlights of the international expert consensus on the primary therapy of early breast cancer 2007. *Ann Oncol* 2007; **18**: 1133–44.
17. Narod SA, Offit K. Prevention and management of hereditary breast cancer. *J Clin Oncol* 2005; **23**: 1656–63.
18. Walsh T, King M. Ten genes for inherited breast cancer. *Cancer Cell* 2007; **11**: 103–5.
19. Boyd NF, Dite GS, Stone J, *et al.* Heritability of mammographic density, a risk factor for breast cancer. *N Engl J Med* 2002; **347**: 886–94.
20. Boyd NF, Guo H, Martin LJ, *et al.* Mammographic density and the risk and detection of breast cancer. *N Engl J Med* 2007; **356**: 227–36.

Index

Note: page numbers in *italics* refer to figures and tables